Register Now for Onlin[e access] to Your Book!

SPRINGER PUBLISHING COMPANY

CONNECT™

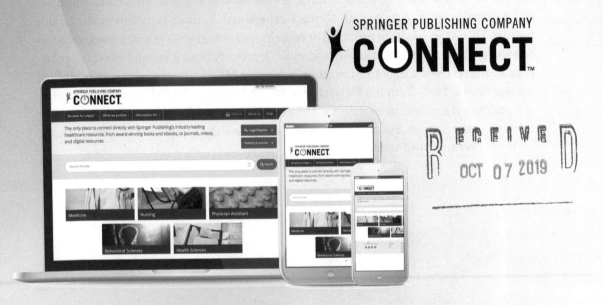

Your print purchase of *Population-Based Nursing, Third Edition,* **includes online access to the contents of your book**—increasing accessibility, portability, and searchability!

Access today at:

http://connect.springerpub.com/content/book/978-0-8261-3674-9 or scan the QR code at the right with your smartphone and enter the access code below.

AS02UM7R

Scan here for quick access.

If you are experiencing problems accessing the digital component of this product, please contact our customer service department at cs@springerpub.com

The online access with your print purchase is available at the publisher's discretion and may be removed at any time without notice.

Publisher's Note: New and used products purchased from third-party sellers are not guaranteed for quality, authenticity, or access to any included digital components.

SPC

SPRINGER PUBLISHING COMPANY

View all our products at springerpub.com

Ann L. Cupp Curley, PhD, RN, recently retired from her position as the Nurse Research Specialist at Capital Health in Trenton, New Jersey, where she was responsible for promoting and guiding the development of nursing research and evidence-based practice. She has an extensive background in nursing education at the undergraduate, graduate, and doctoral levels, and more than 10 years' experience in community and public health nursing. Dr. Curley has been principal or co-principal investigator of many research projects and continues to serve as an advisor on DNP project committees and a research consultant. She received a BSN from Boston College, an MSN in community health/clinical nurse specialist track from the University of Pennsylvania, and a PhD in urban planning and policy development from Rutgers, The State University of New Jersey. Dr. Curley has received many honors, including the Nurse.com Nursing Spectrum Excellence Award for Education and Mentorship.

POPULATION-BASED NURSING

CONCEPTS AND COMPETENCIES FOR ADVANCED PRACTICE

Third Edition

Ann L. Cupp Curley, PhD, RN
Editor

SPRINGER PUBLISHING COMPANY

Copyright © 2020 Springer Publishing Company, LLC

Springer Publishing Company, LLC
11 West 42nd Street
New York, NY 10036
www.springerpub.com
http://connect.springerpub.com

Acquisitions Editor: Adrianne Brigido
Compositor: Exeter Premedia Services Private Ltd.

ISBN: 978-0-8261-3673-2
ebook ISBN: 978-0-8261-3674-9
Instructor's Manual: 978-0-8261-3675-6
DOI: 10.1891/9780826136749

Instructor's Materials: Qualified instructors may request supplements by emailing textbook@springerpub.com.

19 20 21 22 / 5 4 3 2 1

The author and the publisher of this Work have made every effort to use sources believed to be reliable to provide information that is accurate and compatible with the standards generally accepted at the time of publication. Because medical science is continually advancing, our knowledge base continues to expand. Therefore, as new information becomes available, changes in procedures become necessary. We recommend that the reader always consult current research and specific institutional policies before performing any clinical procedure or delivering any medication. The author and publisher shall not be liable for any special, consequential, or exemplary damages resulting, in whole or in part, from the readers' use of, or reliance on, the information contained in this book. The publisher has no responsibility for the persistence or accuracy of URLs for external or third-party Internet websites referred to in this publication and does not guarantee that any content on such websites is, or will remain, accurate or appropriate.

CIP data is on file at the Library of Congress.

Library of Congress Control Number: 2019946289

Contact us to receive discount rates on bulk purchases.
We can also customize our books to meet your needs.
For more information please contact: sales@springerpub.com

Publisher's Note: New and used products purchased from third-party sellers are not guaranteed for quality, authenticity, or access to any included digital components.

Printed in the United States of America.

In Memory of Patty Vitale

Good friends are hard to find . . . and impossible to forget.
—Anonymous

CONTENTS

CONTRIBUTORS

Barbara A. Benjamin, EdD, RN, Adjunct Faculty, University of North Carolina, Chapel Hill

Irina McKeehan Campbell, PhD, MPH, Professor, Department of Health Sciences, School of Health and Human Services, National University, La Jolla, California

Ann L. Cupp Curley, PhD, RN, Research Consultant, Falmouth, Massachusetts

Janna L. Dieckmann, PhD, RN, Clinical Associate Professor, School of Nursing, University of North Carolina at Chapel Hill, Chapel Hill, North Carolina

Alyssa Erikson, PhD, MSN, RN, Associate Professor and Chair, Department of Nursing, California State University Monterey Bay, Seaside, California

Eileen M. Horton, MSN, MSM, RN, NEA-BC, Senior Vice President, Hospital Adminstration and Chief Quality Officer (retired), Capital Health, Trenton, New Jersey

Lucille A. Joel, APN, EdD, FAAN, Distinguished Professor, Rutgers University School of Nursing, Newark, New Jersey

Vera Kunte, DNP, APN, Nurse Research Specialist, Capital Health, Trenton, New Jersey

Barbara A. Niedz, PhD, RN, CPHQ, Assistant Professor, Rutgers University, School of Nursing, Newark, New Jersey

Sonda M. Oppewal, PhD, RN, Professor, School of Nursing, University of North Carolina at Chapel Hill, Chapel Hill, North Carolina

Laura P. Rossi, RN, PhD, Assistant Professor, Simmons University, College of Natural, Health and Behavioral Sciences, School of Nursing; Program Manager, Quality and Patient Safety, Department of Orthopaedic Surgery, Massachusetts General Hospital, Boston, Massachusetts

Patty A. Vitale[†], MD, MPH, FAAP

[†]Deceased

FOREWORD

"What's past is prologue," wrote William Shakespeare in *The Tempest*. Why read *Population-Based Nursing: Concepts and Competencies for Advanced Practice*? In this book, the third edition, there is a lot more to know and learn. If the first two decades of the 21st century have taught us anything it is that what we know as *healthcare* is changing at warp speed. And, as the anniversary of Florence Nightingale's 200th birthday looms large, Shakespeare's words echo in our ears and remind us of needed changes in the practice of the profession of nursing. We inherently know that what has happened in the past sets the scene for the really important morphs yet to be identified and implemented. Those changes will determine nursing's viability in the ever changing national and global health marketplace.

While as in the first and second editions successful strategies that nurses have used to improve population outcomes are paramount, the readers will discover new information in the third edition on how to identify healthcare needs at the population level and how to improve overall population outcomes. *Voila*. Not only that, but introduction of the most common study designs and successful program implementation strategies will lead you to correct design selection, successful implementation and most importantly overall success. Problem solved!

The third edition charts a path toward understanding how to successfully integrate new knowledge into practice. This, as experience teaches us, is no small task. Chapter 6 actually describes how technology can be used to truly enhance population-based nursing and describes the role and importance of APRNs in using data to make decisions that lead to new levels of program development and evaluation. While Clara Barton and Florence Nightingale did not have AI they understood that statistics are needed to measure outcomes. Chapter 8 identifies ways and means to evaluate population outcomes and systems changes. These concepts and roles are explored within the competencies of the APRN. The healthcare marketplace is extremely competitive, and executives and managers are like radar screens looking to identify opportunities to distinguish and validate their organizations. This book helps the new APRN identify the ways and means to achieve such validation.

Nurses need to be part of the highest level of care management and policy decision making in partnership with healthcare policy brokers and healthcare policy makers. In Chapter 10, the emphasis is placed on identifying community needs and assessment of resources. Chapter 11 rounds up by providing specific strategies for program implementation coupled with methods to empower the community to advocate for themselves. In the final chapter global health and cultural issue for population-based nursing theory and practice open one's eyes to recent patterns in international interdisciplinary collaborations including the latest global health competencies. A primer for all practitioners whatever the setting.

This edition targets all of the important aspects in population-based care for the most trusted and recognized of all healthcare professions. Nursing remains, and should remain, a practice centered and caring profession, but current times mandate that nurses discover new and effective strategies for promoting health and providing care. This book gives nurses everything from A to Z describing the role of the APRN in the accreditation process to zeroing in how to eliminate health disparities. By looking back to the lessons and wisdom of the past and opening our minds to the new vistas and parameters of populations and the potential impact of a population-based approach to care it charts the ways and means toward the future. . ., which is now. The past is prologue.

These are nursing's new **Tools of the Trade**.

Patricia A. Polansky, RN, MS
Director, Program Development and Implementation
Center to Champion Nursing in America
RWJF/AARP
Washington, DC

PREFACE

My good friend, colleague, and co-editor Patty Vitale died shortly after we completed the planning for this, the third edition of our book. Patty had enormous energy and zest. Both figuratively and literally she danced her way through life. The joy that she exuded on the dance floor was a reflection of the joy that she had for living. She was dedicated to making the world a better place for children through her work as a pediatrician and an educator. This book is part of the enduring legacy that she left behind.

The original inspiration for this book grew out of our experience while co-teaching an epidemiology course for students enrolled in a doctorate in nursing practice (DNP) program. We found it difficult to find a textbook that addressed the course objectives and was relevant to nursing practice. We decided a population-based nursing textbook, targeted for use as a primary course textbook in a DNP program or as a supplement to other course materials in a graduate community health nursing program, would be of great benefit and value to students enrolled in these programs. This book is the result of that vision. The chapters address the essential areas of content for a DNP program as recommended by the American Association of Colleges of Nursing (AACN), with a focus on the AACN core competencies for population-based nursing. The primary audience for this text is nursing students enrolled in either a DNP program or a graduate community health nursing program. Each chapter includes discussion questions to help students use and apply their newly acquired skills from each chapter.

In this book, the third edition, our goals were to not only update the content of the existing chapters, but also add a chapter on accreditation of population-based programs. We were fortunate that a nurse with extensive experience in accreditation (Eileen Horton) agreed to write the chapter for us. In order to make it easier for readers to enhance their knowledge of the information that is covered in the book, we also decided to add a relevant list of Internet resources to each chapter.

Several events covering a wide range of issues in the healthcare field have occurred over the past few years. These include the attempts by the Trump administration to dismantle the Affordable Care Act and efforts by the 116th Congress to expand the role of public programs in healthcare. Bills being introduced in the House range in scope from broad proposals to create a new national health insurance program for all residents (often referred to as "Medicare for All") to more incremental approaches that would offer a public plan option in addition to current sources of coverage. It appears that the 2020 elections may well turn into a referendum on healthcare and how it should be paid for. States and local governments are increasingly turning to legislation in an attempt to quell outbreaks of measles. As of April 2019, officials at the Centers for Disease Control and Prevention (CDC) had confirmed 695 measles cases across 22 states for the current year, a record high since the disease was thought to have been eliminated in the United States in 2000. According to a UNICEF report, among high-income nations, the United States had the most children who went unvaccinated between 2010 and 2017 (CDC, 2019). There is increasing concern over the usage of electronic cigarettes and hookahs by children. There is also increasing interest in the use of social media to address population health. This edition addresses these as well as other current issues in population-based nursing.

As in the first and second editions, this textbook includes successful strategies that nurses have used to improve population outcomes and reinforces high-level application of activities that require the synthesis and integration of information learned. The goal is to provide readers with information that will help them to identify healthcare needs at the population level and improve population outcomes. In particular, Chapter 1, Introduction to Population-Based Nursing, introduces the concept of population-based nursing and discusses examples of successful approaches and interventions to improve population health. In this edition we use the title "advanced practice registered nurse" (APRN). APRN is the title used in *The Consensus Model for APRN Regulation, Licensure, Accreditation, Certification and Education* (APRN Consensus Workgroup & National Council of State Boards of Nursing APRN Advisory Committee, 2008). This document is the product of the APRN Consensus Work Group and the National Council of State Boards of Nursing (NCSBN).

In order to design, implement, and evaluate interventions that improve the health of populations and aggregates, APRNs need to be able to identify and target outcome measures. Chapter 2, Identifying Outcomes in Population-Based Nursing, explains how to define, categorize, and identify population outcomes using specific examples from practice settings. The identification of outcomes or key health indicators is an essential first step in planning effective interventions and is a requirement for evaluation. The chapter includes a discussion of nurse-sensitive indicators, Healthy People 2020, Healthy People 2030, national health objectives, and health disparities. Emphasis is on the identification of healthcare disparities and approaches that can be used to eliminate or mitigate them. APRNs can advocate needed change at local, regional, state, or national levels by identifying areas for improvement in practice, by comparing evidence needed for effective practice, and by better understanding health disparities. APRNs have an important collaborative role with professionals from other disciplines and community members to work toward eliminating health disparities.

Epidemiology is the basic science of prevention (Gordis, 2014). Evidence-based practice, as it relates to population-based nursing, combines clinical practice and public health through the use of population health sciences in clinical practice (Heller & Page, 2002). Programs or interventions that are designed by APRNs should be evaluated and assessed for their effectiveness and ability to change or improve outcomes. This is true at an individual or population level. Data from these programs should be collected systematically and in such a manner that can be replicated in future programs. Data collection must be organized and analyzed using clearly defined outcomes developed early in the planning process. Best practice requires that data are not just collected; data must also be analyzed, interpreted correctly, and, if significant, put into practice. Understanding how to interpret and report data accurately is critical as it sets up the foundation for evidence-based practice. With that said, it is important to understand the basics of how to measure disease or outcomes, how to present these measures, and to know what types of measures are needed to analyze a project or intervention.

Chapter 3, Epidemiological Methods and Measurements in Population-Based Nursing Practice: Part I, describes the natural history of disease and concepts that are integral to the prevention and recognition (e.g., screening) of disease. Basic concepts that are necessary to understand how to measure disease, and design studies that are used in population-based research, are discussed. Disease measures, such as incidence, prevalence, and mortality rates, are covered, and their relevance to practice is discussed. This chapter also includes information on primary, secondary, and tertiary prevention, and the concept of causality is introduced. A section on survival and prognosis is included. This material broadens the knowledge of readers with information necessary for advanced practice and interpretation of survival data. The basics of data analysis, including the calculation of relative risk, attributable risk, and odds ratio, are presented with examples of how to use these measures. Study design selection is an important part of the planning process for implementing a program. A portion of Chapter 3, Epidemiological Methods and Measurements in Population-Based Nursing Practice: Part I, is dedicated to introducing the most common study designs, because correct design selection is an essential part of sound methodology, successful program implementation, and overall success.

In order for APRNs to lead the field of evidence-based practice, it is critical that they possess skills in analytic methods to identify population trends and evaluate outcomes and systems of care (American Association of Colleges of Nursing [AACN], 2006). They need to carry out studies with strong methodology and be cognizant of factors that can affect study results. Identification and early recognition of factors that can affect the results or outcomes of a study, such as systematic errors (e.g., bias), should be acknowledged because they cannot always be prevented. In Chapter 4, Epidemiological Methods and Measurements in Population-Based Nursing Practice: Part II, the APRN is introduced to the elements of bias with a comprehensive discussion of the complexities of data collection and the fundamentals of developing a database. More in-depth discussion of study designs is covered, as well as a comprehensive review of ways to report on randomized and nonrandomized studies. Critical components of data analysis are discussed, including causality, confounding, and interaction.

In order to provide care at an advanced level, nurses must incorporate the concepts and competencies of advanced practice into their daily practice. This requires that APRNs acquire the knowledge, tools, and resources to know when and how to integrate them into practice. In Chapter 5, Applying Evidence at the Population Level, the APRN learns how to integrate and synthesize information in order to design interventions that are based on evidence to improve population outcomes. Nurses require several skills to become practitioners of evidence-based care. In this chapter, they learn how to identify clinical problems, recognize patient safety issues, compose clinical questions that provide a clear direction for study, conduct a search of the literature, appraise and synthesize the available evidence, and successfully integrate new knowledge into practice.

Information technologies are transforming the way that information is learned and shared. Online communities provide a place for people to support each other and share information. Online databases contain knowledge that can be assessed for information on populations and aggregates, and many websites provide up-to-date information on health and healthcare. Chapter 6, Using Information Technology to Improve Population Outcomes, describes how technology can be used to enhance population-based nursing. It identifies websites that are available and how to evaluate them for quality. It also describes potential ways that technology can be used to improve population outcomes and how to incorporate technology into the development of new and creative interventions. APRNs use data to make decisions that lead to program development, implementation, and evaluation. In Chapter 7, Concepts in Program Design and Development, the APRN learns how to design new programs using organizational theory. Nursing care delivery models that address organizational structure, process, and outcomes are described.

Oversight responsibilities for clinical outcomes at the population level are a critical part of advanced practice nursing. The purpose of Chapter 8, Evaluation of Practice at the Population Level, is to identify ways and means to evaluate population outcomes and systems changes, as well as to address issues of effectiveness and efficiency and trends in care delivery across the continuum. Strategies to monitor healthcare quality are addressed, as are factors that lead to success. These concepts are explored within the role and competencies of the APRN.

The healthcare marketplace is extremely competitive. Administrators are constantly on the look out to identify opportunities to differentiate and validate their organization. Achieving accreditation helps to validate programs and organizations in the context of national and professional standards. Developing programs and working toward program accreditation requires competence in each of the DNP essentials. Chapter 9, The Role of Accreditation in Validating Population-Based Practice/Programs, describes the role of the APRN in the accreditation process.

In order for APRNs to make decisions at the community level, APRNs who work in the community need to be part of the higher level of care management and policy-making and decision-making, in partnership with the community-based consortium of healthcare policy makers. Chapter 10, Building Relationships and Engaging Communities Through Collaboration, describes the tools for successful community collaboration and project development. Emphasis is placed on identifying community needs and assessment of their resources. Specific examples are given to guide APRNs in developing their own community projects.

Chapter 11, Challenges in Program Implementation, identifies barriers to change within communities and the importance of developing and sustaining community partnerships. Specific strategies for program implementation are discussed, as well as the methods to empower the community to advocate for themselves. Specific examples are given in order to guide APRNs in executing a project that has community acceptance and sustainability.

Finally, Chapter 12, Implications of Global Health in Population-Based Nursing, explores the implications of global health for the APRN. Theories of global health, population health, and public/community health are differentiated and compared, to further the understanding of how environmental conditions (e.g., poverty, housing, access to care) affect the health status of individuals and groups. Recent patterns in international interdisciplinary collaborations are reviewed, including the global health competencies developed by the Association of Schools of Public Health (ASPH) and the AACN.

Qualified instructors may obtain access to an instructor's manual for this title by contacting *textbook@springerpub.com*.

Ann L. Cupp Curley

REFERENCES

American Association of Colleges of Nursing. (2006). *The essentials of doctoral education for advanced practice nursing*. Retrieved from http://www.aacn.nche.edu/DNP/pdf/Essentials.pdf

APRN Consensus Workgroup & National Council of State Boards of Nursing APRN Advisory Committee. (2008). *The consensus model for APRN regulation, licensure, accreditation, certification and education*. Retrieved from http://www.aacn.nche.edu/education-resources/APRNReport.pdf

Centers for Disease Control and Prevention. (2019). *CDC media statement: Measles cases in the U.S. are highest since measles was eliminated in 2000*. Retrieved from https://www.cdc.gov/media/releases/2019/s0424-highest-measles-cases-since-elimination.html

Gordis, L. (2014). Epidemiology (5th ed.). Canada: Elsevier Saunders.

Heller, R., & Page, J. (2002). A population perspective to evidence based medicine: "Evidence for population health." *Journal of Epidemiology & Community Health, 56*(1), 45–47. doi:10.1136/jech.56.1.45

ACKNOWLEDGMENTS

I wish to express my thanks to those professional colleagues who provided direction, guidance, and assistance in writing this book. Thank you also to my family and friends for their support throughout this process. I want to give a very special thank you to my husband, Ed, for his unending patience and excellent advice. Thank you to my publisher, Adrianne Brigido, for her valuable advice, assistance, and infinite patience, and to Cindy Yoo and Kris Parrish at Springer Publishing Company for their assistance and expertise throughout the revision of this book. Finally, I could not have completed the text without the help of the library staff of the Health Services Library of Capital Health especially Erika Moncrief, MS, Director of Library Services.

CHAPTER 1

INTRODUCTION TO POPULATION-BASED NURSING

ANN L. CUPP CURLEY

INTRODUCTION

Some of the most significant figures in the history of nursing made their reputations by providing population-based care. Their influence on nursing has been such that their names live on and their achievements continue to be recognized because of their important contributions to nursing and to healthcare. A brief look at the stories of some of these nurses helps to provide a background for understanding population health.

Although she started her career as a teacher, Clarissa (Clara) Barton won her greatest acclaim as a nurse. Horrified by the suffering of wounded soldiers in the American Civil War (many of them were former neighbors and students) and struck by the lack of supplies needed to care for them, she worked to obtain various supplies and put herself at great risk by nursing soldiers on the front lines of several major battles. Her experience would eventually lead to her becoming the founder and first president of the American Red Cross (Evans, 2003).

During the Crimean War, Florence Nightingale used statistical analysis to plot the incidence of preventable deaths among British soldiers. She used a diagram to dramatize the unnecessary deaths of soldiers caused by unsanitary conditions and lobbied political and military leaders in London for the need to reform. She worked to promote the idea that social phenomena could be objectively measured and subjected to mathematical analysis. Along with William Farr, she was one of the earliest healthcare practitioners to collect and analyze data in order to persuade people of the need for change in healthcare practices (Dossey, 2000; Lipsey, 1993).

Mary Breckinridge started the Frontier Nursing Service (FNS) in Kentucky in 1925 and remained its director until her death in 1965. Educated as a nurse and midwife, she devoted her life to improving health in rural areas, especially among women and children. She believed in working with the communities that were served by the FNS and formed and worked with committees composed of community members to help plan and provide care. Similar to Florence Nightingale, she believed in the use of statistics to measure outcomes. From its onset, the FNS was so successful that there was an immediate drop in infant and maternal deaths in the communities served by the FNS (Frontier Nursing University, 2019; January, 2009).

These three nurses all worked to improve the health of at-risk populations. They met with political leaders to advocate changes in polices to benefit those populations, and both Nightingale and Breckinridge used statistical analysis to both support the need for change and to evaluate their interventions. Breckinridge was an early advocate of engaging communities to help address community health issues. They were all pioneers of nursing and, although perhaps not in name, certainly in fact, among the first nurses working in advanced practice.

For decades, community health nurses have recognized the importance and the impact of population-based care, but large segments of nursing practice focused primarily on caring for individual patients. Nursing remains, and should remain, a practice-based and caring profession, but nursing practice is changing. There is an awareness of the need to provide evidence-based care and to design interventions that have a broad impact on the populations that nursing serves, no matter the setting. Population health obligates healthcare professionals to implement standard interventions, based on the best research evidence, to improve the health of targeted groups of people. It also obligates nurses to discover new and effective strategies for providing care and promoting health. Although clinical decision-making related to individual patients is important, it has little impact on overall health outcomes for populations. Interventions at the population level have the potential to improve overall health across communities.

This book addresses the essential areas of content for a doctorate in nursing practice (DNP) as recommended by the American Association of Colleges of Nursing (AACN), with a focus on the AACN core competencies for population-based nursing. The goal is to provide readers with information that will help them to identify healthcare needs at the population level and to improve population outcomes. Although the focus is on the essential components of a DNP program, the intent is to broadly address practice issues that should be the concern of any nurse in an advanced practice role.

This chapter introduces the reader to the concept of population-based nursing. The reader learns how to identify population parameters, the potential impact of a population-based approach to care, and the importance of designing nursing interventions at the population level in advanced nursing practice.

BACKGROUND

For all the scare tactics out there, what's truly scary—truly risky—is the prospect of doing nothing.

—President Barack Obama, *The New York Times*, August 16, 2009

The first two decades of the 21st century have been witness to a growing and contentious debate on healthcare reforms. President Barack Obama's stated goals in pushing for reforming health insurance were to extend healthcare coverage to the millions who lacked health insurance, stop the insurance industry's practice of denying coverage on the basis of pre-existing conditions, and cut overall healthcare costs. Driven by a need for change in how healthcare is paid for, the Patient Protection and Affordable Care Act (ACA) was signed into law by President Obama in 2010. It went into effect over the span of 4 years beginning in 2011. Currently, there are three different "markets" for insurance through the ACA. The federal marketplace is run solely by the federal government. The state marketplace is run solely by the state, and in partnership marketplaces, states run many of the important functions and make key decisions but the marketplace is operated by the federal government. The ACA includes an option that allows states to expand Medicaid eligibility to uninsured adults and children whose incomes are at or below 138% of the federal poverty level (there is also a provision for people living with mental illness).

One of candidate Donald Trump's campaign promises was to repeal the ACA. Since his inauguration, the Trump administration has issued many regulations that have effectively undermined enrollment in the ACA by cutting funding for education, marketing, and outreach. While targeting enrollment, the Trump administration has, for the most part, enforced the law as written although the federal role in enforcement has decreased (Jost, 2018). In December 2018, the U.S. District Court in Fort Worth, Texas, ruled that the individual mandate requiring people to have health insurance is unconstitutional and that the remaining provisions of the ACA are also invalid. In March 2019 the Justice Department sent a letter to the 5th U.S. Circuit Court of Appeals in New Orleans to affirm the judgment issued by the U.S. District Court in Fort Worth, Texas (Robson, 2019). This action signaled a revival of the current administration's efforts to repeal the entire ACA. Three days after this letter was issued an announcement was delivered from the White House that a Republican replacement for the ACA would not be introduced until after the 2020 elections (Pear & Haberman, 2019). As of this writing, the fate of the ACA remains uncertain and the contentious debate surrounding healthcare legislation and reform in the United States continues.

There is ample evidence of a need for healthcare reform in the United States. The gross domestic product (GDP) is the total market value of the output of labor and property located in the United States. It reflects the contribution of the healthcare sector relative to all other production in the United States. In 1960, the health sector's proportion (NHE) of the GDP was 5% (i.e., $5 of every $100 spent in the United States went to pay for healthcare services). By 1990, this figure had grown to 12% and by 1996, 14%. A report issued by the Committee on the Budget of the U.S. Senate in 2008 warned that unless changes were made in how the United States provides care to its citizens, the GDP for the healthcare sector would grow to 25% by 2025 and 49% by 2089 (Orszag, 2008). In 2017, the NHE was $3.5 trillion and accounted for 17.9% of the GDP. The Centers for Medicare & Medicaid Services (CMS) published its forecast of healthcare costs for 2018 to 2027. It estimates that health spending will grow 0.8 percentage point faster than the GDP per year over the 2018 to 2027 period and, as a result, the health share of GDP is expected to rise from 17.9% in 2017 to 19.4% by 2027. According to the CMS, income growth, the aging of the U.S. population, and the rising costs of medical goods and services are the three major factors driving healthcare costs at this time (CMS, 2019). The Organization for Economic Cooperation and Development (OECD) provides a global picture of healthcare spending. It reports that U.S. expenditures for healthcare as reflected by the GDP is the highest among OECD countries and nearly double the average for OECD countries. One interesting fact that can be gleaned from that report is that the OECD attributes the difference in costs (U.S. costs as compared to other countries) is due to private health sector prices, primarily pharmaceuticals (OECD, 2019).

The rising cost of healthcare is reflected in the insurance industry. According to the Henry J. Kaiser Family Foundation (2019a), the average annual premium for employer-sponsored family health coverage in 2017 was $18,687 and the average annual contribution from employees was $5,218.

Unfortunately, although the United States ranks first in spending on healthcare among industrialized nations, it ranks lower than most industrialized countries in important health indicators. Two commonly used indicators for measuring a country's health are infant mortality and life expectancy at birth. Worldwide, the United States ranked 43rd for life expectancy at birth (life expectancy at birth in the United States is 80 years) and 55th for infant mortality (infant mortality rate in the United states is 5.87 per 1,000 live births) in 2017 (Central Intelligence Agency [CIA], n.d.). A report issued by the Institute of Medicine (IOM, 2010) argues that the system used in the United States for gathering and analyzing health measures is part of the problem. A second problem is the inadequate system used in the United States for gathering, analyzing, and communicating information on the underlying factors that lead to chronic health conditions and other risk factors that contribute to poor health. Readers can refer to Chapter 12, Implications of Global Health in Population-Based Nursing, for a more detailed description of how the United States ranks among other countries in relation to health indicators.

Health insurance is an important factor in any discussion about healthcare. The United States is the only industrialized country in the world without universal care. In 2017, 20% of people in the United States who were uninsured went without needed medical care. People who are uninsured are less likely than those who are insured to receive preventive care (The Henry J. Kaiser Family Foundation, 2019b). The Commonwealth Fund, a private foundation whose stated mission is to promote a high-performing healthcare system, commissioned a survey of U.S. adults that was conducted by Princeton Survey Research Associates (Collins, Doty, Robertson, & Garber, 2011). The survey looked at the effect of health insurance coverage on healthcare-seeking behaviors. They found that among uninsured women aged 50 to 64, 48% say they did not see a doctor when they were sick, did not fill a prescription, or skipped a test, treatment, or follow-up visit because they could not afford it. The survey results also showed that only 67% of uninsured adult respondents had their blood pressure checked within the past year compared to 91% of insured adults. Additionally, only 31% of uninsured women aged 50 to 64 reported having a mammogram in the past 2 years, compared to 79% of women with health insurance.

The ACA has had an impacted on insurance rates. The number of uninsured adults decreased from 19.3% in 2013 to 18.4% during the first quarter of 2014 and to 12.4% in 2018. The Commonwealth Fund's Biennial Health Insurance Survey assesses the extent and quality of coverage for U.S. working-age adults. The 2018 results reveal that, for the most part, fewer adults are uninsured today compared to 2010, and the duration of coverage gaps people experience has shortened significantly. Unfortunately, more people who have coverage are more underinsured now than they were in 2010, with the greatest increase occurring among those in employer plans. Although the ACA expanded and improved coverage options for people without access to a job-based health plan, it has had little impact on employer plans (Collins, Bhupal, & Doty, 2019). For complete results of the survey go to: www.commonwealthfund.org/publications/issue-briefs/2019/feb/health-insurance-coverage-eight-years-after-aca.

Differences in insurance rates are being observed based on the choices made by states as they relate to the ACA. In 2018, adults aged 18 to 64 in states with a federal market-place were more likely to be uninsured than those in states with a state-based market-place or states with a hybrid marketplace. In Medicaid expansion states, the percentage of uninsured adults decreased from 18.4% in 2013 to 8.7% in the first 3 months of 2018. In nonexpansion states, the percentage of uninsured adults decreased, from 22.7% in 2013 to 17.5% in 2015. The percentage of people who were uninsured in these states increased from 17.5% in 2015 to 19.0% in 2017, and there was no significant change between 2017 and the first 3 months of 2018 (18.4%) (Cohen, Martinez, & Zammitti, 2018).

Enough time has passed since the enactment of the ACA that researchers have been able to examine the impact of Medicaid expansion on health outcomes. As of 2019, 37 states including the District of Columbia have opted to expand Medicaid (Massachusetts and Wisconsin, which are included in these numbers, expanded Medicaid before enact-ment of the ACA). Bhatt and Beck-Sagué (2018) compared infant mortality rates before and after the adoption of Medicaid expansion. They found that the infant mortality rate in the United States declined nationally by 11.9% from 6.7 (2010) to 5.9 (2016) deaths per 1,000 live births. These declines were more modest in non–Medicaid expansion (11.0%) than in Medicaid expansion (15.2%) states. The mean infant mortality rate in non-Medicaid expansion states rose slightly (6.4 to 6.5) from 2014 to 2016, whereas in Medicaid expansion states, it declined from 5.9 to 5.6 per 1,000 live births. Mazurenko, Balio, Agarwal, Carroll, and Menachemi (2018) analyzed 77 published, peer-reviewed studies. They found expansion of Medicaid under the ACA was linked to increases in health coverage, use of health services and quality of care. Among their findings was that health insurance gains were largest for adults without a college degree; use of primary care, mental health services, and preventive care among Medicaid enrollees went up; and reliance on emergency departments decreased. In another study, researchers found that counties in states where Medicaid expanded had 4 fewer deaths per 100,000 resi-dents each year from cardiovascular causes after expansion, compared with counties in non-expansion states (Khatana et al., 2019).

Our healthcare system is complex, and there is no simple solution to lowering costs and improving access. The goal of this textbook is not to provide an overarching solution to the issues of cost, but to propose that nurses can contribute to improving the cost-effectiveness and efficiency of care through the provision of evidence-based treatment guidelines to identified populations with shared needs, and by advocating for policies that address the underlying factors that impact health and healthcare. To do this, we must change the way that we deliver healthcare and become politically active. In an ideal world, healthcare policies are created based on valid and reliable evidence and population need and demand. The ideal premise is that there is equitable distribution of healthcare services and that the appropriate care is given to the right people at the right time and at a reasonable cost. For 20 years, the American Nurses Association (ANA) has been advocating for healthcare reforms that would guarantee access to high-quality healthcare for all. The ANA supports the ACA and was an advocate for the public option. In 2016 the organization sent a letter to President Trump that advocated for "universal access to a standard package of essential healthcare services" (ANA, 2019, para 5). It is a function of individual choice to either support or not support health-care reforms. The actions of professional organizations are driven by membership. Regardless of your political alliance, involvement in professional organizations as well as in local, state, and national political activities (even if only minimally as a regis-tered and active voter) is part of the professional responsibility of advanced practice registered nurses (APRNs).

DEFINING POPULATIONS

The AACN definition of advanced practice nursing includes recognizing the importance of identifying and managing health outcomes at the population level (AACN, 2004). In 2006, the AACN specified that graduates of DNP programs have competency in meeting "the needs of a panel of patients, a target population, a set of populations, or a broad community" (AACN, 2006, p. 10). A core component of DNP education is clinical pre-vention (health promotion and disease prevention at individual and family levels) and population health (focus of care at aggregate and community levels and examination of environmental, occupational, cultural, and socioeconomic dimensions of health) (AACN, 2006; Allan et al., 2004). Regardless of whether DNP graduates practice with a focus on clinical prevention or population health, the ability to define, identify, and analyze outcomes is imperative for improving the health status of individuals and popu-lations (AACN, 2006).

The goal of population-based nursing is to provide evidence-based care to targeted groups of people with similar needs in order to improve outcomes. Population-based nursing uses a defined population or aggregate as the organizing unit for care. The Merriam-Webster Dictionary ("Population," 2019, para. 1) defines a population as "the whole number of people or inhabitants in a country or region." A second definition is given as "a body of persons or individuals having a quality or characteristic in common" (para. 1). Subpopulations may be referred to as *aggregates*. Many different parameters can be used to identify or categorize subpopulations or aggregates. They may be defined by ethnicity (e.g., African American or Hispanic), religion (e.g., Roman Catholic or

Muslim), or geographical location (e.g., Boston or San Diego). Aggregates can also be defined by age or occupation. People with a shared diagnosis (e.g., diabetes) or a shared risk factor (e.g., smoking) comprise other identifiable aggregates. Sometimes people may choose to describe themselves as members of a particular group (e.g., conservative or liberal). One person may belong to more than one such group (e.g., White, younger than 18 years, current smoker).

A community is composed of multiple aggregates. The most common aggregate used in population-based nursing is the high-risk aggregate. A high-risk aggregate is a subgroup or subpopulation of a community that shares a high-risk factor among its members, such as a high-risk health condition (e.g., congestive heart failure) or a shared high-risk factor (e.g., smoking and sedentary behavior). The aggregate concept can be used to target interventions to specific aggregates or subpopulations within a community (Porche, 2004). The implementation of standard or proven (evidence-based) strategies to prevent illness and/or improve the health of targeted groups of people can have the effect of ameliorating health problems at the population and/or aggregate level. Making change at the population level may impact the health of a community not only in the present but for generations to come. As we learn how to approach and target populations using evidence, we improve our chance of long-term success and can strive to make lifelong changes in the health of a group of people.

USING DATA TO TARGET POPULATIONS AND AGGREGATES AT RISK

The collection and analysis of data provide healthcare professionals and policy makers with a starting point for identifying, selecting, and implementing interventions that target specific populations and aggregates. Many of the leading causes of death in the United States are preventable. One in three American adults has cardiovascular disease, and it is the leading cause of death among both men and women in the country, killing on average one American every 40 seconds (Boston Scientific, 2019). On the basis of data from 2016, the Centers for Disease Control and Prevention (CDC) has identified, in descending order, the 10 leading causes of death in the United States. They are heart disease, cancer, accidents (unintentional injuries), chronic lower respiratory diseases, stroke (cerebral vascular diseases), Alzheimer's disease, diabetes, influenza and pneumonia, renal diseases, and intentional self-harm (e.g., suicide) (CDC, 2017a). Several factors, such as the physical environment, healthcare systems, personal behaviors, and the social environment, can have a deleterious impact on individual and community health. The negative consequences of these factors are researched and well documented.

Smoking

Life expectancy for smokers is at least 10 years shorter than for nonsmokers. It is a leading cause of preventable morbidity and mortality, causing nearly one of every five deaths annually in the United States. This figure includes heart attack deaths and lung cancer deaths among nonsmokers who are exposed to secondhand smoke. It is estimated that smoking contributes $170 billion to healthcare costs in the United States (CDC, 2019a).

The CDC used the *2017 National Health Interview Survey* (NHIS) to estimate adult smoking prevalence rates in the United States. The findings indicate that 19.3% of U.S. adults use a tobacco product every day or some days. Smoking rates are higher among men, younger adults, non-Hispanic adults, those living in the Midwest and South, those with less education and income, and LGBT (lesbian, gay, bisexual, and transgender) adults (CDC, 2019b). Although higher rates are seen in younger adults, a reduction in smoking by school-age children should result in reductions in tobacco-related deaths in the future, but new data reveal that tobacco rates among American youth are increasing (CDC, 2019c). This is particularly bad news coming on the heels of the 2012–2013 National Adult Tobacco Survey, which had revealed the lowest smoking rates for high school students since 1991. The current rise in smoking use among school age children is attributed to an increase in E-cigarette use (CDC, 2014, 2019c).

Technology has contributed to many positive advances in healthcare. E-cigarettes are not one of them. E-cigarettes are metal tubes that heat liquid into an inhalable vapor that contains nicotine. Between 2017 and 2018, E-cigarette use increased from 11.7% to 20.8% among high school students and from 3.3% to 4.9% among middle school students. During the same time period, no change was found in the use of other tobacco products (including cigarettes) (CDC, 2019d). As of December 2018, 50 states have enacted laws that restrict the use of E-cigarettes by youth. The minimum legal age to purchase E-cigarettes in these 50 states varies but falls within a narrow range (19 to 21). Go to publichealthlawcenter.org/sites/default/files/States-with-Laws-Restricting-Youth-Access-to-ECigarettes-Dec2018.pdf for specific information about youth access to E-cigarettes in the United States (Public Health Law Center, n.d.). Canada passed the Tobacco and Vaping Products Act in May, 2018. This act regulates the manufacture, sale, labeling and promotion of tobacco products and vaping products sold in Canada and includes restrictions on the sale of tobacco products to youth (Government of Canada, 2018). For more information on this Act go to www.canada.ca/en/health-canada/services/health-concerns/tobacco/legislation/federal-laws/tobacco-act.html. APRNs need to keep abreast of new behaviors that can impact health. Being informed about risky behaviors is of primary importance for APRNs to be effective in planning and delivering evidence-based education and in lobbying for changes to protect the public's health.

Another very popular trend is the use of hookahs. Hookahs are water pipes used to smoke specially flavored tobaccos. Youth are drawn toward this social trend in which groups of people share a hookah usually in a café setting. Although hookahs have been around for hundreds of years, they are not a safe alternative to smoking. Hookah use rates among youth remained relatively constant from 2011 to 2018. In 2018 1.2% of middle schoolers (1% in 2011) and 4.1% of high school students (4.1% in 2011) reported that they had used a hookah within the past 30 days (CDC, 2018a). The tobacco and smoke from hookahs have toxic properties and have been linked to various cancers, including lung and oral cancers. Many of the same effects of cigarette smoking are found with smoking hookahs. As with any potential threat to health, education of our youth and adult populations regarding the deleterious effects of hookahs is paramount to reducing the potential morbidity and mortality of long-term exposure to these flavored tobaccos. More recently, newer electronic forms of hookahs have been introduced, and little research has been conducted to determine the long-term health effects of these products. Regardless, the use of hookahs is another health behavior that an APRN can attempt to modify by evidence-based prevention education. For more on the effects of hookahs, refer to the CDC's site (www.cdc.gov/tobacco/data_statistics/fact_sheets/tobacco_industry/hookahs/index.htm#overview).

There is huge potential for cost savings by preventing smoking-related illnesses, and one cannot overlook the effects of secondhand smoke on the health of family members and coworkers. It is well known that secondhand smoke has long-lasting effects on the unborn fetus, infant, and child. These effects can manifest as preterm births (Been et al., 2014), increased respiratory infections and higher risk of asthma exacerbations (Abreo, Gebretsadik, Stone, & Hartert, 2018), sudden infant death (CDC, 2018b), and a lower intelligence quotient (Ling & Heffernan, 2016). Thus, it is important to recognize not only the direct effects of smoking on health but also the indirect effects on fetuses, infants, children, and family members. The effects of secondhand smoke are not specific to smoking cigarettes. Exposure to hookah smoke is also associated with very similar effects on fetuses, infants, and family members. Education of pregnant mothers is just as important as with other family members as they may not realize the negative effects of secondhand exposure to hookah or cigarette smoke.

As with other smoking-related diseases, the cessation of smoking early on can reverse or ameliorate the potential long-term harmful effects of secondhand smoke exposure. These data provide a starting point for targeting specific high-risk groups for intervention based on parameters such as age, education, income, and geographical location. Another pertinent fact is that many insurance companies are now charging higher premiums for smokers than for nonsmokers. This has led to increasing interest in cessation programs, but whether this will have a long-term impact on smoking rates is unknown. The recent increase in tobacco use by youth in the United States (largely attributed to the use of E-cigarettes) represents a troubling trend. Smoking cessation and smoking prevention programs are areas that offer opportunities for improving the health of people in the United States and for saving money. Other health problems, such as obesity, are also significant public health concerns.

Obesity

In 2009, researchers published their analysis of the cost of obesity in the United States, taking into account separate categories for inpatient, outpatient, and prescription drug spending. They estimated that the medical costs of obesity may have been as high as $147 billion/year by 2008 (including $7 billion in Medicare prescription drug costs). According to their findings, the annual medical costs for people who are obese were $1,429 higher than those for normal-weight people (Finkelstein, Trogdon, Cohen, & Dietz, 2009).

As part of *Healthy People 2020*, the United States set an objective to decrease the proportion of obese adult Americans (20 years of age or older) to 30.5%. H*ealthy People 2020* use the baseline of 33.9%, which was the percentage of persons aged 20 years and older who were obese in 2005 to 2008. The target objective for children (aged 2 to 19 years) is 14.5%. The baseline data for this objective is 16.1%, which was the percentage of children who were considered obese in 2005 to 2008 (HealthyPeople.gov, 2019). For the years 2015–2016 the prevalence of obesity among adults in the U.S. was 39.8%. This represents an increase from the *Healthy People* baseline. The highest rates were found among Hispanics (47.0%) and non-Hispanic Blacks (46.8%) followed by non-Hispanic Whites (37.9%) and non-Hispanic Asians (12.7%). Young adults had the lowest prevalence rate (35.7%) and middle-aged adults had the highest (42.8%; CDC, 2018c). The CDC (2018d) reports that the prevalence of obesity among children (aged 2–19) in the United States is 18.5% (an increase over the *Healthy People* baseline data). The prevalence rate is lowest for children aged 2 to 5 (13.9%) and highest for children aged 12 to 19 (20.6%). It is most common for Hispanic (25.8%) and non-Hispanic Blacks (22.0%). It is lowest for non-Hispanic Whites (14.1%) and non-Hispanic Asians (11.0%).

Obesity is associated with increased morbidity and mortality rates. Abdelaal, le Roux, and Docherty (2017) have summarized the most important comorbidities of obesity. They point out that obesity can cause both psychosocial (depression) and metabolic (diabetes) dysfunction and identified 13 specific domains that account for morbidity and mortality in obesity. Cardiovascular disease (CVD) and cancer account for the greatest mortality risk associated with obesity even when controlling for demographic and behavioral characteristics. Although people are familiar with the association between heart disease and obesity, many are just learning about the relationship between obesity and cancer. Obesity is associated with an increased risk for many cancers, including esophageal, pancreatic, colon and rectal, breast (after menopause), endometrial, kidney, thyroid, and gallbladder. It has been estimated that the percentage of cases attributed to obesity (although it varies) may be as high as 54% for some cancers (National Cancer Institute, 2017).

Jacobs et al. (2010) published a study that helps to illustrate the complexity of understanding risk factors and their relationship to the development of poor health. They studied the association between waist circumference and mortality among 48,500 men and 56,343 women 50 years or older. They determined that waist circumference as a measure of abdominal obesity is associated with higher mortality independent of body mass index (BMI). They note that waist circumference is associated with higher circulating levels of inflammatory markers, insulin resistance, type 2 diabetes, dyslipidemia, and coronary heart disease. In recent years, the constellation of these factors has been described as the *metabolic syndrome*. Metabolic syndrome is a complex syndrome that encompasses many conditions and risk factors, particularly abdominal obesity, high blood pressure, abnormal cholesterol and triglyceride levels, and insulin resistance, and is known to be associated with an increased risk of stroke, heart disease, and type 2 diabetes (Grundy, 2016). The increasing prevalence of metabolic syndrome is becoming a tremendous public health concern, and more evidence is appearing in the literature to better define the treatment as well as preventive measures needed to reduce the incidence. Although it is ill defined in children and adolescents, it is clear that early interventions to reduce obesity and sedentary behavior and to improve nutrition can have long-term effects and can improve overall life expectancy. Metabolic syndrome, similar to many conditions, demonstrates the complexity of interactions that occur in disease development and that no one factor in and of itself can be targeted alone. Our understanding of obesity is also becoming more complex, as new studies have identified independent associations between sitting time/sedentary behaviors and increasing all-cause and cardiovascular disease mortality risk. This phenomenon highlights the importance of exercising and avoiding prolonged, uninterrupted periods of sitting time (Patel, Maliniak, Rees-Punia, Matthews, & Gapstur, 2018). The APRN needs to take into consideration the many facets of health and disease, genetics and environment, including human attitudes, attributes, and behavior when determining how to implement a population-based intervention.

Diabetes Mellitus

One cannot talk about the epidemic of obesity and not mention its concomitant relationship to diabetes mellitus (DM). The number of American adults treated for DM more than doubled between 1996 and 2007 (from about 9 to 19 million). This includes an increase from 1.2 to 2.4 million among people aged 18 to 44 years. During this time period, the treatment costs for DM climbed from $18.5 to $40.8 billion (Soni, 2010). In 2017, the American Diabetes Association released the results of the *National Diabetes Statistics* report (CDC, 2017b). The report highlights the importance of tracking morbidity rates and the need to be aware of trends in order to target groups for interventions. The percentage of Americans with DM aged 65 and older is estimated to be as high as 25.2% (accounting for approximately 12 million seniors), which includes those who are undiagnosed. Approximately 24% of Americans under the age of 20 have been diagnosed with diabetes. The incidence rate of diabetes in 2015 was 6.7 per 1,000 or 1.5 million new cases. According to the American Diabetes Association (2018) the total costs of diagnosed diabetes in the United States in 2017 was $327 billion.

The rise in both incidence and prevalence rates for DM is closely tied to rising obesity levels, which is a preventable risk factor. This upward trend in the incidence rate for DM provides a clear direction for targeting prevention measures toward younger populations. There is, in fact, a huge potential for improving the health of populations by targeting children using primary prevention measures that go well beyond reducing diabetes rates. Implications for early interventions beginning in pregnancy and continuing through infancy and early childhood are clear. Evidence is increasing that early feeding patterns (e.g., breastfeeding versus formula feeding) as well as parental obesity and parental eating patterns are linked to the increased likelihood of developing obesity in children, which puts them at an increased risk for type 2 DM (Owen, Martin, Whincup, Smith, & Cook, 2005). There are many opportunities for APRNs to apply evidence-based, primary prevention interventions to improve the long-term outcomes of children at the beginning of pregnancy and at birth and thereafter. This approach may include targeting high-risk aggregates (e.g., parents with obesity and type 2 DM) and then expanding to communities through educational campaigns or changes in health policy.

Health and the Social Environment

Most of the information discussed earlier exemplifies the biological and environmental factors that contribute to poor health in adults. However, it is becoming more apparent that social (e.g., psychological) factors starting as early as conception (e.g., maternal stress) may play a more significant role in adult health than was once thought. Having a comprehensive understanding of the underlying causes of adult diseases (including social, psychological, biological, and environmental) is necessary to successfully approach the problems seen in populations. Without this comprehensive understanding, it may be difficult to successfully implement a primary prevention program (the goal of which is to prevent disease before it occurs).

Stress is a regular part of day-to-day life, and small amounts of stress are normal and necessary for developing coping skills. However, exposure to prolonged and severe stressors, such as abuse, neglect, or being a witness to or victim of violence, can lead to changes that occur in the brain and can lead to short-term and even long-term poor health outcomes. This type of stress is termed *toxic stress*. The effects of toxic stress are being rigorously studied, and in particular, studies looking at adverse childhood events (ACE) were some of the first to show a correlation between toxic stress exposures and high-risk behaviors and poor health outcomes in adults. The ACE study is an ongoing, joint project of the CDC and Kaiser Permanente that looks retrospectively at the relationships among several categories of childhood trauma. Childhood trauma exposures were broken down into three categories: abuse (e.g., physical or sexual), neglect (e.g., emotional or physical), and household dysfunction (e.g., having an incarcerated household member, family member with mental health issue and/or drug and alcohol problems, domestic violence, or parental divorce or separation). An ACE score is calculated based on past exposures to the subparts of each of the aforementioned categories. The higher the ACE score, the stronger the relationship to high-risk behaviors or poor health outcomes (CDC, 2016). In one widely cited ACE study (Felitti et al., 1998), people who experienced a score of four or more categories of ACEs, compared with those who had no history of exposure, had a four- to 12-fold increased risk for alcoholism, drug abuse, depression, and suicide attempts. They also experienced a two- to four-fold increase in smoking and self-reported poor health. Subsequent research provides additional evidence to support the link between childhood trauma and adverse events and poor health outcomes. For additional information on the effects of childhood stress, refer to the CDC publication at www.cdc .gov/violenceprevention/childabuseandneglect/acestudy/index.html.

Many additional studies have been conducted that demonstrate the destructive effects of exposure to *toxic stress*. Smyth, Heron, Wonderlich, Crosby, and Thompson (2008) completed a study of students entering college directly from high school to investigate the association between adverse events in childhood and eating disturbances. They found that childhood adverse events predicted eating disturbances in college. Childhood adverse events have also been linked to drug abuse and dependence

(Messina et al., 2008) and greater use of healthcare and mental health services (Cannon, Bonomi, Anderson, Rivara, & Thompson, 2010). Building on earlier studies that linked smoking in adulthood with ACEs, Brown et al. (2010) discovered a relationship between a history of ACEs and the risk of dying from lung cancer. Researchers have identified similar outcomes in studies carried out with populations in other countries. A study conducted in Saudi Arabia, where beating and insults are often an acceptable parenting style, identified a correlation between beating and insults (once or more per month) and an increased risk for cancer, cardiac disease, and asthma (Hyland, Alkhalaf, & Whalley, 2012). Scott, Smith, and Ellis (2012) completed a study in New Zealand, which found that adults who had a history of child protection involvement had increased odds of a diagnosis of asthma. McKelvey, Saccente, and Swindle (2019) examined the associations between ACEs in infancy and toddlerhood and obesity and related health indicators in middle childhood. Across all outcomes examined, children with four or more ACEs had the poorest health and were more likely to be obese when compared to children with no ACE exposure.

More and more studies are being conducted to look at the relationship of sustained exposure to toxic stress to a variety of poor health outcomes and high-risk behaviors. These behaviors include such things as cutting, hypervigilance, promiscuity, eating disorders, poor school performance, depression, violence, suicidal ideation/attempts, and justice system involvement. These are just a few of the many behaviors found to be associated with sustained exposure to toxic stress. Studies such as these illustrate the importance of understanding the social determinants of poor health and the potential for doing good and preventing harm to aggregates and populations by targeting exposures to such things as child abuse and neglect for prevention, early recognition, and intervention.

Population Strategies in Acute Care

Targeting evidence-based interventions toward aggregates in the acute care population also has the potential to improve health outcomes broadly. How can we improve the quality of care for our acute care patients by taking a population-based approach? When nurses apply evidence-based interventions to identified aggregates, they can improve outcomes more effectively than when interventions are designed on a case-by-case (individualized) basis. The following examples illustrate this point.

Several organizations, including the Association for Professionals in Infection Control and Epidemiology and the CDC, proposed a call to action to move toward elimination of healthcare–associated infections. The CDC and Agency for Healthcare Research and Quality (AHRQ) have published evidence-based recommendations for preventing central venous catheter-related bloodstream infections (CR-BSIs). These recommendations include hand hygiene, use of maximal barrier precautions, use of chlorhexidine gluconate for insertion site preparation, and avoidance of catheter changes. Catheters impregnated with antimicrobial agents are recommended when infection rates are high and/or catheters will be in place for a long time. Using these guidelines, hospitals have made good progress in reducing the incidence rate of CR-BSIs. In a report released by the CDC, CR-BSIs fell 50% between 2008 and 2014 (Thompson, 2018).

Another intervention that uses standard, evidence-based protocols to improve long-term outcomes addresses the treatment of stroke in an acute care setting. It was found that stroke patients taken to hospitals that follow specific treatment protocols have a better chance of surviving than patients taken to hospitals without specific stroke treatment protocols. A study evaluated the outcomes of the first 1 million stroke patients treated at hospitals enrolled in the *Get With the Guidelines* (GWTG-S) stroke program that was started by the American Heart Association (AHA) in 2003. The American Stroke Association (ASA) guidelines require that hospitals follow seven specific evidence-based steps for treating stroke patients. Between 2003 and 2009, hospitals that followed these protocols lowered the risk of death by 10% for patients with ischemic stroke (Fonarow et al., 2011). The program grew from 24 participating hospitals in 2003 to more than 2,000 hospitals by the end of 2017. It is estimated that 80% of all ischemic stroke patients are now discharged from hospitals that participate in the GWTG-S program. It is notable that stroke declined from the nation's third to the fourth leading cause of death in 2008 and continued to decline to the fifth leading cause of death in 2013 where it remained in 2017 (AHA & ASA, 2018). For more information on stroke centers see Chapter 9, The Role of Accreditation in Validating Population-Based Practice/Programs.

Surveillance of poor health outcomes in acute care facilities is one way in which APRNs can identify causative factors and design interventions to reduce costs and improve care. For example, recognizing the causative factors that lead to increased rehospitalization rates and superutilization of emergency departments could be the first step in designing an intervention. The AHRQ analyzed data from the Healthcare Cost and Utilization Project from 2010 to examine 30-day rehospitalization rates for specific diseases and procedures. Approximately 25% of all U.S. hospital patients are readmitted within 1 year for the same conditions that led to their original hospitalization. Although superutilizers constitute just 2.6% to 6.1% of all patients seen in an emergency department, they account for 10.5% to 26.2% of all visits. Medicare and Medicaid patients have both higher 30-day readmission rates and higher emergency department superutilization rates than both uninsured and privately insured patients. Some specific diagnoses and procedures have higher rates for these two events also. For example, among Medicare patients diagnosed with congestive heart failure, 25% were readmitted to hospitals within 30 days and among privately insured the rate was 20% (AHRQ, 2018).

Readmissions and superutilization of services are costly in dollars to both consumers and hospitals and negatively impact the quality of life for patients. Better outpatient care could prevent unnecessary repeat hospital admissions and reduce superutilization of services. Identifying and targeting populations who are at high risk for either event offers great return on investment.

Chronic Conditions

Noncommunicable diseases (NCDs) are the main cause of illness and disability in the United States and are responsible for the greater part of healthcare costs according to the CDC. About 60% of U.S. adults have at least one chronic condition, and 40% have two or more chronic conditions. Most chronic conditions result from preventable risk factors such as smoking, poor diet, sedentary behavior, and excessive alcohol consumption (CDC, 2019e). The U.S. Department of Health and Human Services (DHHS) created and supports the *Initiative on Multiple Chronic Conditions*. Its strategic framework includes goals to foster healthcare and public health system changes to improve the health of those with multiple chronic conditions (MCC). Two additional goals are to equip care providers with tools, information, and other interventions to help people with MCC and to support targeted research about individuals with MCC and effective interventions. The intention of the framework is to create change in how chronic illnesses are addressed in the United States. from an individual approach to one that uses a population-focused approach (DHHS, 2015).

The problem of chronic diseases is not restricted to the United States. The World Health Organization (WHO) has published a report that documents the global problem of NCDs. NCDs now account for more deaths than infectious diseases even in poor countries. Director-General Dr. Margaret Chan of WHO is quoted as saying, "[F]or some countries, it is no exaggeration to describe the situation is an impending disaster; a disaster for health, society, most of all for national economies" (WHO, 2011, p. ii). Chronic diseases, such as heart disease, stroke, cancer, chronic respiratory diseases, and diabetes, are the leading causes of global mortality. WHO estimates that NCDs kill 40 million people each year and account for 70% of deaths worldwide. Nearly 40% of these deaths occur in people younger than 70 (WHO, 2019). Millions of people die each year as a result of modifiable risk factors that underlie the major NCDs. The writers of a report by WHO contend that 8% of premature heart disease, stroke, and diabetes can be prevented. Ten action points, including banning smoking in public places, enforcing tobacco advertising bans, restricting access to alcohol, and reducing salt in food, are listed. All of these actions require a population approach to be effective (WHO, 2019).

A survey conducted by the AHA lends an interesting perspective to this argument. They surveyed 1,000 people in the United States. The AHA found that only 30% of respondents knew the AHA's recommended limits for daily wine consumption. Drinking too much alcohol of any kind can increase blood pressure and lead to heart failure. The survey results also found that most respondents do not know the source of sodium content in their diets and are confused by low-sodium food choices. A majority of the respondents (61%) believe that sea salt is a low-sodium alternative to table salt when in fact it is chemically the same (AHA, 2011). A poll conducted in 2017 by the American Society of Clinical Oncology (ASCO) revealed that only 31% of Americans are aware that obesity is a risk factor for cancer and just 30% recognize alcohol consumption as a risk factor (ASCO, 2017). These surveys reinforce the idea that people require more understanding of nutrition and the relationship between nutrition and health. It also reinforces the argument that interventions to improve health must be addressed at the community or population level.

Interventions that are evidence-based and population appropriate can reduce the underlying causes of chronic disease. This approach has the potential to lower the mean level of risk factors and shift outcomes in a favorable direction. An example that receives a lot of attention is sodium intake. Excess sodium in the diet can put people at risk for stroke and heart disease. The CDC has reported that 9 of 10 Americans consume more salt than is recommended. Only 5.5% of adults follow the recommendation to limit sodium intake to less than 2,300 mg a day. Most sodium does not come from salt added to foods at the table but from processed foods. These foods include grain-based frozen meals, soup, and processed meat. Sodium content can vary across brands, making it difficult to monitor intake. A cheeseburger from a fast food restaurant for example can have between 370 mg and 730 mg of sodium. Reducing dietary salt could greatly reduce the yearly number of U.S. cases of coronary heart disease, stroke, and heart attacks, with a savings of up to $18 billion in healthcare costs each year (CDC, 2019f).

This discussion illustrates the need to promulgate laws and develop policies that can effect positive health outcomes. It also illustrates the difficulty involved in planning interventions when evidence is sometimes contradictory, and causation is not only multifactorial but sometimes outside of the control of the people whose health is compromised. Changing individual behavior is difficult and has little impact on population health. Using the power of legislation and regulation to make changes in the environment, such as banning smoking in public places, improving air quality, and reducing the amount of sodium in processed foods, has enormous potential for improving the overall health of populations.

The basic sciences of public health (particularly epidemiology and biostatistics) provide tools for the APRN working with specialized populations and the means to find evidence for effective and efficient interventions. The care of specialized groups is the core of advanced practice. *Evidence-based practice* is defined as "a life-long problem-solving approach to the delivery of healthcare that integrates the best evidence from well-designed studies (i.e., external evidence) and integrates it with a patient's preferences and values and a clinician's expertise, which includes internal evidence gathered from patient data" (Melnyk, Gallagher-Ford, Long, & Fineout-Overholt, 2014, p. 5).

Population-based nursing requires APRNs to plan, implement, and evaluate care in the population of interest. The evaluation of outcome measures in populations begins with an identification of the health problems, the needs of defined populations, and the differences among groups. The rates calculated from these numbers can help the APRN to identify risk factors, target populations at risk, and lay the foundation for designing interventions. Prevention is best carried out at the population level, whether at the level of direct care or through the support and promotion of policies. For example, an evidence-based program to prevent hospital readmissions for congestive heart failure can lead to improved health and decreased health-related costs. The promulgation of policies and regulations to support primary prevention measures, such as decreased sodium in prepared foods, could potentially lead to decreased rates of hypertension and heart disease. Interventions that are appropriate at the individual level and applied at the population level can result in a far-reaching effect.

Outcomes measurement refers to collecting and analyzing data using predetermined outcomes indicators for the purposes of making decisions about healthcare (ANA, 2015).

Outcomes research in APRN practice is research that focuses on the effectiveness of nursing interventions. Outcomes measurement in population-based care begins with the identification of the population and the problem, followed by the generation of a clinical question related to outcomes. It is a measure of the process of care. An outcomes measure should be clearly quantifiable, be relatively easy to define, and lend itself to standardization.

In outcomes measurement, the APRN is ultimately concerned with whether a population benefits from an intervention. The APRN also needs to be concerned with the question of quality, efficacy (Does the intervention work under ideal conditions?), and effectiveness (Does it work under real-life situations?). Other important considerations are efficiency (cost benefit), affordability, accessibility, and acceptability.

SUMMARY

The Robert Wood Johnson Foundation and the IOM issued a report to respond to the need to transform the nursing profession. The committee developed four key messages:

1. Nurses should practice to the full extent of their education and should achieve higher levels of education and training.

2. The education system for nurses should be improved so that it provides seamless academic progression.

3. Nurses should be full partners with physicians and other healthcare professionals.

4. Healthcare in the United States should be redesigned for effective workforce planning and policy making (IOM, 2011).

To improve population health, APRNs need to practice to the full extent of their education, be active in the political arena, and work collaboratively with other healthcare professionals. To promote health, APRNs can use epidemiological methods to identify aggregates at risk, analyze problems of highest priority, design evidence-based interventions, and evaluate the results. An important concept in the field of population health is attention to the multiple determinants of health outcomes and the identification of their distribution throughout the population. These determinants include medical care, public health interventions, characteristics of the social environment (e.g., income, education, employment, social support, culture), physical environment (e.g., housing, air, and water quality), genetics, and individual behavior. A final note about the use of "APRN" in this book: *The Consensus Model for APRN Regulation: Licensure, Accreditation, Certification & Education* was completed and published in 2008 by the APRN Consensus Work Group and the National Council of State Boards of Nursing APRN Advisory Committee. The title "APRN" is used throughout this book to refer to certified nurse anesthetists, certified nurse midwives, clinical nurse specialists, and certified nurse practitioners. The model was created through a collaborative effort of more than 40 organizations in order to "align the interrelationships among licensure, accreditation, certification, and education to create a more uniform practice across the country" (American Nurses Credentialing Center [ANCC], 2014). The goal for implementation of the model was 2015. As of 2019 many states have adopted portions of the model but there are variations from state to state. APRNs can check the status of the model in their state by going to: www.ncsbn.org/5397.htm (NCSBN, 2019).

EXERCISES AND DISCUSSION QUESTIONS

Exercise 1.1 Using the following table as an example, list the parameters that describe the population(s) to whom you provide care.

POPULATION	FRAMING DEFINITIONS	PARAMETERS
Patients who have been diagnosed with congestive heart failure (CHF) and who live in the community	Adult (18 years of age and older) patients discharged from an urban medical center with a primary diagnosis of CHF	P1 = diagnosis P2 = age P3 = location/service area
Population of New Jersey	All permanent residents of New Jersey	P1 = geographical location P2 = permanent residency

Exercise 1.2 PolitiFact is a website created by the *St. Petersburg Times* (now the *Tampa Bay Times*) and a winner of the 2009 Pulitzer Prize (www.politifact.com). It was created to help people find the truth in American politics. Reporters and editors from the newspaper check statements by members of Congress, the White House, lobbyists, and interest groups and rate them on a *Truth-O-Meter*. Find a statement that is being circulated about the ACA, and then check the Truth-O-Meter to determine the veracity of the statement.

Exercise 1.3 Identify two or three population-based and health-related interventions at your institution or in your community. Determine whether the approach has been successful in changing outcomes and/or reducing health-related costs. Identify the aggregate population and what parameters were used in this intervention. Identify any changes in policy associated with these interventions.

Exercise 1.4 This chapter includes a brief description of the health effects of E-cigarettes. Design an educational program for a school-age aggregate that addresses the negative health effects of E-cigarettes. First, research the health effects of E-cigarettes and select three to five health effects to address. Identify your target population and design an educational intervention for your target population. What outcomes will you look at to determine whether your intervention works? What approach will you use to engage your target population? Does your state regulate the purchase of E-cigarettes by youth?

Exercise 1.5 The relationship between obesity and cancer is described and discussed in this chapter. Conduct a search to answer the following questions. The incidence rates for six cancers associated with obesity are increasing in young Americans. Identify them. What is the prevalence rate of obesity in people younger than 18 in your state? Which children are at highest risk for obesity in your state? Are there any prevention programs in your state that address this issue? Are they effective? Has your state passed and enacted any laws designed to decrease obesity? Are they effective? If they are not effective, explain why you believe they are not working.

REFERENCES

Abdelaal, M., le Roux, C. W., & Docherty, N. G. (2017). Morbidity and mortality associated with obesity. *Annals of Translational Medicine, 5*(7), 161. doi:10.21037/atm.2017.03.107

Abreo, A., Gebretsadik, T., Stone, C. A., & Hartert, T. V. (2018). The impact of modifiable risk factor reduction on childhood asthma development. *Clinical & Translational Medicine, 7*(1), 1. doi:10.1186/s40169-018-0195-4

Agency for Healthcare Research and Quality. (2018). 30-day readmission rates to U.S. hospitals. Retrieved from https://www.ahrq.gov/data/infographics/readmission-rates.html

Allan, J., Barwick, T., Cashman, S., Cawley, J. F., Day, C., Douglass, C. W., . . . Wood, D. (2004). Clinical prevention and population health: Curriculum framework for health professions. *American Journal of Preventive Medicine, 27*(5), 471–476. doi:10.1016/s0749-3797(04)00206-5

American Association of Colleges of Nursing. (2004). *AACN position statement on the practice doctorate in nursing*. Washington, DC: Author.

American Association of Colleges of Nursing. (2006). *The essentials of doctoral education for advanced practice nursing*. Washington, DC: Author. Retrieved from https://www.aacnnursing.org/DNP/DNP-Essentials

American Diabetes Association. (2018). *Statistics about diabetes*. Retrieved from http://www.diabetes.org/diabetes-basics/statistics

American Heart Association. (2011). *Most Americans don't understand health effects of wine and sea salt, survey finds*. Dallas, TX: Author. Retrieved from https://www.prnewswire.com/news-releases/most-americans-dont-understand-health-effects-of-wine-and-sea-salt-survey-finds-120595304.html

American Heart Association & American Stroke Association. (2018). *Twenty years of progress*. Retrieved from https://www.strokeassociation.org/-/media/stroke-files/about-the-asa/asa-20th-anniv-report-ucm_498858.pdf?la=en

American Nurses Association. (2015). *Nursing: Scope and standards of practice* (3rd ed.). Washington, DC: Author.

American Nurses Association. (2019). Health system reform. Retrieved from https://www.nursingworld.org/practice-policy/health-policy/health-system-reform

American Nurses Credentialing Center. (2018). *APRN Faculty Tool Kit*. Retrieved from https://www.nursingworld.org/~48cd5b/globalassets/docs/ancc/faculty-toolkit-presentation.pdf

American Society of Clinical Oncology. (2017). *National survey reveals most Americans are unaware of key cancer risk factors*. Retrieved from https://www.asco.org/about-asco/press-center/news-releases/national-survey-reveals-most-americans-are-unaware-key-cancer

APRN Consensus Work Group & the National Council of State Boards of Nursing APRN Advisory Committee. (2008). *Consensus model for APRN regulation: Licensure, accreditation, certification & education*. Retrieved from https://www.ncsbn.org/Consensus_Model_for_APRN_Regulation_July_2008.pdf

Been, J. V., Nurmatov, U. B., Cox, B., Nawrot, T. S., van Schayck, C. P., & Sheikh, A. (2014). Effect of smoke-free legislation on perinatal and child health: A systematic review and meta-analysis. *Lancet (London, England), 383*(9928), 1549–1560. doi:10.1016/S0140-6736(14)60082-9

Bhatt, C. B., & Beck-Sagué, C. M. (2018). Medicaid expansion and infant mortality in the United States. *American Journal of Public Health, 108*(4), 565–567. doi:10.2105/AJPH.2017.304218

Boston Scientific. (2019). *Heart disease facts*. Retrieved from http://www.your-heart-health.com/content/close-the-gap/en-US/heart-disease-facts.html

Brown, D., Anda, R., Felitti, V., Edwards, V., Malarcher, A., Croft, J., & Giles, W. (2010). Adverse childhood experiences are associated with the risk of lung cancer: A prospective cohort study. *BMC Public Health, 10*, 20. Retrieved from EBSCO*host*.

Cannon, E., Bonomi, A., Anderson, M., Rivara, F., & Thompson, R. (2010). Adult health and relationship outcomes among women with abuse experiences during childhood. *Violence and Victims, 25*(3), 291–305. Retrieved from EBSCO*host.*

Centers for Disease Control and Prevention. (2014). *Cigarette smoking among U.S. high school students at lowest level in 22 years* [Press Release]. Retrieved from http://www.cdc.gov/media/releases/2014/p0612-YRBS.html?s_cid=ostltsdyk_cs_506

Centers for Disease Control and Prevention. (2016). Adverse childhood experiences (ACE). Retrieved from https://www.cdc.gov/violenceprevention/childabuseandneglect/acestudy/index.html

Centers for Disease Control and Prevention. (2017a). *Leading causes of death.* Retrieved from https://www.cdc.gov/nchs/fastats/leading-causes-of-death.htm

Centers for Disease Control and Prevention. (2017b). *National diabetes statistics report, 2017.* Retrieved from https://www.cdc.gov/diabetes/pdfs/data/statistics/national-diabetes-statistics-report.pdf

Centers for Disease Control and Prevention. (2018a). *Smoking and tobacco use–hookahs.* Retrieved from http://www.cdc.gov/tobacco/data_statistics/fact_sheets/tobacco_industry/hookahs/index.htm#overview

Centers for Disease Control and Prevention. (2018b). *Health effects of secondhand smoke.* Retrieved from https://www.cdc.gov/tobacco/data_statistics/fact_sheets/secondhand_smoke/health_effects/index.htm

Centers for Disease Control and Prevention. (2018c). *Adult obesity facts.* Retrieved from https://www.cdc.gov/obesity/data/adult.html

Centers for Disease Control and Prevention. (2018d). *Childhood obesity facts.* Retrieved from https://www.cdc.gov/obesity/data/childhood.html

Centers for Disease Control and Prevention. (2019a). *Smoking and tobacco use.* Retrieved from https://www.cdc.gov/tobacco/data_statistics/fact_sheets/index.htm

Centers for Disease Control and Prevention. (2019b). *Smoking and tobacco use: Current cigarette smoking among adults in the United States.* Retrieved from https://www.cdc.gov/tobacco/data_statistics/fact_sheets/adult_data/cig_smoking/index.htm

Centers for Disease Control and Prevention. (2019c). *Tobacco use by youth is rising. Vital Signs.* Retrieved from https://www.cdc.gov/vitalsigns/youth-tobacco-use/?s_cid=osh-stu-home-slider-005

Centers for Disease and Control and Prevention. (2019d). *Youth and tobacco use.* Retrieved from https://www.cdc.gov/tobacco/data_statistics/fact_sheets/youth_data/tobacco_use/index.htm

Centers for Disease Control and Prevention. (2019e). *About chronic diseases.* Retrieved from https://www.cdc.gov/chronicdisease/about/index.htm

Centers for Disease Control and Prevention. (2019f). *Salt.* Retrieved from https://www.cdc.gov/salt/index.htm

Centers for Medicare & Medicaid Services. (2019). *NHE fact sheet.* Retrieved from https://www.cms.gov/research-statistics-data-and-systems/statistics-trends-and-reports/nationalhealthexpenddata/nhe-fact-sheet.html

Central Intelligence Agency. (n.d.). *The world factbook.* Retrieved from https://www.cia.gov/library/publications/the-world-factbook/rankorder/2091rank.html

Cohen, R. A., Martinez, M. E., & Zammitti, E. P. (2018). Health insurance coverage: Early release of estimates from the National Health Interview Survey, January-March 2018. Retrieved from https://www.cdc.gov/nchs/data/nhis/earlyrelease/Insur201808.pdf

Collins, S., Bhupal, H., & Doty, M. (2019). *Health insurance coverage eight years after the ACA.* Retrieved from https://www.commonwealthfund.org/publications/issue-briefs/2019/feb/health-insurance-coverage-eight-years-after-aca

Collins, S., Doty, M., Robertson, R., & Garber, T. (2011). *How the recession has left millions of workers without health insurance, and how health reform will bring relief: Findings from the Commonwealth Fund Biennial Health Insurance Survey of 2010.* Retrieved from https://www.commonwealthfund.org/publications/fund-reports/2011/mar/help-horizon-how-recession-has-left-millions-workers-without

Dossey, B. (2000). *Florence Nightingale: Mystic, visionary, healer.* Springhouse, PA: Springhouse Corporation.

Evans, G. D. (2003). Clara Barton: Teacher, nurse, Civil War heroine, founder of the American Red Cross. *International History of Nursing Journal, 7*(3), 75–82.

Felitti, V., Anda, R., Nordenberg, D., Williamson, D., Spitz, A., Edwards, V., . . . Marks, J. (1998). Relationship of childhood abuse and household dysfunction to many of the leading causes of death in adults: The adverse childhood experiences (ACE) study. *American Journal of Preventative Medicine, 14,* 245–258. doi:10.1016/s0749-3797(98)00017-8

Finkelstein, E., Trogdon, J., Cohen, J., & Dietz, W. (2009). Annual medical spending attributable to obesity: Payer-and service-specific estimates. *Health Affairs, 28*(5). Retrieved from http://content.healthaffairs .org/content/28/5/w822.full.pdf

Fonarow, G., Smith, E., Saver, J., Reeves, M., Bhatt, D., Grau-Sepulveda, M., . . . Schwamm, L. (2011). Timeliness of tissue-type plasminogen activator therapy in acute ischemic stroke: Patient characteristics, hospital factors, and outcomes associated with door-to-needle times within 60 minutes. *Circulation, 123*(7), 750–758. Retrieved from EBSCO*host*.

Frontier Nursing University. (2019). *Historical timeline.* Retrieved from https://frontier.edu/about-frontier/ history

Government of Canada. (2018). Tobacco and Vaping Products Act. Retrieved from https://www.canada.ca/ en/health-canada/services/health-concerns/tobacco/legislation/federal-laws/tobacco-act.html

Grundy, S. M. (2016). Metabolic syndrome update. *Trends in Cardiovascular Medicine, 26*(4), 364–373. doi:10.1016/j.tcm.2015.10.004

HealthyPeople.gov. (2019). *Nutrition and weight status (Healthy People 2020).* Retrieved from https://www .healthypeople.gov/2020/topics-objectives/topic/nutrition-and-weight-status/objectives

Hyland, M. E., Alkhalaf, A. M., & Whalley, B. (2012). Beating and insulting children as a risk for adult cancer, cardiac disease and asthma. *Journal of Behavioral Medicine, 36*(6), 632–640. doi:10.1007/ s10865-012-9457-6

Institute of Medicine. (2010). *For the public's health: The role of measurement in action and accountability.* Retrieved from http://www.nationalacademies.org/hmd/Reports/2010/For-the-Publics-Health-The-Role -of-Measurement-in-Action-and-Accountability.aspx

Institute of Medicine. (2011). *Initiative on the future of nursing.* Retrieved from http://www.thefutureofnurs- ing.org/recommendations

Jacobs, E., Newton, C., Wang, Y., Patel, A., McCullough, M., Campbell, P., . . . Gapster, S. (2010). Waist circumference and all-cause mortality in a large U.S. cohort. *Archives of Internal Medicine, 170*(15), 1293–1301. doi:10.1001/archinternmed.2010.201

January, A. M. (2009). Friday at Frontier Nursing Service. *Public Health Nursing, 26*(2), 202–203. doi:10.1111/j.1525-1446.2009.00771.x

Jost, T. S. (2018). *The Affordable Care Act under the Trump administration.* Retrieved from The Commonwealth Fund website https://www.commonwealthfund.org/blog/2018/affordable-care-act- under-trump-administration

Khatana, S. A., Bhatla, A., Nathan, A. S., Giri, J., Shen, C., Kazi, D. S., & Groeneveld, P. W. (April, 2019). 3— *Association of medicaid expansion with cardiovascular mortality—A quasi-experimental analysis.* Paper presented at American Heart Association, Quality of Care & Outcomes Research, Arlington, VA.

Ling, J., & Heffernan, T. (2016). The cognitive deficits associated with second-hand smoking. *Frontiers in Psychiatry, 7*, 46. doi:10.3389/fpsyt.2016.00046

Lipsey, S. (1993). *Mathematical education in the life of Florence Nightingale.* Retrieved from http://www .agnesscott.edu/lriddle/women/night_educ.htm

Mazurenko, O., Balio, C. P., Agarwal, R., Carroll, A. E., & Menachemi, N. (2018). The effects of Medicaid expansion under the ACA: A systematic review. *Health Affairs (Project Hope), 37*(6), 944–950. doi:10.1377/ hlthaff.2017.1491

McKelvey, L. M., Saccente, J. E., & Swindle, T. M. (2019). Adverse childhood experiences in infancy and toddlerhood predict obesity and health outcomes in middle childhood. *Childhood Obesity, 15*(3), 206–215. doi:10.1089/chi.2018.0225

Melnyk, B. M., Gallagher-Ford, L., Long, L. E., & Fineout-Overholt, E. (2014). The establishment of evidence-based practice competencies for practicing registered nurses and advanced practice nurses in real-world clinical settings: Proficiencies to improve healthcare quality, reliability, patient outcomes, and costs. *Worldviews on Evidence-Based Nursing, 11*(1), 5–15. doi:10.1111/wvn.12021

Messina, N., Marinelli-Casey, P., Hillhouse, M., Rawson, R., Hunter, J., & Ang, A. (2008). Childhood adverse events and methamphetamine use among men and women. *Journal of Psychoactive Drugs, 40* (Suppl. 5), 399–409. Retrieved from EBSCO*host*.

National Cancer Institute. (2017). *Obesity and cancer.* Retrieved from http://www.cancer.gov/cancertopics/ factsheet/Risk/obesity

NCSBN. (2019). *APRN collaboration consensus status.* Retrieved from https://www.ncsbn.org/5397.htm

Obama, B. (2009, August 16). Why we need healthcare reform. *The New York Times*, WK9.

Organisation for Economic Co-operation and Development. (2019). Health expenditure. Retrieved from http://www.oecd.org/els/health-systems/health-expenditure.htm

Orszag, P. R. (2008). *Growth in healthcare costs. Statement before the Committee on the Budget United States Senate.* Retrieved from http://www.cbo.gov/ftpdocs/89xx/doc8948/01-31-HealthTestimony.pdf

Owen, C. G., Martin, R. M., Whincup, P. H., Smith, G. D., & Cook, D. G. (2005). Effect of infant feeding on the risk of obesity across the life course: A quantitative review of published evidence. *Pediatrics, 115*(5), 1367–1377.

Patel, A. V., Maliniak, M. L., Rees-Punia, E., Matthews, C. E., & Gapstur, S. M. (2018). Prolonged leisure time spent sitting in relation to cause-specific mortality in a large U.S. cohort. *American Journal of Epidemiology, 187*(10), 2151–2158. doi:10.1093/aje/kwy125

Pear, R., & Haberman, M. (2019, April 2). Trump retreats on health care after McConnell warns it won't happen. *The New York Times.* Retrieved from https://www.nytimes.com/2019/04/02/us/politics/obamacare-donald-trump.html

Population. (2019). *Merriam Webster Dictionary.* Boston, MA: Houghton Mifflin. Retrieved from https://www.merriam-webster.com/dictionary/population

Porche, D. J. (2004). *Public and community health nursing practice.* Thousand Oaks, CA: Sage.

Public Health Law Center. (n.d.). *Youth access to e-cigarettes.* Retrieved from https://publichealthlawcenter.org/sites/default/files/States-with-Laws-Restricting-Youth-Access-to-ECigarettes-Dec2018.pdf

Robson, N. (2019). *In reversal, DOJ now says whole ACA unconstitutional.* Retrieved from The National Law Journal website https://www.law.com/nationallawjournal/2019/03/25/in-reversal-doj-now-says-whole-aca-unconstitutional/?slreturn=20190305094315

Scott, K., Smith, D., & Ellis, P. (2012). A population study of childhood maltreatment and asthma diagnosis: Differential associations between child protection database versus retrospective self-reported data. *Psychosomatic Medicine, 74*(8), 817–823. doi:10.1097/PSY.0b013e3182648de4

Smyth, J., Heron, K., Wonderlich, S., Crosby, R., & Thompson, K. (2008). The influence of reported trauma and adverse events on eating disturbance in young adults. *International Journal of Eating Disorders, 41*(3), 195–202. Retrieved from EBSCO*host.*

Soni, A. (2010, December). *Trends in use and expenditures for diabetes among adults 18 and older, U.S. civilian noninstitutionalized population, 1996 and 2007.* Agency for Healthcare Research and Policy. Retrieved from http://www.meps.ahrq.gov/mepsweb/data_files/publications/st304/stat304.pdf

The Henry J. Kaiser Family Foundation. (2019a). *Average annual family premium per enrolled employee for employer based health insurance.* Retrieved from https://www.kff.org/other/state-indicator/family-coverage/?currentTimeframe=0&sortModel=%7B%22colId%22:%22Location%22,%22sort%22:%22asc%22%7D

The Henry J. Kaiser Family Foundation. (2019b). *Key facts about the uninsured population.* Retrieved from https://www.kff.org/uninsured/fact-sheet/key-facts-about-the-uninsured-population

Thompson, W. H. (2018). Management of catheter-related bloodstream infections. *Critical Care Alert, 26*(2), 9–13.

U.S. Department of Health and Human Services. (2015). HHS initiative on multiple chronic conditions. Retrieved from https://www.hhs.gov/ash/about-ash/multiple-chronic-conditions/index.html

World Health Organization. (2011). *WHO report: Deaths from noncommunicable diseases rise, hitting developing countries hard.* Retrieved from https://www.who.int/pmnch/media/news/2011/20110427_who_ncd_rise/en

World Health Organization. (2019). *Noncommunicable diseases and their risk factors.* Retrieved from http://www.who.int/chp/en

INTERNET RESOURCES

Centers for Disease Control and Prevention, ACESs
https://www.cdc.gov/violenceprevention/childabuseandneglect/acestudy/index.html

Centers for Disease Control and Prevention, Smoking and Tobacco Use
https://www.cdc.gov/tobacco/data_statistics/fact_sheets/index.htm

Centers for Disease Control and Prevention, Smoking and Tobacco Use / Hookahs
https://www.cdc.gov/tobacco/data_statistics/fact_sheets/tobacco_industry/hookahs/index.htm#overview

Canada / *Tobacco and Vaping Products Act*
https://www.canada.ca/en/health-canada/services/health-concerns/tobacco/legislation/federal-laws/
tobacco-act.html

Findings: Commonwealth Fund's Biennial Health Insurance Survey
https://mail.yahoo.com/d/folders/1/messages/AFZhsg8SqrtiXK3xhQOlmKQk0ws

Public Health Law Center, Youth Access to E-cigarettes
https://publichealthlawcenter.org/sites/default/files/States-with-Laws-Restricting-Youth-Access-to-
ECigarettes-Dec2018.pdf

U.S. Department of Health and Human Services (DHHS) / DHHS initiative on multiple chronic conditions
https://www.hhs.gov/ash/about-ash/multiple-chronic-conditions/index.html

CHAPTER 2

IDENTIFYING OUTCOMES IN POPULATION-BASED NURSING

ALYSSA ERIKSON | SONDA M. OPPEWAL

INTRODUCTION

Nurses have a long and rich history of wanting to do the most good for the most people. Today, it is imperative that advanced practice registered nurses (APRNs) continue that tradition by delivering care that improves the health of populations. By assessing community, aggregate, family, and individual factors and conditions that have a strong influence on health, APRNs are better equipped to deliver effective and evidence-based care. Identifying population-level healthcare needs and healthcare disparities can improve equity in health outcomes at all levels.

The American Association of Colleges of Nursing's (AACN) definition of advanced practice nursing includes the importance of identifying and managing health outcomes at the population level (AACN, 2004). In 2006, the AACN specified in *Essential II: Organizational and Systems Leadership for Quality Improvement and Systems Thinking* that graduates of doctorate in nursing practice (DNP) programs have competency in meeting "the needs of a panel of patients, a target population, a set of populations, or a broad community" (p. 10). A core component of DNP education is clinical prevention (health promotion and disease prevention at individual and family levels) and population health (focus of care at aggregate and community levels and examination of environmental, occupational, cultural, and socioeconomic dimensions of health) (AACN, 2006; Zenzano et al. 2011). Regardless of whether DNP graduates practice with a focus on clinical prevention or population health, the ability to define, identify, and analyze outcomes is imperative for improving the health status of individuals and populations (AACN, 2006; U.S. Department of Health and Human Services [DHHS], 2018a).

The purpose of this chapter is to explore how APRNs can identify determinants of health and define population outcomes. Specific examples from various settings, such as acute care, primary care, long-term care, and the community, are given, as well as outcomes related to health disparities and national health objectives. The identification of factors that lead to certain outcomes or key health indicators is an essential first step in planning effective interventions and is used later in the evaluation process. By comparing outcomes, APRNs can advocate for needed resources and changes in policies at local, regional, state, and/or national levels by identifying areas for improvement in practice, by comparing evidence needed for effective practice, and by better understanding health disparities.

Health disparities are not fair or socially just. They are preventable. They reflect an uneven distribution of social determinants and environmental, economic, and political factors. Health disparities can be defined as the differences identified in incidence or prevalence of illness, health outcomes, mortality, injury, or violence, or differences in opportunities to reach optimal health equity due to disadvantages based on ethnicity, socioeconomic status, gender, sexual orientation, geographic location, or other reasons (Penman-Aguilar, Bouye, & Liburd, 2016). Health equity is both a process and an outcome that is defined as "reducing and ultimately eliminating disparities in health and its determinants that adversely affect excluded or marginalized groups" (Braverman, Arkin, Orleans, Proctor, & Plough, 2017). Along with professionals from other disciplines and community members, APRNs play an important collaborative role in the work required to eliminate health inequities and healthcare disparities.

IDENTIFYING AND DEFINING POPULATION OUTCOMES

Background

One of the earliest records of observed outcomes by nurses dates back to 1854 during the Crimean War at the Scutari Hospital in Turkey under Florence Nightingale's leadership and pioneering work. Nightingale, credited as the founder of modern nursing, documented a decrease in mortality among the British soldiers after providing more nutritious food, cleaning up the environment, and improving the sewage system (Fee & Garofalo, 2010). Despite these exemplary nursing outcomes in the 1850s, variation and challenges with outcome documentation persisted as the nursing profession matured. By the mid-1990s, documentation of nursing outcomes started to improve (Griffiths, 1995; Hill, 1999; Lang & Marek, 1991; van Maanen, 1979). Early work in nursing outcomes focused on costs, and it was clear that a more comprehensive model that included other types of outcomes was needed to advance healthcare and reflect the various outcomes that result from nursing interventions (Nelson, Batalden, Plume, & Mohr, 1996). Today, nursing interventions are based on evidence using models of practice that include standards and synchronization with other systems to deliver quality of care, patient safety, and optimal population health outcomes (Institute of Medicine [IOM], 2015; Patrician et al., 2013; Xiao, Widger, Tourangeau, & Berta, 2017). Health reform efforts to improve quality and access to care and to reduce costs spurred more work to examine outcomes while also examining their relationship to indicators of structure and process. The Patient-Centered Outcomes Research Institute (PCORI), for example, developed out of the Patient Protection and Affordable Care Act of 2010 (ACA) and uniquely engages patients and the healthcare community on research projects (Newhouse, Barksdale, & Miller, 2015).

Defining, Categorizing, and Identifying Outcomes

Health outcomes are usually defined as an end result that follows some kind of healthcare provision, treatment, or intervention and may describe a patient's condition or health status (Jones, 2016; Kleinpell, 2007; Kleinpell & Gawlinski, 2005). Using a population perspective, a health outcome can be measured using public health metrics, such as mortality and life expectancies, that are used to demonstrate the contribution of certain diseases to population mortality. New trends also emphasize the inclusion of qualitative metrics that are based on subjective data, such as self-perceived health status, psychological state, or ability to function, that can illustrate collective social well-being (Boothe, Sinha, Bohm, & Yoon, 2013; Parrish, 2010).

Evaluating population-based outcomes and their impact on population health involves looking at what to assess and how to assess it. Establishing the impact takes time and requires using an evaluation that is able to link interventions to long-term outcomes such as reducing disease morbidity and mortality at the population level. APRNs can best determine the effectiveness of an intervention and long-term impact by focusing on an accurate assessment and interpretation of data that are generated or collected using individual, population, and community health indicators (Anderson & McFarlane, 2015).

Classifying and categorizing outcomes can be done in several ways. Outcomes may be classified into categories by describing "who" is measured, such as individuals, aggregates, communities, populations, or organizations; by identifying the "what" or the type of outcome, such as care, patient, or performance-related outcomes (Kapu, Sicoutris, Broyhill, D'Agostino, & Kleinpell, 2017; Kleinpell & Gawlinski, 2005); and by determining the "when" or the time it takes to achieve an outcome, such as short-term, intermediate, or long-term outcomes (Rich, 2015). Table 2.1 provides examples of various outcomes using these different classification systems. Each outcome type is listed by beneficiary and has a related example of the type of measurement, the potential outcome, and the potential impact of that outcome. Many of them also include a time frame for the outcome.

The Donabedian (1980) framework is frequently used in nursing and healthcare to evaluate quality of care and relies on the examination of three components: *structure, process,* and *outcome. Structure* refers to healthcare resources, such as the number and type of health and social service agencies, and can also include utilization indicators. *Process* describes how the healthcare is delivered. *Outcome* refers to the change in health status related to the intervention provided (Donabedian, 1980). This framework is particularly useful in describing the health of a community. It is based on the concept of community as client and focuses on the health of the collective or population instead of the individual (Gibson & Thatcher, 2016).

TABLE 2.1 Examples of Outcomes, Measures, and Impact by Beneficiary, Type, and Time Frame

BENEFICIARY (WHO?)	MEASURE	POTENTIAL OUTCOME	IMPACT
Individual outcomes	BP measurement	Decreased BP	The degree to which perceived health status is improved by BP management
Aggregate outcomes	Weekly weights of participants in an exercise class	Reduced mean weight for exercise class members each week	Sustained weight maintenance using BMI parameters
Community outcomes	A town's seat belt usage per 100 drivers ≥18 years of age computed yearly	Increased yearly rate of a town's seat belt usage per 100 drivers ≥18 years of age	Decrease in the town's percentage of automobile accident injuries/fatalities in drivers ≥18 years of age
Population outcomes	Reported number of infant deaths within 1 year of birth per 1,000 infants	Decreased infant mortality rate compared to previous year	Five-year decrease in infant mortality rate
TYPE (WHAT?)	**MEASURE**	**POTENTIAL OUTCOME**	**IMPACT**
Care-related outcomes	Annual rate of hospital-acquired infections determined from hospital infectious disease reports	Decreased hospital-acquired infections rate from previous year	Decreased length of stay and decreased mortality in patients with hospital-acquired infections
Patient-related outcomes	Observation of insulin injection administration technique	Correct demonstration by patient of safe insulin administration technique	Decreased hemoglobin A1C and decreased incidence of microvascular complications
Performance-related outcomes	Chart review for completed checklist of asthma best-practices protocol	Nursing staff adherence to asthma best-practices protocol	Decreased hospital readmissions due to asthma
TIME FRAME (WHEN?)	**MEASURE**	**POTENTIAL OUTCOME**	**IMPACT**
Short-term outcomes	Self-report of nipple discomfort among first-time breast-feeding mothers in a postpartum unit	Absence of nipple discomfort among first-time breast-feeding mothers 1 week after hospital discharge from a postpartum unit	Improved breast-feeding rates among women discharged from a postpartum unit
Intermediate outcomes	Self-report of tobacco usage by first-time outpatient clinic users during the calendar year	An increase in smoking-cessation rates among outpatient clinic users during the calendar year	Decrease in smoking-related illnesses among outpatient clinic users during the calendar year
Long-term outcomes	Incidence rate of HIV in an urban African American population	Annual reduction of incidence rate of HIV in an urban African American population	Annual reduction of morbidity and mortality related to HIV in an urban African American population

BMI, body mass index; BP, blood pressure.

Using Donabedian's framework, a community's health can be described in terms of its *structure* by the number and type of health and social agencies present, its healthcare workforce, health services utilization indicators, and the community's educational and socioeconomic levels in relation to demographic measures of ethnicity, gender, and age. A community's health *process* can measure healthcare delivery methods and how well community members work together to build capacity and solve their problems, which reflects the ability to share power and resources and to respond to needs and changes (Minkler & Wallerstein, 2012). Community health *outcomes* can include measures associated with vital statistics (e.g., births, deaths, marriages, divorces, fetal deaths, and induced termination of pregnancies); morbidity or illness data and trends; social determinants of health such as housing, unemployment, and poverty rates; health risk profiles of aggregates by specific areas, neighborhood safety, access to fresh fruits and vegetables, as well as physical activity venues such as parks, playgrounds, and neighborhood sports fields (Anderson & McFarlane, 2015). Other indicators of a community's health status may include the number of premature deaths, quality of life, disabilities, risk factors, and injuries. Community health outcomes models are used to assess the interaction between the physical and the social environments (the built environment) and the impact on health at the individual, population, and community levels (DeGuzman & Kulbok, 2012). Guided by these models of practice and research, APRNs can work in partnership with community members to identify what they see as relevant and important, build social capital, use outcome data to advocate for changes in policy, and then continue to work in partnership to identify strategies to intervene, monitor, and improve those outcomes (Bigbee & Issel, 2012; Loyo et al., 2012; Payán et al., 2017).

Vital Statistics

Vital statistics provide important outcome measures that APRNs can monitor and compare over time and analyze by demographic variables to detect such things as health disparities. In the United States, the National Center for Health Statistics (NCHS) located within the Centers for Disease Control and Prevention (CDC) collects information from a variety of sources, such as birth and death certificates, health records, surveys, physical exams, and laboratory testing (Rothwell, 2015). Personnel from local health departments review the data from death certificates, including demographic data, looking at the immediate cause of death and any contributing factors of death, and recording multiple causes of death. Local data are sent to a state office for collation and then sent to the NCHS, which provides this information to the public on its website (www. cdc.gov/nchs) and in an annual publication, *Vital Statistics of the United States* (Friis & Sellers, 2015). APRNs can access national and global health statistics from multiple agency sources, including government agencies, to identify health trends and patterns. However, due to the lack of agencies and/or resources in certain populations or regions, health information might not be available or might be limited in scope. *Partners in Information Access for the Public Health Workforce* is a collaborative project among U.S. government agencies, public health organizations, and health science libraries that provides a list of extensive web links for sources of data that healthcare providers can use to identify local issues and develop interventions to improve health (U.S. National Library of Medicine [NLM], 2018).

Behavioral Risk Factor Surveillance System (BRFSS)

In the early 1980s, personal health behaviors became a key source of information that paved the way in understanding risk behavior and its impact on morbidity and mortality. The Behavioral Risk Factor Surveillance System (BRFSS; www.cdc.gov/brfss), a system established to collect state-level data, also allows states to estimate prevalence for regions that can be compared across states (CDC, 2014). The data generated by this surveillance system have been pivotal in assessing and addressing urgent or emerging health issues. Examples of emergent health issues include man-made and natural disasters, influenza vaccine shortages, and increasing incidence of preventable diseases such as influenza or measles. The ability to reach cell phone users has expanded BRFSS's accessibility to populations that were not accessible by prior data-collection methods. This ability has increased representation and generated higher quality information.

Social Determinants of Health

Social determinants of health and disparities data are areas that APRNs can also use to inform and guide their practice to develop socioculturally appropriate interventions. Social determinants that lead to health disparities are recognized situations related to where people are born, grow up, work, live, and the systems of care available to them to deal with illness and disease (DHHS, 2018a; World Health Organization [WHO], 2011). Examples of social determinants that are related to health inequalities include poverty, educational level, racism, income, and poor housing. These inequalities can lead to poor quality of life, poor self-rated health, multiple morbidities, limited access to resources, unnecessary risks and vulnerabilities, and premature death. To expand our understanding of the association between social determinants and health outcomes, theoretical models are being tested to examine the interaction between the social environment (physical, chemical, biological, behavioral, and/or life events) and genetics and its application to population health, such as examining the interplay of social environments, genetics and Black-White disparities and their contribution to infant mortality (El-Sayed, Paczkowski, Rutherford, Keyes, & Galea, 2015).

Another example of social determinants of health and inequalities is that people living at or below 100% of the federal poverty level (FPL) have decreased access to healthcare compared to those at or above 400% of the FPL, which can then negatively impact health status (Agency for Healthcare Research and Quality [AHRQ], 2017). These social and economic conditions may limit a person's ability to be employed, access healthcare services, and receive timely quality care. This is evident in rural populations who experience place-based health disparities due to limited local healthcare services, lack of technological infrastructure to support health promotion interventions, and potential job-associated exposures (e.g., chemicals in agriculture work; Weinstein, Geller, Negussie, & Baciu, 2017).

A problem encountered repeatedly by healthcare practitioners is the lack of available census data and statistics about key issues in the health and healthcare of people with unauthorized status. APRNs may be able to access health information needed by working together with other sectors outside of health, such as housing, labor, education, and community-based or faith-based organizations that offer services to immigrant communities. This involves the collection, documentation, and use of data that can be used to monitor health inequalities in exposures, opportunities, and outcomes.

Morbidity and Mortality Data

APRNs are often responsible for reviewing morbidity and mortality trends and can use this information to advocate for improved health policy and additional resources, or to develop innovative interventions. Provisional weekly updates of reportable diseases can be accessed electronically through the *Morbidity and Mortality Weekly Report* (*MMWR*), published by the CDC. Morbidity data are less standardized in general than mortality data because state legislatures and local agencies decide what illnesses must be reported to the CDC. Reporting of cases of infectious diseases and related conditions is an important step in controlling and preventing the spread of communicable disease. The list of reportable or notifiable diseases can change as some diseases may become eradicated and other, new diseases and conditions are discovered such as the 2014-2016 Ebola outbreak in the United States. The accuracy of morbidity data is diminished if healthcare providers fail to report a disease or illness for fear of violating an individual's privacy or because they may not be aware of reporting requirements or because the healthcare provider misdiagnosed the illness (Macha & McDonough, 2012). It is imperative that APRNs educate themselves on the reporting requirements in their state. Certain diseases with easy and/ or rapid transmission are more likely to harm a population's health. Infectious or communicable diseases, such as certain sexually transmitted infections (STIs) or other diseases, such as rabies, rubella, plague, measles, tetanus, and food-borne illnesses, can lead to significant morbidity and mortality if not reported promptly (Friis & Sellers, 2015).

Another way to evaluate population morbidity is derived from population surveys that are conducted to determine the frequency of acute and chronic illnesses and disability as well as other population characteristics. The U.S. National Health Interview Survey (NHIS) is an example of a morbidity survey that was first authorized by Congress in 1956 for the purpose of informing the U.S. population about various health measures and indicators. In an effort obtain a representative national sample, the NHIS continuously surveys households throughout the year on a variety of health topics, such as physical and mental health status, chronic conditions, and access to and use of healthcare services. One finding from the 2017 data indicated a disparity in health insurance coverage, with Hispanic persons more likely to be without coverage than non-Hispanic Black and non-Hispanic White persons (Schiller, Clark, & Norris, 2018). The NHIS debuted a redesign in 2019 to improve its content and structure. The redesign emphasized content with a strong link to public health, such as intermediate health outcomes for leading causes of morbidity/mortality. It also targeted major federal health promotion initiatives, and healthcare access and utilization (CDC, 2018).

The NHIS is one sector of the data collection program at the NCHS, housed within the CDC. The NCHS works with public and private partners to collect data that provide reliable and valid evidence on a population's health status, influences on health, and health outcomes (CDC, 2017). APRNs can review these data to identify health disparities among subgroups based on ethnicity and/or socioeconomic status, monitor trends with health status and with healthcare delivery systems, support research endeavors, identify health problems, evaluate health policies, and access important information that can be used to improve policies and health services.

In addition to population surveys such as the NHIS, the NCHS collects data using other surveys with each method yielding information that is readily available on the Internet for use by healthcare providers, researchers, and educators. First, the *National Vital Statistics System* provides information about state and local vital statistics, including teen birth rates, prenatal care, birth weights, risk factors related to poor pregnancy outcomes, infant mortality rates, life expectancy, and leading causes of death (www.cdc.gov/nchs/nvss). Second, the *National Health and Nutrition Examination Survey* (NHANES) is conducted through mobile examination centers held at randomly selected sites throughout the United States. Data are obtained from interviews (e.g., environmental exposures, risk factors), and additional data are collected from physical examinations, diagnostic procedures, laboratory tests, and indicators of growth and development, including weight, diet, and nutrition (www.cdc.gov/nchs/nhanes.htm). Third, *The National Healthcare Surveys* obtain data using a collection of surveys targeted toward various healthcare providers and healthcare settings (www.cdc.gov/nchs/dhcs). A variety of data is collected, including information regarding patient safety and safety indicators, clinical management of specific health conditions, disparities in healthcare utilization and health quality, and information about the use of healthcare innovations. All these survey data are collated and made available for policy makers, practitioners, and researchers and all provide useful outcome information for APRNs. Additional surveys can be found on the NCHS website, but the aforementioned surveys are most useful for analyzing outcomes data.

Morbidity and mortality trends and other health-related survey data can be used by APRNs to advocate for improved health policy and additional resources, or to develop innovative interventions. For example, if an APRN notices an increase over the past year of closed head injuries in teenagers because of motor vehicle crashes (MVCs), the APRN can design a plan of care that targets risk factors associated with teenage driving and MVCs. The APRN may review emergency department (ED) records of teenage drivers in car accidents to assess factors such as seat belt usage, distracted driving behaviors, blood alcohol levels, drug screening, prior ED visits for accidents, and age at the time of the incident. The APRN may also approach high schools in order to collaborate with school nurses for the purpose of developing peer training programs. High school students could be trained as peer teachers to encourage classmates to wear seat belts, avoid entering a car with an impaired driver, say no to drug and alcohol usage, and eliminate use of electronic devices, such as cellular phones, while driving. Nurse educators could encourage teachers to integrate the importance of wearing seat belts in their classes by discussing the potential for traumatic brain injury in MVCs, especially in unrestrained drivers. Review of the biomechanics of accidents in a physics or science class might provide teens with knowledge that is both beneficial and relatable and may reinforce the dangers of unrestrained driving. Additionally, the hospital could partner with a high school and pilot an educational program with adolescents to reduce texting while driving (Unni et al., 2017). Or school nurses could implement an online educational tool, like *Let's Choose Ourselves*, to address adolescent drivers' inattention and distraction (McDonald, Brawner, Fargo, Swope, & Sommers, 2017).

After developing and implementing appropriate interventions, the APRN should reassess (e.g., in 6 months, 1 year) seat belt usage and repeat ED visits for MVCs, and revaluate whether there have been any positive drug screens, elevated blood alcohol concentrations, or documented distracted driving related to MVCs. Re-evaluation of these data can help to identify those interventions that work. It may also lead to changes in school policy and/or curriculum to modify behavior, thereby reducing MVCs among teens. Statewide policy changes that the APRN can advocate for include legislation whereby any detectable blood alcohol concentration is illegal, more stringent and enforced driving fines for unrestrained passengers and drivers, and graduated driving license laws that increase driving supervision time, restrict passengers, and limits nighttime driving (Williams, 2017). Although this is just one example of how surveillance by an APRN could lead to the development of interventions to improve outcomes in a population, one can see the potential value of community collaboration and the use of such outcomes to identify a need for change and to evaluate the impact of interventions.

Identifying Outcomes

How do APRNs decide what outcomes to study? There are a variety of outcomes that exist in relation to cost, clinical and functional data, social conditions, and community and environmental indicators. Often, outcomes will reflect the desired or anticipated effects of the intervention that are related to the problem or population of interest. Another way to select outcomes is by reviewing available epidemiological and social epidemiological data for outcomes that may be of interest or relevance to an APRN's intervention or study (Galea & Link, 2013; Macha & McDonough, 2012; Minkler & Wallerstein, 2012). Using the earlier example of designing an intervention to reduce teenage MVCs, an APRN could seek out epidemiological data from the *National Highway Traffic Safety Administration's* (NHTSA) *Fatality Analysis Reporting System* and review annual data and trends for fatalities in drivers age 15 to 19 (crashstats.nhtsa.dot.gov).

Outcomes can also be identified using County Health Rankings & Roadmaps (CHR&R), a user-friendly web-based data source. It allows an APRN to compare similarly sized counties on various measures, such as premature death, low birthweight, or drug overdose deaths (www.countyhealthrankings.org). McCullough and Leider (2017) used data from the CHR&R and U.S. Census Bureau to examine the relationship among county wealth, health, and social services spending, and health outcomes.

There is no shortage of usable resources for identifying outcomes. *The Community Guide* is a helpful resource (available at www.thecommunityguide.org). It provides evidence-based recommendations for public health interventions, analyses from systematic reviews to determine program and policy effectiveness, information on whether an intervention might work in one's community, and information about the intervention's costs and benefits. APRNs can review topics or areas of focus and strategies that work for various outcomes. For example, systematic reviews are available on adolescent health. By spending a few minutes exploring the website, one can find numerous outcomes such as number of self-reported risk behaviors, including engagement in any sexual activity, frequency of sexual activity, number of partners, frequency of unprotected sexual activity, use of protection to prevent STIs, use of protection to prevent pregnancy, and self-reported or clinically documented STIs. Other community-guide topics are listed in Table 2.2 with example outcomes adapted from the website.

Trust for America's Health (TFAH) is another resource to inform APRNs' outcome identification (www.tfah.org). The TFAH's work is centered on three main principles (prevention, protection, and communities) and is a resource for issues such as public health funding, obesity, substance abuse and misuse, and health disparities. It also allows an APRN to examine state level data and rankings on key health indicators (e.g., percentage of the population with hypertension, the number of cases of tuberculosis, and the percentage of asthma in high school students).

Outcome Monitoring

After identifying outcomes, monitoring of measures to assess effectiveness of interventions is increasingly important and, in many cases, is a necessity to justify program implementation or program funding. For example, outcome monitoring is used to assess quality of healthcare by examining the association between the level of improved health services and the desired health outcomes of individuals and populations (IOM, 2015). This is best done by having a quality-improvement (QI) plan that systematically and consistently implements improvement strategies to address areas that are deficient and not meeting benchmarks. The Institute for Healthcare Improvement (IHI) is a useful resource for determining a QI plan and provides a toolkit with 10 tools (e.g., Plan Study Do Act [PDSA] worksheet) to guide QI projects (www.ihi.org/resources/Pages/Tools/Quality-Improvement-Essentials-Toolkit.aspx).

Outcomes are an expected part of what APRNs must collect when their focus is on populations. When combined with an evidence-based practice approach, outcomes can help provide standards or parameters for developing innovative interventions, instituting approaches more likely to impact the problem, and/or developing new practice guidelines or protocols. Through working with populations, APRNs contribute to meeting the IHI (2018) Triple Aim: (a) improve the patient experience, (b) improve the health of the population, and (c) reduce the per capita cost of health. For example, an APRN working in a community-based clinic with a Hispanic population may gather information on factors related to an increased rate of type 2 diabetes mellitus, such as hypertension, obesity or acculturation. An assessment can be made to determine if differences in

TABLE 2.2 Community Guide Topics and Outcome Examples

TOPICS	OUTCOME EXAMPLES
Adolescent health	Alcohol, tobacco, and drug usage; injury, violence, and suicide rates; BMI, physical activity, and educational attainment
Asthma	Symptom-free days, quality-of-life scores, school absenteeism, environmental mold remediation, medication usage, hospital admissions
Birth defects	Folic acid daily intake, daily alcohol consumption, medications, vaccinations
Cancer	Cigarette smoking, physical activity, nutrition, screening test results
Cardiovascular disease	Blood pressure, physical activity, cholesterol levels, BMI
Diabetes	Hemoglobin A1C, incidence of skin infections, obesity, peripheral neuropathy, renal insufficiency
Health communication and health information technology	Use of reliable digital and mobile technology for HI or appointment reminders, health literacy level, communication by provider of understandable HI, difficulty using HI
Health equity	Use of school-based health centers, use of interpreter services or number of bilingual providers, access to healthcare, employment rates
HIV/AIDS, STIs, and pregnancy	Abstinence, condom use, incidence of STIs or pregnancy
Mental health	Depression scale scores, hospital admissions, attendance at school or work, suicidal ideation or attempts
Motor vehicle crashes	Use of child safety seats, use of seat belts, blood alcohol concentration, use of phone while driving, moving violations
Nutrition	Daily intake of fruits and vegetables, BMI, soda intake, fat intake, fiber intake
Obesity	Daily physical activity; sedentary time in front of the TV, computer, or electronic screen; weight loss; BMI
Oral health	Dental caries; incidence of oral or throat cancer; use of helmets, face masks, and mouth guards in contact sports; reduced or discontinued use of chewing tobacco
Physical activity	Muscle strength and endurance activities, moderate- or vigorous-intensity aerobic physical activity
Tobacco	Out-of-pocket costs for cessation therapies, creation of smoke-free policies, retail tobacco sales to youth
Vaccination	Number of infectious cases, hospitalizations, deaths from vaccine-preventable disease, immunization rates, immunization failures
Violence	Number of violence-related hospitalizations and deaths, participation in therapeutic foster care, school-based violence prevention programs, reduction of nonaccidental trauma in infants and toddlers
Worksite health	Stair usage by employees, gym membership by employees, use of weight management counseling by employees

BMI, body mass index; HI, health information.

Source: Adapted from U.S. Department of Health and Human Services, Community Preventive Services Task Force (2019). *The community guide.* Retrieved from https://www.thecommunityguide.org

health outcomes exist based on social support, family structures, barriers to obtaining medications or durable medical equipment, or other variables of interest. Once these outcomes are assessed, actions can be taken to address the issues that may contribute to poor health outcomes or increased incidence, such as implementing a community health worker (CHW) intervention (Chang et al., 2018). A reassessment of outcomes is necessary after an intervention to determine if a change has occurred.

Outcomes can also be used to measure quality of care in an outpatient setting. APRNs in an outpatient pediatric oncology practice who administer chemotherapy through a central venous catheter may set a goal to reduce catheter-related bloodstream infections by employing a before and after hands-on simulation education program for parents and nurses emphasizing aseptic techniques before, during, and after infusion. The success of the intervention can be measured by comparing outcomes such as number of positive cultures and prolonged hospitalizations, and rates of bloodstream infection before and after implementation of the educational intervention.

Nurse-Sensitive Quality Indicators

As documented evidence of patient safety concerns grew in the United States and at a time when healthcare costs were increasing and healthcare quality was being questioned, various nursing organizations started to focus on establishing a coordinated system for evaluating patient safety. In 1994, the American Nurses Association (ANA) developed Nursing's Safety and Quality Initiative, which initiated studies of patient safety with the goal of advocating healthy change. It was clear that nurse managers and administrators needed sound data for comparing their hospital units with similar units across the nation as a means of improving quality by developing and refining quality-improvement initiatives and monitoring progress. The indicators needed to be specific or sensitive to nursing care rather than ones that reflected medical care or institutional care. The indicators would have to be highly correlated with nursing quality and be measurable with a high degree of reliability and validity. Furthermore, the indicator must not pose undue hardships on personnel tasked with collecting the data. Donabedian's (1982) framework of focusing on structure, process, and patient-centered outcomes was used for identifying and honing the indicators. *Structure* indicators included staff mix and nursing care hours per patient day; *process* indicators included maintenance of skin integrity and nurse satisfaction; and patient-focused *outcomes* included nosocomial infections, patient fall rates, patient satisfaction with pain management, patient education, nursing care, and overall care (Montalvo, 2007).

The National Database of Nursing Quality Indicators® (NDNQI®) was created in 1998 by the ANA as part of the initiative to make changes to improve safety and quality of care, to help educate nurses about measurement, and to invest in research studies that examined safe and high-quality patient care. The NDNQI helped standardize information that was submitted by hospital units throughout the United States on indicators related to nursing structure (staffing level, educational level), process measures, and outcome measures. Hospitals use these results to compare their performance with those of other hospitals with similar demographic makeup and patient population. Originally housed and managed by the University of Kansas Medical Center (KUMC) School of Nursing through a contractual agreement with the American Nurses Credentialing Center (ANCC), NDNQI was purchased by Press Ganey Associates in 2014. Technical assistance and continuing education are provided by liaisons to ensure that reliable and valid data-collection methods are used by hospital personnel. This database provides a wealth of information on a quarterly and annual basis of more than 2,000 facilities in the United States (Press Ganey Associates, n.d.). In addition to hospital indicators, nurse-sensitive indicators for community-based healthcare settings also exist. The ability to collect and compare data on nurse-sensitive indicators and the ability to develop new indicators over time enhance the NDNQI initiative and provide APRNs with important information to help measure, compare, and improve the health and safety of populations.

Standardized Language in Nursing

The use of standardized language is important in any field to ensure a level of communication that is both consistent and effective in ensuring quality outcomes. Specifically, in nursing and other health professions, standardized language is critical for patient safety and quality of care. By establishing a uniform nursing language in electronic health records, research, and the development of evidence-based practice, APRNs have a stronger foundation to communicate and improve patient outcomes and standards of care. The North American Nursing Diagnosis Association (NANDA) was developed in the 1970s to classify and standardize nursing diagnoses. Now referred to as NANDA International or NANDA-I, the nursing diagnoses include a name or label, signs and symptoms or defining characteristics, and risk factors associated with the diagnosis. The NANDA-I definitions and classifications have been recently updated to reflect new trends in nursing healthcare (www.nanda.org). Members of NANDA-I worked with nursing researchers at the University of Iowa to develop the Nursing Interventions Classification (NIC) and the Nursing Outcomes Classification (NOC). NANDA-I, NIC, and NOC, now referred to as NNN, collectively reflect a standardized way of communicating with defined terms within and across various national and international settings (Smith & Craft-Rosenberg, 2010). As APRNs contribute to the body of evidence-based practice and collaborate with others to generate more evidence of effective practice, their work may benefit from reviewing and using the NNN language for diagnoses, nursing interventions, and patient outcomes (Kautz & Van Horn, 2008). It is imperative that APRNs use standardized language in their research and in their practice so that outcomes can be compared in similar ways with larger databases for evaluation and research purposes.

NATIONAL HEALTHCARE OBJECTIVES

AHRQ's National Healthcare Quality Report

Since 2003, the AHRQ has partnered with members of the DHHS to report on healthcare quality improvement by publishing the *National Healthcare Quality and Disparities Report (QDR)*. The intent of this report is to respond to the status of healthcare quality in the United States, identify where improvement is most needed, and describe how the quality of healthcare that is given to Americans changes over time. This report includes more than 250 measures of quality and disparities and uses the Three Aims for Improving Healthcare as its framework, which are (a) better care, (b) healthy people/healthy community, and (c) affordable care (AHRQ, 2017). Findings from the 2016 report reveal that healthcare for Americans is improving in some areas and worsening in others. The QDR examines quality through six priority areas; person-centered care, patient safety, healthy living, effective treatment, care coordination, and care affordability. The priority area of person-centered care saw the largest number of measures improve and the priority area of care affordability saw the least. Some areas of care that improved included a decrease in uninsured rates, a decrease in hospital admissions with central venous catheter-related blood infections, and an improvement in provider-patient communication. Examples of areas where the quality of care worsened include a lower percentage of women ages 21 to 65 that received a Pap smear in the last 3 years and an increase in the percentage of children ages 12 to 19 who are obese.

A key finding related to disparities is that some disparities narrrowed between 2000 and 2015, but still existed. On many measures, poor and low-income households demonstrated worse care than high-income households. A second key finding is in the differences in quality-of-care outcomes based on geography, with Southern and Southwestern states, several Western states, and one Midwestern state performing poorly in delivering overall quality care compared to Mideast and Northeast states. Hospital care has been improving since the Centers for Medicare & Medicaid Services (CMS) started reporting on quality measures. These measures can be found on the Hospital Compare website (www.medicare.gov/hospitalcompare/search.html). A third key finding is a difference in quality of care for Blacks, Hispanics, and Asians compared with Whites among states. The report details initiatives to address survey findings, such as Project ECHO and the Language Access Portal (AHRQ, 2017). In addition to the annual QDR report, AHRQ's website has useful information that APRNs can use to identify and monitor outcomes (www.qualityindicators.ahrq.gov). Other tools, referred to as indicators, can be used by APRNs to identify outcomes or measures of the quality of healthcare. The inpatient quality indicators were designed to help hospitals identify possible issues and problems in need of quality improvement by using hospital administrative data to analyze morbidity and mortality rates for specific conditions and procedures, hospital- and area-level procedure utilization rates, and number of procedures (for select procedures). In addition to the inpatient quality indicators, other sets of quality indicators are available, including preventive quality indicators, patient safety indicators, and pediatric quality indicators.

Healthy People 2020

Healthy People 2020, released by the DHHS in early December 2010, serves as a blueprint or road map for the United States to achieve health promotion and disease prevention objectives that are designed to improve the health of all Americans. The *Healthy People* initiative started in 1979 when the surgeon general released a report that focused on promoting health and preventing disease for all Americans. It was followed by *Healthy People 2000* in 1989 and, 10 years later, *Healthy People 2010*. With leadership provided by the DHHS, an appointed advisory committee and numerous public and private groups, local and state policy makers and officials, and numerous organizations (voluntary, advocacy, faith-based, and for-profit businesses), input is solicited regionally, statewide, and nationally to help craft the vision, mission, and overarching goals. These groups and organizations also develop strategies to improve health and prevent disease with the ultimate goal of helping Americans live longer and healthier lives. The resulting objectives, whether on the county, state, or national level, are intended for use by broad audiences and stakeholders to help motivate, guide, and focus action for a healthier nation.

Compared to previous national health promotion blueprints, the *Healthy People 2020* framework emphasizes the importance of a variety of influences on health, such as personal (e.g., genetic, biological, psychological), organizational or institutional (e.g., Head Start or employee health programs), environmental (e.g., social and physical), and policy level (e.g., smoking bans in public places, seat belt laws). It moves beyond an individual-level approach to interventions and guides the creation of policies to promote the social and physical environments that are conducive to health. Another change in the 2020 version is the reorganization of objectives so that they can be retrieved by three broad categories: interventions, determinants, and objectives and information (with a feature for users to be able to retrieve information by local, state, or national level). Some of the 2020 objectives were retained from *Healthy People 2010* because they were not met, some objectives were modified, and some were entirely new to *Healthy People 2020*. Improvements to *Healthy People 2020* made it more web user-friendly, such that users can easily retrieve, search, and interact with the database. Hence, APRNs and other users are able to tailor information available from *Healthy People 2020* for their specific use and needs.

Table 2.3 provides a summary of the *Healthy People 2020* initiatives with its vision, mission, goals, foundation health measures, and topic areas. Each topic area has a list of objectives with data sources, baseline, and target measures to achieve. The *Healthy People* website is continually improved to ease access of the data and to make sense of the findings. Features of *Healthy People 2020* are additional topic-related clinical recommendations, evidence-based interventions, a program planning tool, eLearning, and other resources and links with consumer health information. Social determinants of health is extensively described, along with related objectives and an interventions and resources webpage. Information about *Healthy People 2020* can be found at www .healthypeople.gov.

Healthy People 2030 is under development by the Secretary's Advisory Committee with considerable input from stakeholders. Its framework is publicly available and includes an updated vision, mission, foundational principles, overarching goals, and plan of action. New objectives are being identified and will be available for public comment before its launch in 2020. (For more information on the development of *Healthy People 2030* go to www.healthypeople.gov/2020/About-Healthy-People/Development-Healthy-People-2030.)

TABLE 2.3 Vision, Mission, Goals, Foundation Health Measures, and Topic Areas of *Healthy People 2020*

VISION	A SOCIETY IN WHICH ALL PEOPLE LIVE LONG, HEALTHY LIVES
Mission	*Healthy People 2020* strives to: ■ Identify nationwide health-improvement priorities ■ Increase public awareness and understanding of the determinants of health, disease, and disability and the opportunities for progress ■ Provide measurable objectives and goals that can be used at the national, state, and local levels ■ Engage multiple sectors to take actions to strengthen policies and improve practices that are driven by the best available evidence and knowledge ■ Identify critical research, evaluation, and data-collection needs
Overarching goals	Attain high-quality, longer lives free of preventable disease, disability, injury, and premature death ■ Achieve health equity, eliminate disparities, and improve the health of all groups ■ Create social and physical environments that promote good health for all ■ Promote quality of life, healthy development, and healthy behaviors across all life stages
Foundation Health Measures	
General health status	■ Life expectancy ■ Healthy life expectancy ■ Physical and mental unhealthy days ■ Limitation of activity ■ Chronic disease prevalence ■ International comparison (where available)
Disparities and inequity	Disparities/inequity to be assessed by the following: ■ Race/ethnicity ■ Gender ■ Socioeconomic status ■ Disability status ■ LGBT status ■ Geography
Social determinants of health	Determinants can include the following: ■ Social and economic factors ■ Natural and built environments ■ Policies and programs
Health-related quality of life and well-being	Well-being/satisfaction ■ Physical, mental, and social health-related quality of life ■ Participation in common activities category
Healthy People 2020 Topic Areas	
■ Access to health services ■ Adolescent health ■ Arthritis, osteoporosis, and chronic back conditions ■ Blood disorders and blood safety ■ Cancer ■ Chronic kidney diseases ■ Dementias, including Alzheimer's disease	

(continued)

TABLE 2.3 Vision, Mission, Goals, Foundation Health Measures, and Topic Areas of *Healthy People 2020* **(continued)**

- Diabetes
- Disability and health
- Early and middle childhood
- Educational and community-based programs
- Environmental health
- Family planning
- Food safety
- Genomics
- Global health
- Healthcare-associated infections
- Health communication and health information technology
- Health-related quality of life and well-being
- Hearing and other sensory or communication disorders
- Heart disease and stroke
- HIV
- Immunization and infectious diseases
- Injury and violence prevention
- LGBT health
- Maternal, infant, and child health
- Medical product safety
- Mental health and mental disorders
- Nutrition and weight status
- Occupational safety and health
- Older adults
- Oral health
- Physical activity
- Preparedness
- Public health infrastructure
- Respiratory diseases
- Sexually transmitted diseases
- Sleep health
- Social determinants of health
- Substance abuse
- Tobacco use
- Vision

LGBT, lesbian, gay, bisexual, and transgender

Source: Adapted from the U.S. Department of Health and Human Services. (2018b). *Healthy People 2020*: Disparities. Retrieved from https://www.healthypeople.gov/2020/about/foundation-health-measures/Disparities

Health Disparities

Healthy People 2010 included two overarching goals: to increase years of healthy living and to eliminate health disparities. These goals were retained for *Healthy People 2020* as evidence continues to mount that the United States has issues related to equity of healthcare access, quality of care, and health status. The midcourse review of *Healthy People 2020* as well as many governmental and nongovernmental reports and independent studies document these disparities (AHRQ, 2017; Armstrong et al., 2018; IOM, 2015; DHHS, 2018b).

By monitoring potential differences among groups, health professionals will have the tools to recognize why and where population disparities are occurring. This in turn will (one hopes) lead to creative strategies to reduce health disparities and improve equity in health and the delivery of healthcare.

There are numerous dimensions of disparities or differences related to health that can adversely affect groups of people because of specific characteristics or obstacles. It is widely recognized now that the social determinants of health, such as housing, education, access to public transportation, access to safe water, access to fresh food, and the built environment, are all related to a population's health. In addition to ethnicity, other characteristics also contribute to the presence of disparities or the achievement of good health such as gender; sexual orientation; geographic location; working environment; cognitive, sensory, or physical disability; and socioeconomic status. The outcomes identified in the objectives of *Healthy People 2020* are intended to improve the health of all groups of people and bridge those gaps. *Healthy People 2020* and *Healthy People 2030* will assess health disparities in U.S. populations by tracking morbidity and mortality outcomes in relation to factors found to be associated with disparities.

Online Resources

APRNs have numerous online resources they can access to improve quality and timely access to healthcare, and decrease health disparities. Kleinpell and Kapu (2017) describe 13 resources for quality measures that are relevant to APRN practice, such as the Nurse Practitioner Outcomes Toolkit through the American Association of Nurse Practitioners (AANP). The National Partnership for Action (NPA) to End Health Disparities (minorityhealth.hhs.gov/npa/) was started by the Office of Minority Health to mobilize individuals and groups to work to improve quality and eliminate health disparities. Established in 1988, the Office of Minority Health and Health Disparities (OMHD) is housed within the CDC. Resources available from this office can be used by APRNs to determine how minority populations compare with the U.S. population as a whole. Such disparities are complicated to analyze and explain as they go beyond differences in genetics, biological characteristics, and health behaviors (microlevel properties). Racist and discriminatory behaviors and policies, cultural barriers, lack of access to care, and interaction with the environment (macrolevel properties) play a major role in creating the problem (see Chapter 11, Challenges in Program Implementation).

National Quality Partners™ (www.qualityforum.org/National_Quality_Partners. aspx) includes key private and public stakeholders who have agreed to work on major health priorities of patients and families, palliative and end-of-life care, care coordination, patient safety, and population health. Another excellent resource can be found on the site of the Association of American Medical Colleges (AAMC). It has compiled the report *The State of Health Equity Research: Closing Knowledge Gaps to Address Inequities* (available at www.aamc.org/initiatives/research/healthequity/402654/closingknowledgegaps. html). The AAMC and AcademyHealth worked together to review all U.S. health disparities–focused health services research funded during the 5-year period between 2007 and 2011. Their purpose was to determine where such research is taking place and who is funding it, identify gaps in populations and health outcomes, and assess trends in the funding of solution-focused health equity research (AAMC, 2014).

Established in 2000 and housed within the National Institute of Health (NIH), is the National Institute on Minority Health and Health Disparities (NIMHD). It supports researchers who address issues of health inequity. Its website highlights successful initiatives and programs (www.nimhd.nih.gov/programs/edu-training), such as the Transdisciplinary Collaborative Center for Health Disparities Research Program, which funds regional coalitions. APRNs can contact the principal investigators or other research staff to obtain information, to explore collaborative endeavors with researchers, to participate with community-based participatory research, to assist with translational research studies, and to share expertise with the aim of decreasing health disparities among vulnerable populations.

Also within the NIH, is the National Cancer Institute's Division of Cancer Control and Population Sciences (DCCPS), which has a variety of resources available, including funding opportunities, reports and health surveys, data sets, tool kits for research projects, and cross-cutting areas such as health disparities, patient-centered communication, and care coordination (cancercontrol.cancer.gov). There is also a health disparities calculator (HD*Calc). HD*Calc is statistical software that can be downloaded and used to generate and calculate 11 disparity measurements (seer.cancer.gov/hdcalc).

Examples of Health Disparities

Even a cursory review of reports and studies available through government agencies and various other organizations as well as peer-reviewed journals reveals many examples of healthcare disparities in the United States. The following are just a few examples.

Despite advances in diabetes prevention and treatment, American Indian/Alaska Natives (AI/AN) have a higher age-adjusted percentage of people with diabetes mellitus (as compared to Whites), followed by non-Hispanic Blacks and Hispanics (CDC, 2017; Subica, Agarwal, Sullivan, & Link, 2017). African Americans 65 years and younger continue to have a higher death rate than Whites (851.9 per 100,000 compared to 735.0 per 100,000) for all-cause mortality (CDC, 2017). Gu, Yue, Desai, and Argulian (2017) found poorer hypertension control in African Americans and Hispanics compared to Whites in analyzing data from 2003 to 2012. Even though the infant mortality rate in the United States has declined in recent years, and even when controlling for socioeconomic factors, the African American infant mortality rate is more than double that of rates for Whites or Hispanics (El-Sayed et al., 2015; Gregory, Drake, & Martin, 2018).

Examples of studies that explore gender inequities include a literature review of 11 studies on acute coronary syndromes in older adults that found that women had a higher in-hospital mortality rate than men (Gillis, Arslanian-Engoren, & Struble, 2014). Researchers in the area of health literacy have found disparities based on the literacy level of the client and the ability of the provider to facilitate patient understanding of treatment and management of a disease. Studies on the impact of health literacy on health outcomes have found that there is poor access to care, lower health-related quality of life, and lower health knowledge among people with low health litreracy (Cajita, Cajita, & Hae-Ra, 2016; Hälleberg, Nilsson, Dahlberg, & Jaensson, 2018; Levy & Janke, 2016).

Evidence-based nursing interventions can be successful in addressing such disparities (AHRQ, 2017; Schneiderman et al., 2014). One research team successfully integrated a diabetes education program within a faith-based framework for use in African American churches to support health behavior changes (Whitney et al., 2017). To address the higher prevalence of diabetes in Hispanic/Latino populations, researchers in the Diabetes Among Latinos Best Practices Trial (DIALBEST) randomly assigned a group of Latinos with type 2 diabetes to community-health workers (CHWs). They received culturally and linguistically appropriate services (CLAS) through education sessions on nutrition, blood glucose monitoring, medication adherence and other topics. The researchers found that subjects in the CHWs group had improved HbA1C at 3, 6, 12, and 18 months post intervention, but there was no change in serum lipid levels, hypertension, or weight (Pérez-Escamilla et al., 2015). Similar findings were found across 53 studies in a scoping review on CHWs' role in diabetes management (Egbujie et al., 2018). Policies are being written and adopted at all levels of government to address healthcare disparities. Some of these policies can be reviewed on the National Conference of State Legislatures (NCSL) website at www.ncsl.org/research/health/population-groups/health-disparities.aspx.

In summary, health disparities are deplorable, and effective strategies to reverse this trend are urgently needed. Although much research has been done to better understand healthcare disparities, researchers suggest that a multidimensional approach is needed; a history of institutionalized racism and individual racism that is embedded in every aspect of life of ethnic minorities must be recognized and properly addressed (Hardeman, Murphy, Karbeah, & Kozhimannil, 2018). For the purpose of eliminating health disparities, the National Stakeholder Strategy for Achieving Health Equity, a product of the National Partnership for Action, established guidelines for the development and continuous assessment of the impact of policies and programs to improve the health of vulnerable populations and achieve health equity. Healthcare workers need cultural competency training, communication needs to improve between providers and patients, strategies to improve community relations are needed, and adherence to non-discriminatory health policies is also necessary to bridge the gaps in providing equity and quality care to eliminate health disparities. (See report at www.minorityhealth.hhs.gov/npa/files/Plans/NSS/CompleteNSS.pdf.)

It is critical that APRNs advocate for the elimination of health disparities, as this work is of vital importance and urgently needed. And from an ethical standpoint, working to eliminate health disparities is the *right thing to do*. By recognizing health disparities and developing a better understanding of how process and status impact the outcome of interest, APRNs are better prepared to develop effective interventions to eliminate or reduce health disparities. Such strategies may include advocating better health insurance coverage for poor and immigrant populations; incorporating social determinants of health into a broader framework of care delivery; assessing the interaction among social environments, genetics, and population health; encouraging minority participation in research studies with community-based participatory research and specifically with practice-based research networks; using linguistically and culturally appropriate communication and written handouts; promoting and facilitating community partnerships; and implementing strategies to graduate a diverse nursing workforce (Gates, 2018; Quinones, Talavera, Castaneda, & Saha, 2015; Sentell et al., 2014; Williams & Purdie-Vaughns, 2016).

APRNs have successfully tested interventions to decrease health disparities, and by careful and thorough review of the current literature and resources available, they have the tools to develop additional effective and culturally sensitive interventions and to identify outcomes in order to achieve better and more equitable health outcomes.

SUMMARY

APRNs have a critical role in improving population health by intervening at every level from the individual to the community. Before an effective intervention can take place, it is imperative that realistic and measurable outcomes are first identified and defined so that they can be measured and analyzed. Outcomes may be classified by the beneficiary of the health intervention and by type such as care, patient, or performance-related, and also by time frame of achievement. Outcomes may also be categorized by clinical or disease-specific outcomes, function, cost-effectiveness, self-perception health status, and satisfaction outcomes. A commonly used framework to classify outcomes is Donabedian's framework of structure, process, and outcomes. This framework has been used for describing a community's health as well as for classifying nurse-sensitive indicators. Outcomes are an important part of the standardized language that nursing leaders and researchers continue to refine and operationalize as a means of improving healthcare.

The national healthcare objectives in *Healthy People 2020* and updated in *Healthy People 2030* provide a blueprint of health promotion and disease prevention objectives that are designed to improve the health of all people in the United States. Building on the goal of *Healthy People*, APRNs can use these web-based resources to identify outcomes and compare them with national and state data that can be further analyzed by stratifying for a population's ethnicity, race, income, education, and/or gender. Federal agencies, such as the AHRQ, the CDC Office of Minority Health and Health Disparities, and the NIH's NIMHD, provide ready access to a plethora of information and resources that can be used to identify and define outcomes.

APRNs have a tremendous opportunity to access and use available data to contribute to the current body of knowledge that forms the basis for evidence-based practice. By selecting and using well-defined indicators and comparing those to national norms, APRNs can provide important information on trends or patterns of quality of care. This information has the potential to stimulate the development of creative and innovative programs or interventions to improve health outcomes. Evidence of improved outcomes will help APRNs to justify and advocate for change through policy, practice, and research, with the ultimate goal of providing quality care for all.

EXERCISES AND DISCUSSION QUESTIONS

Exercise 2.1 An APRN is working in a community clinic providing postnatal care to a diverse population of families. The APRN knows that there is an ethnic disparity for infant mortality.

1. Where could the APRN go to find information on infant mortality disparities?
2. What is the ethnic disparity in infant mortality?
3. What social determinants of health are associated with infant mortality?
4. How might an APRN participate in local efforts to reduce infant mortality rates on a population level?

Exercise 2.2 An APRN who is interested in reducing opiate-related overdoses in high schools develops an online training program to teach all school employees to administer Narcan® (naxolone).

1. What are related Leading Health Indicators found in *Healthy People 2020*?
2. In examining the Community Guide topics, which ones are most relevant to this scenario?
3. What outcomes might the APRN monitor for effectiveness of the program?
4. What other population level strategies could the APRN implement to address the issue?

Exercise 2.3 APRNs should not only recognize health disparities, they should also make it part of their practice to develop strategies to reduce or eliminate them. Review information from *Healthy People 2020* and the CDC Office of Minority Health and Health Disparities websites.

1. What health disparities can you find that are relevant to your county or state?
2. What culturally and linguistically appropriate services (CLAS) interventions could an APRN implement in his or her specific practice that are consistent with the National CLAS Standards?
3. What outcomes could an APRN monitor related to the health disparities/state issue?
4. Which objectives in *Healthy People 2020/2030* could help this effort?

Exercise 2.4 Diabetes affects a growing number of Americans. An APRN working in a local hospital is part of a collaborative of community agencies strategically addressing diabetes from a community perspective.

1. What social determinants of health should the community look at in relation to risk or incidence of diabetes?
2. What resources could the APRN use to identify different outcomes related to diabetes?

3. What outcomes related to diabetes are of most interest to community members?

4. Using the AHRQ's Healthcare Quality and Disparities Report Data Query (nhqrnet.ahrq.gov/inhqrdr/data/submit), what related national and state level data are available to the APRN?

REFERENCES

Agency for Healthcare Research and Quality. (2017). *National healthcare quality and disparities reports.* Retrieved from https://www.ahrq.gov/research/findings/nhqrdr/index.html

American Association of Colleges of Nursing. (2004). *AACN position statement on the practice doctorate in nursing.* Washington, DC: Author.

American Association of Colleges of Nursing. (2006). *The essentials of doctoral education for advanced nursing practice.* Retrieved from http://www.aacn.nche.edu/DNP/pdf/Essentials.pdf

Anderson, E. T., & McFarlane, J. (2015). *Community as partner: Theory and practice in nursing* (7th ed.). New York, NY: Lippincott Williams & Wilkins.

Armstrong, S., Wong, C. A., Perrin, E., Page, S., Sibley, L., & Skinner, A. (2018). Association of physical activity with income, race/ethnicity, and sex among adolescents and young adults in the United States: Findings from the National Health and Nutrition Examination Survey, 200–2016. *JAMA Pediatrics, 172*(8), 732–740. doi:10.1001/jamapediatrics.2018.1273

Association of American Medical Colleges. (2014). *The state of health equity research: Closing knowledge gaps to address inequities.* Retrieved from https://www.aamc.org/initiatives/research/healthequity/402654/closingknowledgegaps.html

Bigbee, J. L., & Issel, L. M. (2012). Conceptual models for population-focused public health nursing interventions and outcomes: The state of the art. *Public Health Nursing, 29*(4), 370–379. doi:10.1111/j.1525-1446.2011.01006.x

Boothe, V. L., Sinha, D., Bohm, M., & Yoon, P. W. (2013). Community health assessment for population health improvement; resource of most frequently recommended health outcomes and determinants. *CDC Stacks Public Health Publications.* Retrieved from http://stacks.cdc.gov/view/cdc/20707

Braverman, P., Arkin, E., Orleans, T., Proctor, D., & Plough, A. (2017). *What is health equity? And what difference does a definition make?* Princeton, NJ: Robert Wood Johnson Foundation. Retrieved from https://www.rwjf.org/content/dam/farm/reports/issue_briefs/2017/rwjf437393

Cajita, M. I., Cajita, T. R., & Hae-Ra, H. (2016). Health literacy and heart failure. *Journal of Cardiovascular Nursing, 31*(2), 121–130. doi:10.1097/JCN.0000000000000229

Centers for Disease Control and Prevention. (2014). *Behavioral Risk Factor Surveillance System (BRFSS).* Retrieved from http://www.cdc.gov/brfss/about/about_brfss.htm

Centers for Disease Control and Prevention. (2017). *National health care surveys.* Retrieved from http://www.cdc.gov/nchs/dhcs.htm

Centers for Disease Control and Prevention. (2018). *2019 questionnaire redesign.* Retrieved from https://www.cdc.gov/nchs/nhis/2019_quest_redesign.htm

Chang, A., Patberg, E., Cueto, V., Hua, L., Singh, B., Kenya, S., & . . . Carrasquillo, O. (2018). Community health workers, access to care, and service utilization among Florida Latinos: A randomized controlled trial. *American Journal of Public Health, 108*(9), 1249–1251. doi:10.2105/AJPH.2018.304542

DeGuzman, P. B., & Kulbok, P. A. (2012). Changing health outcomes of vulnerable populations through nursing's influence on neighborhood built environment: A framework for nursing research. *Journal of Nursing Scholarship, 44*(4), 341–348. doi:10.1111/ j.1547-5069.2012.01470.x

Donabedian, A. (1980). *Explorations in quality assessment and monitoring.* Ann Arbor, MI: Health Administration Press.

Donabedian, A. (1982). *The criteria and standards of quality.* Ann Arbor, MI: Health Administration Press.

Egbujie, B. A., Delobell, P. A., Levitt, N., Puone, T., Sanders, D., & van Wyk, B. (2018). Role of community health workers in type 2 diabetes mellitus self-management: a scoping review. *PLOS One, 13*(6), e0198424. doi:10.1371/journal.pone.0198424

El-Sayed, A. M., Paczkowski, M., Rutherford, C. G., Keyes, K. M., & Galea, S. (2015). Social environments, genetics, and Black-White disparities in infant mortality. *Paediatric & Perinatal Epidemiology, 29*(6), 546–551. doi:10.1111/ppe.12227

Fee, E., & Garofalo, M. E. (2010). Florence Nightingale and the Crimean war. *American Journal of Public Health, 100*(9), 1591. doi:10.2105/AJPH.2009.188607

Friis, R. H., & Sellers, T. A. (2015). *Epidemiology for public health practice* (5th ed.). Boston, MA: Jones & Bartlett.

Galea, S., & Link, B. G. (2013). Six paths for the future of social epidemiology. *American Journal of Epidemiology, 178*(6), 843–849. doi:10.1093/aje/kwt148

Gates, S. A. (2018). What works in promoting and maintaining diversity in nursing programs. *Nursing Forum, 53*(2), 190–196. doi:10.1111/nuf.12242

Gibson, M. E., & Thatcher, E. J. (2016). Community as client: Assessment and analysis. In M. Stanhope & J. Lancaster (Eds.), *Public health nursing: Population-centered health care in the community* (9th ed., pp. 396–421). St. Louis, MO: Mosby.

Gillis, N. K., Arslanian-Engoren, C., & Struble, L. M. (2014). Acute coronary syndromes in older adults: A review of the literature. *Journal of Emergency Nursing, 40*(3), 270–275. doi:10.1016/j.jen.2013.03.003

Gregory, E. C. W., Drake, P., & Martin, J. A. (2018). Lack of change in perinatal mortality in the United States, 2014-2016. *NCHS Data Brief, No 316*. Retrieved from https://www.cdc.gov/nchs/data/databriefs/db316.pdf

Griffiths, P. (1995). Progress in measuring nursing outcomes. *Journal of Advanced Nursing, 21*(6), 1092–1100. doi:10.1046/j.1365-2648.1995.21061092.x

Gu, A., Yue, Y., Desai, R. P., & Argulian, E. (2017). Racial and ethnic differences in antihypertensive medication use and blood pressure control among U.S. adults with hypertension: The National Health and Nutrition Examination Survey, 2003 to 2012. *Circulation: Cardiovascular Quality and Outcomes, 10*(1), doi:10.1161/circoutcomes.116.003166

Hålleberg, N. M., Nilsson, U., Dahlberg, K., & Jaensson, M. (2018). Association between functional health literacy and postoperative recovery, health care contacts, and health-related quality of life among patients undergoing day surgery: Secondary analysis of a randomized clinical trial. *JAMA Surgery, 153*(8), 738–745. doi:10.1001/jamasurg.2018.0672

Hardeman, R. R., Murphy, K. A., Karbeah, J., & Kozhimannil, K. B. (2018). Naming institutionalized racism in the public health literature: A systematic literature review. *Public Health Reports, 133*(3), 240–249. doi:10.1177/0033354918760574

Hill, M. (1999). Outcomes measurement requires nursing to shift to outcome-based practice. *Nursing Administration Quarterly, 24*(1), 1–16. doi:10.1097/00006216-199910000-00003

Institute for Healthcare Improvement. (2018). *Triple Aim for Populations*. Retrieved from http://www.ihi.org/Topics/TripleAim/Pages/default.aspx

Institute of Medicine. (2015). *Vital signs: Core metrics for health and health care progress*. Washington, DC: National Academies Press.

Jones, T. (2016). Outcome measurement in nursing: Imperatives, ideals, history, and challenges. *Online Journal of Issues in Nursing, 21*(2), 1. doi:10.3912/OJIN.Vol21No02Man01

Kapu, A. N., Sicoutris, C., Broyhill, B. S., D'Agostino, R., & Kleinpell, R. M. (2017). Measuring outcomes in advanced practice nursing: Practice-specific quality metrics. In R. Kleinpell (Ed.), *Outcome assessment in advanced practice nursing* (4th ed., pp. 1-18). New York, NY: Springer Publishing Company.

Kautz, D. D., & Van Horn, E. R. (2008). An exemplar of the use of NNN language in developing evidence-based practice guidelines. *International Journal of Nursing Terminologies and Classifications, 19*(1), 14–19. doi:10.1111/j.1744-618X.2007.00074.x

Kleinpell, R. M. (2007). APRNs: Invisible champions? *Nursing Management, 38*(5), 18–22. doi:10.1097/01.LPN.0000269815.74178.de

Kleinpell, R., & Gawlinski, A. (2005). Assessing outcomes in advanced practice nursing practice: The use of quality indicators and evidence-based practice. *AACN Clinical Issues, 16*(1), 43–57. doi:10.1097/00044067-200501000-00006

Kleinpell, R., & Kapu, A. N. (2017). Quality measures for nurse practitioner practice evaluation. *Journal of The American Association Of Nurse Practitioners, 29*(8), 446–451. doi:10.1002/2327-6924.12474

Lang, N. M., & Marek, K. D. (1991). The policy and politics of patient outcomes. *Journal of Nursing Quality Assurance, 5*(2), 7–12.

Levy, H., & Janke, A. (2016). Health literacy and access to care. *Journal of Health Communication, 21*(Suppl 1), 43–50. doi:10.1080/10810730.2015.1131776

Loyo, H. K., Batcher, C., Wile, K., Huang, P., Orenstein, D., & Milstein, B. (2012). From model to action: Using a system dynamics model of chronic disease risks to align community action. *Health Promotion Practice, 14*(1), 53–61. doi:10.1177/1524839910390305

Macha, K., & McDonough, P. (Eds.). (2012). *Epidemiology for advanced nursing practice*. Sudbury, MA: Jones & Bartlett.

McDonald, C. C., Brawner, B. M., Fargo, J., Swope, J., & Sommers, M. S. (2017). Development of a theoretically grounded, web-based intervention to reduce adolescent driver attention. *The Journal of School Nursing, 34*(4), 270–280. doi:10.1177/1059840517711157

McCullough, J. M., & Leider, J. P. (2017). Associations between county wealth, health and social service spending, and health outcomes. *American Journal of Preventive Medicine, 53*(5), 592–598. doi:10.1016/j.amepre.2017.05.005

Minkler, M., & Wallerstein, N. (2012). Improving health through community organization and community building: Perspectives from health education and social work. In M. Minkler (Ed.), *Community organizing and community building for health and welfare* (3rd ed., pp. 37–58). New Brunswick, NJ: Rutgers University Press.

Montalvo, I. (2007). The National Database of Nursing Quality Indicators® (NDNQI®). *Online Journal of Issues in Nursing, 12*(3), doi:10.3912/OJIN.Vol12No03Man02

Nelson, E. C., Batalden, P. B., Plume, S. K., & Mohr, J. J. (1996). Improving health care, Part 2: A clinical improvement worksheet and users' manual. *Joint Commission Journal on Quality Improvement, 22*(8), 531–548. doi:10.1016/s1070-3241(16)30254-1

Newhouse, R., Barksdale, D. J., & Miller, J. A. (2015). The Patient-Centered Outcomes Research Institute: Research done differently. *Nursing Research, 64*(1), 72–77. doi:10.1097/NNR.0000000000000070

Parrish, R. G. (2010). Measuring population health outcomes. *Preventing Chronic Disease, 7*(4), A71. Retrieved from https://www.cdc.gov/pcd/issues/2010/jul/10_0005.htm

Patrician, P. A., Dolansky, M. A., Pair, V., Bates, M., Moore, S. M., Splaine, M., & Gilman, S. C. (2013). The Veterans Affairs National Quality Scholars program: A model for interprofessional education in quality and safety. *Journal Nursing Care Quality, 28*(1), 24–32. doi:10.1097/NCQ.0b013e3182678f41

Payán, D. D., Sloane, D. C., Illum, J., Vargas, R. B., Lee, D., Galloway-Gilliam, L., & Lewis, L. B. (2017). Catalyzing implementation of evidence-based interventions in safety net settings: A clinical–community partnership in south Los Angeles. *Health Promotion Practice, 18*(4), 586–597. doi:10.1177/1524839917705418

Penman-Aguilar, A., Bouye, K., & Liburd, L. (2016). Strategies for reducing health disparities – Selected CDC-sponsored interventions, United States, 2016. *Morbidity and Mortality Weekly Report, 65*(1), 2–3. doi:10.15585/mmwr.su6501a2

Pérez-Escamilla, R., Damio, G., Chhabra, J., Fernandez, M. L., Segura-Pérez, S., Vega-López, S., . . . D'Agostino, D. (2015). Impact of a community health workers-led structured program on blood glucose control among Latinos with type 2 diabetes: The DIALBEST trial. *Diabetes Care, 38*(2), 197–205. doi:10.2337/dc14-0327

Press Ganey Associates. (n.d.). *National Database of Nursing Quality Indicators® (NDNQI®)*. Retrieved from http://www.nursingquality.org/#intro

Quinones, A. R., Talavera, G. A., Castaneda, S. F., & Saha, S. (2015). Interventions that reach into communities – promising directions for reducing racial and ethnic disparities in healthcare. *Journal of Racial and Ethnic Health Disparities, 2*(3), 336–40. doi:10.1007/s40615-014-0078-3

Rich, K. A. (2015). Evaluating outcomes of innovations. In N. A. Schmidt & J. M. Brown (Eds.), *Evidence-based practice: Appraisal and application of research* (3rd ed., pp. 484–503). Sudbury, MA; Jones & Bartlett.

Rothwell, C. J. (2015). *About the national center for health statistics*. Retrieved from https://www.cdc.gov/nchs/about/index.htm

Schiller, J. S., Clarke, T. C., & Norris, T. (2018). *Early release of selected estimates based on data from the January–September 2017 National Health Interview Survey*. Retrieved from https://www.cdc.gov/nchs/data/nhis/earlyrelease/EarlyRelease201803.pdf

Schneiderman, N., Llabre, M., Cowie, C. C., Barnhart, J., Carnethon, M., Gallo, L. C., . . . Avilés-Santa, M. L. (2014). Prevalence of diabetes among Hispanics/Latinos from diverse backgrounds: the Hispanic community health study/study of Latinos (HCHS/SOL). *Diabetes Care, 37*(8), 2233–2239. doi:10.2337/dc13-2939

Sentell, T., Zhang, W., Davis, J., Baker, K. K., & Braun, K. L. (2014). The influence of community and individual health literacy on self-reported health status. *Journal of General Internal Medicine, 29*(2), 298–304. doi:10.1007/s11606-013-2638-3

Smith, K. J., & Craft-Rosenberg, M. (2010). Using NANDA, NIC, and NOC in an undergraduate nursing practicum. *Nurse Educator, 35*(4), 162–166. doi:10.1097/NNE.0b013 e3181e33953

Subica, A. M., Agarwal, N., Sullivan, G., & Link, B. G. (2017). Obesity and associated health disparities among understudied multiracial, Pacific Islander, and American Indian adults. *Obesity, 25*(12), 2128–2136. doi:10.1002/oby.21954

Unni, P., Estrade, C. M., Chung, D. H., Riley, E. B., Worsely-Hynd, L., & Stinson, N. (2017). A multiyear assessment of a hospital program to promote teen motor vehicle safety. *The Journal of Trauma and Acute Care Surgery, 83*(5S), S190–S196. doi:10.1097/TA.0000000000001521

U.S. Department of Health and Human Services. (2018a). *Healthy People 2020.* Retrieved from http://www.healthypeople.gov

U.S. Department of Health and Human Services. (2018b). *Healthy People 2020: Disparities.* Retrieved from https://www.healthypeople.gov/2020/about/foundation-health-measures/Disparities

U.S. Department of Health and Human Services, Community Preventive Services Task Force (2019). The community guide. Retrieved from https://www.thecommunityguide.org

U.S. National Library of Medicine. (2018). *About partners in information access for the public health workforce.* Retrieved from https://www.nlm.nih.gov/nichsr/partners.html?_ga=2.260215309 .129585028.1534454264-809822319.1534454264

van Maanen, H. M. T. (1979). Perspectives and problems on quality of nursing care: An overview of contributions from North America and recent developments in Europe. *Journal of Advanced Nursing, 4*(4), 377–389. doi:10.1111/j.1365-2648.1979.tb00872.x

Williams, A. F. (2017). Graduated driving licensing (GDL) in the United States in 2016: A literature review and commentary. *Journal of Safety Research, 63,* 29–41. doi:10.1016/j.jsr.2017.08.010

Williams, D. R., & Purdie-Vaughns, V. (2016). Needed interventions to reduce racial/ethnic disparities in health. *Journal of Health Politics, Policy and Law, 41*(4), 627–651. doi:10.1215/03616878-3620857

Whitney, E., Kindred, E., Pratt, A., O'Neal, Y., Harrison, R. C. P., & Peek, M. E. (2017). Culturally tailoring a patient empowerment and diabetes education curriculum for the African-American church. *The Diabetes Educator, 43*(5), 441–448. doi:10.1177/0145721717725280

Weinstein, J. N., Geller, A., Negussie, Y., & Baciu, A. (2017). *Communities in action: Pathways to health equity.* Washington (DC): The National Academies Press. Retrieved from https://www.ncbi.nlm.nih.gov/books/NBK425844

World Health Organization. (2011). *Rio political declaration on social determinants of health.* Retrieved from http://www.who.int/sdhconference/declaration/Rio_political_declaration.pdf?ua=1

Xiao, S., Widger, K., Tourangeau, A., & Berta, W. (2017). Nursing process health care indicators. *Journal of Nursing Care Quality, 32*(1), 32–39. doi:10.1097/ncq.0000000000000207

Zenzano, T., Allan, J. D., Bigley, M. B., Bushardt, R. L., Garr, D. R., Johnson, K., . . . Stanley, J. M. (2011). The roles of healthcare professionals in implementing clinical prevention and population health. *American Journal of Preventative Medicine, 40*(2), 261–267. doi:10.1016/j.amepre.2010.10.023

INTERNET RESOURCES

Agency for Healthcare Research and Quality (AHRQ): www.qualityindicators.ahrq.gov

Association of American Medical Colleges (AAMC) *"The State of Health Equity Research: Closing Knowledge Gaps to Address Inequities"*: www.aamc.org/initiatives/research/healthequity/402654/closing knowledgegaps.html

CMS, "Hospital Compare": https://www.medicare.gov/hospitalcompare/search.html

County Health Rankings and Roadmaps: http://www.countyhealthrankings.org

Healthy People 2020: https://www.healthypeople.gov

Healthy People 2030 Development Plan: https://www.healthypeople.gov/2020/About-Healthy-People/ Development-Healthy-People-2030

Institute for Healthcare Improvement/Quality Improvement Essentials Toolkit: http://www.ihi.org/ resources/Pages/Tools/Quality-Improvement-Essentials-Toolkit.aspx

NANDA International: www.NANDA.org

National Cancer Institute, Division of Cancer Control & Population Sciences: http://cancercontrol.cancer.gov

National Cancer Institute, Health Disparities Calculator: http://seer.cancer.gov/hdcalc

National Center for Health Statistics (NCHS): http://www.cdc.gov/nchs

National Center for Health Statistics / National Vital Statistics Program: www.cdc.gov/nchs/nvss

National Center for Statistics and Analysis (NCSA) Motor Vehicle Traffic Crash Data Resource Page: https://crashstats.nhtsa.dot.gov

National Conference of State Legislature (NCSL): http://www.ncsl.org/research/health/population-groups/health-disparities.aspx

National Health and Nutrition Examination Survey (NHNES): www.cdc.gov/nchs/nhanes.htm

National Quality Partners': https://www.qualityforum.org/National_Quality_Partners.aspx

National Stakeholder Strategy for Achieving Health Equity: https://www.minorityhealth.hhs.gov/npa/files/Plans/NSS/CompleteNSS.pdf

NIH, National Institute on Minority Health and Health Disparities: https://www.nimhd.nih.gov/programs/edu-training

The Behavioral Risk Factor Surveillance System (BRFSS): http://www.cdc.gov/brfss

The Community Guide: www.thecommunityguide.org

The National Healthcare Surveys: www.cdc.gov/nchs/dhcs

The National Partnership for Action (NPA) to End Health Disparities: https://minorityhealth.hhs.gov/npa

Trust for America's Health: https://www.tfah.org

CHAPTER 3

EPIDEMIOLOGICAL METHODS AND MEASUREMENTS IN POPULATION-BASED NURSING PRACTICE: PART I

PATTY A. VITALE | ANN L. CUPP CURLEY

INTRODUCTION

Evidence-based practice as it relates to population-based nursing combines clinical practice and public health through the use of population health sciences in clinical practice (Heller & Page, 2002). Epidemiology is the science of public health. It is concerned with the study of the factors determining and influencing the frequency and distribution of disease, injury, and other health-related events and their causes (Gordis, 2014). In addition to epidemiology, an understanding of other scientific disciplines, such as biology and biostatistics, is also important for identifying associations and determining causation when looking at exposures and outcomes as they relate to population health.

Population-based care focuses on populations at risk, analysis of aggregate data, evaluation of demographic factors, and recognition of health disparities. It is concerned with the patterns of delivery of care and outcome measurements at the population or subpopulation level. The purpose of this chapter is to provide readers with an understanding of the natural history of disease and the approaches that are integral for the prevention of disease. It addresses the Doctor of Nursing Practice competencies specified in *Essential III: Clinical Scholarship and Analytical Methods for Evidence-Based Practice* (American Association of Colleges of Nursing [AACN], 2006). We introduce basic concepts that are necessary to understand how to measure disease outcomes and select study designs that are best suited for population-based research. Emphasis is placed on measuring disease occurrence with a fundamental discussion of how to calculate incidence, prevalence, and mortality rates. Successful advanced practice nursing in population health depends upon the ability to recognize the difference between the individual and population approaches to the collection and use of data and the ability to assess needs and evaluate outcomes at the population level. Concepts surrounding survival data are also discussed along with strategies to guide advanced practice registered nurses (APRNs) on how to calculate and interpret survival data.

THE NATURAL HISTORY OF DISEASE

The natural history of disease refers to the progression of a disease from its *preclinical state* (prior to symptoms) to its *clinical state* (from onset of symptoms to cure, control, disability, or death). Disease is not something that occurs suddenly, but rather it is a multifactorial process that is dynamic and occurs over time. It evolves and changes and is sometimes initiated by events that take place years, even decades, before symptoms first appear. Many diseases have a natural life history that can extend over a very long period of time. The natural history of disease is described in stages. Understanding the different stages allows for a better understanding of the approach to the prevention and control of disease.

Stage of Susceptibility

The stage of susceptibility refers to the time prior to disease development. In the presence of certain risk factors, genetics, or environment, disease may develop and the severity can vary among individuals. Risk factors are those factors that are associated with an increased likelihood of disease developing over time. The idea that individuals could modify "risk factors" tied to heart disease, stroke, and other diseases is one of the key findings of the Framingham Heart Study (National Heart, Lung, and Blood Institute and Boston University, 2018). Started in 1948 and still in operation, this study is one of the most important population studies ever carried out in the United States. Before Framingham, for example, most healthcare providers believed that atherosclerosis was an inevitable part of the aging process. Although not all risk factors are amenable to change (e.g., genetic factors), the identification of risk factors is important and fundamental to disease prevention.

Preclinical Stage of Disease

During the preclinical phase, the disease process has begun but there are no obvious symptoms. Although there is no clear manifestation of disease, because of the interaction of biological factors, changes have started to occur. During this stage, however, the changes are not always detectable. Screening technologies have been developed to detect the presence of some diseases before clinical symptoms appear. The Papanicolaou (Pap) smear is an example of an effective screening method for detecting cancer in a premalignant state to improve mortality related to cervical cancer. The use of the Pap smear as a screening tool facilitates early detection and treatment of premalignant changes of the cervix prior to development of malignancy.

Clinical Stage of Disease

In the clinical stage of disease, sufficient physiologic and/or functional changes occur, leading to the development of recognizable symptoms of disease. It might also be accurately referred to as the treatment stage. For some people, the disease may completely resolve (either spontaneously or with medical intervention), whereas for some it will lead to disability and/or death. It is for this reason that the clinical stage of disease is sometimes subdivided for better medical management. Staging systems used in malignancies to better define the extent of disease involvement are an example of a system that can help guide the type of treatment modality selected based on the stage. In many cases, staging can provide an estimate of prognosis. Another example is the identification of disability as a specific subcategory of the treatment stage. Disability occurs when a clinical disease leaves a person either temporarily or permanently disabled. When people become disabled, the goal of the treatment is to mitigate the effects of disease and to help these individuals to function to their optimal abilities. This is very different from the goal for someone who can be treated and restored to the level of functioning that he or she enjoyed prior to the illness.

The Nonclinical Disease Stage

This nonclinical or unapparent disease stage can be broken into four subparts. The first subpart is the *preclinical stage*, which, as mentioned earlier, is the acquisition of disease prior to development of symptoms and is destined to become disease. The second subpart is the *subclinical stage* that occurs when someone has the disease but it is not destined to develop clinically. The third subpart is the *chronic or persistent stage of disease*, which is disease that persists over time. And finally, there is the fourth subpart or *latent stage* in which one has disease with no active multiplication of the biologic agent (Gordis, 2014).

The Iceberg Phenomenon

For most health problems, the number of identified cases is exceeded by the number of unidentified cases. This occurrence, referred to as the "iceberg phenomenon," makes it difficult to assess the true burden of disease. Many diseases do not have obvious symptoms, as stated earlier, and may go unrecognized for many years. Unrecognized diseases, such as diabetes, hypertension, and mental illness, create a significant problem with identifying populations at risk and estimating service needs. Complications also arise when patients are not recognized or treated during an early stage of a disease when interventions are most effective. Additionally, patients who do not have symptoms or do not recognize their symptoms do not seek medical care and, in many cases, even if they do have a diagnosis, do not take their medications as they perceive that they are healthy when they are asymptomatic.

PREVENTION

Understanding the natural history of disease is as important as understanding the causal factors of disease because it provides the APRN with the knowledge that is required to design programs or interventions that target populations at risk. Understanding how disease develops is fundamental to the concept of prevention and provides a framework for disease prevention and control. The primary goal of prevention is to prevent disease before it occurs. The concept of prevention has evolved to include measures taken to interrupt or slow the progression of disease or to lessen its impact. There are three levels of prevention.

Primary Prevention

Primary prevention refers to the process of altering susceptibility or reducing exposure to susceptible individuals and includes general health promotion and specific measures designed to prevent disease prior to a person getting the disease. Interventions designed for primary prevention are carried out during the stage of susceptibility and can include things such as providing immunizations to change a person's susceptibility. Actions taken to prevent tobacco usage are another example of primary prevention. Tobacco use is one of the 12 leading health indicators used by Healthy *People 2020* to measure health. Cigarette smoking is the leading cause of preventable mortality in the United States (Centers for Disease Control and Prevention [CDC], 2018a), and prevention or cessation of smoking can reduce the development of many smoking-related diseases. Taxes on cigarettes, education programs, and support groups to help people stop smoking and the creation of smoke-free zones are all examples of primary prevention measures. The CDC linked a series of tobacco control efforts by Minnesota to a decrease in adult smoking prevalence rates. From 1999 to 2010, Minnesota implemented a series of antismoking initiatives, including a statewide smoke-free law, cigarette tax increases, media campaigns, and statewide cessation efforts. Adult smoking prevalence decreased from 22.1% in 1999 to 16.1% in 2010 (CDC, 2011). In 2013, Minnesota increased the tax on a pack of cigarettes an additional $1.60. Following this increase, smoking decreased by 33% among Minnesota's 11th graders and by 10% among adult residents. Smokers reported that the tax increase did influence their smoking behaviors (Minnesota Department of Health, 2018). This is an excellent example of a successful statewide primary prevention effort to reduce smoking prevalence through a variety of initiatives.

Secondary Prevention

The early detection and prompt treatment of a disease at the earliest possible stage are referred to as *secondary prevention*. The goals of secondary prevention are to either identify and cure a disease at a very early stage or slow its progression to prevent complications and limit disability. Secondary prevention measures are carried out during the preclinical or presymptomatic stage of disease. Screening programs are designed to detect specific diseases in their early stages while they are curable and to prevent or reduce morbidity and mortality related to a later diagnosis of disease. Examples of secondary prevention include the Pap smear, mentioned earlier, as well as annual testing of cholesterol levels, mammography, and rapid HIV testing of asymptomatic individuals.

Tertiary Prevention

Tertiary prevention strategies are implemented during the middle or late stages of clinical disease and refer to measures taken to alleviate disability and restore effective functioning. Attempts are made to slow the progression or to cure the disease. In cases in which permanent changes have taken place, interventions are planned and designed to help people lead a productive and satisfying life by maximizing the use of remaining capabilities (rehabilitation). Cardiac rehabilitation programs that provide physical and occupational therapies to postoperative cardiac patients are an example of tertiary prevention.

CAUSATION

The Epidemiological Triangle

The relationship between risk factors and disease is complex. Research studies may describe a relationship between a risk factor and disease, but how do we know that this relationship is causal? An understanding of causation is important if APRNs want to effectively impact the health of populations. The *epidemiological triangle* is a model that has historically been used to explain causation. The model consists of three interactive factors: the causative agent (those factors for which presence or absence cause disease—biologic, chemical, physical, nutritional), a susceptible host (things such as age, gender, race, immune status, genetics), and the environment (including diverse elements such as water, food, neighborhood, pollution). A change in the agent, host, and environmental balance can lead to disease (Harkness, 1995). The underlying assumptions of this model are that causative factors can be both intrinsic and extrinsic to the host and that the cause of disease is related to interaction among these three factors. This model was developed initially to explain the transmission of infectious diseases and was particularly useful when the focus of epidemiology was on acute diseases. It is less helpful for understanding and explaining the more complicated processes associated with chronic disease. With the rise of chronic diseases as the primary cause of morbidity and mortality, a model that recognizes multiple causative factors was needed to better understand this complex interaction.

The Web of Causation

The dynamic nature of chronic diseases calls for a more sophisticated model for explaining causation than the epidemiological triangle. Introduction of the *web of causation* concept first appeared in the 1960s when chronic diseases overtook infectious diseases as the leading cause of morbidity and mortality in the United States. The foundation of this concept is that disease develops as the result of many antecedent factors and not as a result of a single, isolated cause. Each factor is itself the result of a complex pattern of events that can be best perceived as interrelated in the complex configuration of a web. The use of a web is helpful for visualizing how difficult it is to untangle the many events that can precede the onset of a chronic illness.

Critics have argued that this model places too much emphasis on epidemiological methods and too little on theories of disease causation. As theories evolved about the relationship between smoking and cancer, the U.S. Surgeon General appointed a committee to review the evidence. This committee developed a set of guidelines for judging whether an observed association is causal. These guidelines include temporal relationship, strength of the association, dose–response relationship, replication of the findings, biologic plausibility, consideration of alternative explanation, cessation of exposure, consistency with other knowledge, and specificity of the association (Gordis, 2014). For a more detailed discussion on this model, see Chapter 4, Epidemiological Methods and Measurements in Population-Based Nursing Practice.

METHODS OF ANALYSIS

Successful population-based approaches depend on the ability to recognize the difference between the collection and use of data from individuals and populations and the ability to assess needs and evaluate outcomes at the population level. Several of the more recent theories of causation can be helpful in determining whether an exposure is causally related to the development of disease. In particular, calculating the strength of association using statistics is one of several criteria that can be used to determine causality. However, statistics must be used with caution. Health is a multidimensional variable: Factors that affect health, and that interact to affect health, are numerous. Many relationships are possible. There are problems inherent in the use of statistics to explain differences among groups. Although statistics can describe disparities, they cannot explain them. It is left to the researchers to explain the differences. In addition to statistics, one must also be aware of the validity and reliability of the data. There are problems associated with the categorizing and gathering of statistics that can have an effect on how the data should be interpreted. In order to be successful in research, one must do more than just collect data: One must look at the theoretical issues associated with explaining the relationship among the variables. Additionally, even if a relationship is found to be statistically significant, that does not ensure that it is clinically significant. Recognizing limitations in research and in practice are the most important steps prior to making conclusions in any setting. Therefore, it is important that APRNs have a commitment to higher standards with an emphasis placed on adherence to careful and thorough procedural and ethical practice.

Methods derived from epidemiology can be useful in identifying the etiology or the cause of a disease. Among the important steps in this process are the identification of risk factors and their impact in a population, determining the extent of a disease and/or adverse events found in a population, and evaluating both existing and new preventive and therapeutic measures and modes of healthcare delivery. Applying strong epidemiologic methods with a sound application and interpretation of statistics are the foundation for evidence-based practice. The integration of evidence can lead to the creation of good public policy and regulatory decisions.

Descriptive Epidemiology

Rates

Knowledge of how illness and injury are distributed within a population can provide valuable information on disease etiology and can lay the foundation for the introduction of new prevention programs. It is important to know how to measure disease in populations, and rates are a useful method for measuring attributes over time such as disease and injury in any population. Rates can also be used to identify trends and evaluate outcomes and can allow for comparisons within and between groups. The *Morbidity and Mortality Weekly Report* (*MMWR*; located at www.cdc.gov/mmwr) is a publication of the CDC and contains updated information on incidence and prevalence of many diseases and conditions. These rates provide healthcare providers with up-to-date information on the risks and burdens of various diseases and conditions (CDC, 2018b). The information obtained from the *MMWR* can be used to identify trends and provide policy makers with information for designating resources. The following is an example of such information:

> Drinking sugar sweetened beverages (SSBs) is associated with several adverse health consequences including obesity, type 2 diabetes, and cardiovascular disease. In 2013 the Behavioral Risk Factor Surveillance System (a telephone survey) investigated self-reported SSB intake in the United States.In this survey of adults aged 18 years of age and older an SSB was identified as regular soda, fruit drink, sweet tea, and sports or energy drink intake. The results revealed that the overall age-adjusted prevalence of SSB intake once or more per day is 30% and ranges from 18% in Vermont to 47.5% in Mississippi. It is most prevalent among adults aged 18 to 24 years (43.3%), men (34.1%), non-Hispanic Blacks (39.9%), unemployed adults (34.4%) and persons with less than a high school education (42.4%). (This excerpt is adapted from an issue of *MMWR* published on February 26, 2016 [Park, Xu, Town, & Blanck, 2016].)

By publishing rates in percentages and comparing those rates among groups, it highlights the disparity between different demographic profiles related to SSB intake. Information such as this can be useful to both clinicians and policy makers who make decisions about interventions and services.

When calculating rates, the numerator is the number of events that occur during a specified period of time and is divided by the denominator, which is the average population at risk during that specified time period. This number is multiplied by a constant—either 100, 1,000, 10,000, or 100,000—and is expressed per that number. The purpose of expressing rates per 100,000, for example, is to have a constant denominator, and it allows investigators to compare rates among groups with different population sizes. To put it simply, the rate is calculated as follows:

$$\text{Rate} = \text{Numerator/denominator} \times \text{Constant multiplier}$$

In order to calculate rates, the APRN must first have a clear and explicit definition of the patient population and of the event. An important consideration when calculating rates is that anyone represented in the denominator must have the potential to enter the group in the numerator, and all persons represented in the numerator must come from the denominator.

Rates can be either crude or specific. Crude rates apply to an entire population without any reference to any characteristics of the individuals within it. For example, to calculate the crude mortality rate, the numerator is the total number of deaths during a specific period of time divided by the denominator, which is the average number of people in the population during that specified period of time (including those who have died). Typically, the population value for a 1-year period is determined using the mid-year population.

Specific rates can also be calculated for a population that has been categorized into groups. Suppose that an APRN wants to calculate the number of new mothers who initiate breastfeeding in a specific hospital in 2018. The formula would be:

$$\frac{\text{Total number of breastfeeding infants in community hospital in 2018}}{\text{Total number of live births in the same community hospital in 2018}} \times \text{Constant multiplier}$$

In order to compare rates in two or more groups, the events in the numerator must be defined in the same way, the time intervals must be the same, and the constant multiplier must be the same. Rates can be used to compare two different groups, or one group during two different time periods. Returning to the example about breastfeeding, the breastfeeding rates could be compared in the same hospital, but at two different times, before and after implementation of a planned intervention to increase breastfeeding rates.

Formulae for the rates discussed in this chapter can be found in Exhibit 3.1.

EXHIBIT 3.1

LIST OF USEFUL FORMULAE

Calculating Rates

Incidence rate describes the occurrence of *new* disease cases in a community over a period of time relative to the size of the population at risk.

$$\text{Incidence rate} = \frac{\text{Number of new cases during a specified period}}{\text{Population at risk during the same specified period}} \times \text{Constant multiplier}$$

(continued)

EXHIBIT 3.1

Prevalence rate is the number of *all* existing cases of a specific disease in a population *at a given point in time* relative to the population at risk.

$$\text{Prevalence rate} = \frac{\text{Number of existing cases at a specified period}}{\text{Population at risk at the same specified period}} \times \text{Constant multiplier}$$

Crude rates summarize the occurrence of births (crude birth rate) or deaths (crude death rate). The numerator is the number of events and the denominator is the average population size (usually estimated as a midyear population).

$$\text{Crude death rate} = \frac{\text{Number of deaths in a population during a specified period}}{\text{Population estimate during same specified period}} \times \text{Constant multiplier}$$

Specific rates are used to overcome some of the biases seen with crude rates. They are used to control for variables such as age, race, gender, and disease.

$$\text{Age-specified death rate} = \frac{\text{Number of deaths for a specified age group during a specified time}}{\text{Population estimate for the specified age group during same specified time}} \times \text{Constant multiplier}$$

Case fatality rate is used to measure the percentage of people who die from a certain disease. This rate tells you how fatal or severe a disease is compared to other diseases.

$$\text{Case fatality rate} = \frac{\text{Number of individuals dying after disease onset or diagnosis}}{\text{Number of individuals with the specified disease}} \times 100$$

Proportionate mortality ratio is useful for determining the leading causes of death.

$$\text{Proportionate mortality ratio} = \frac{\text{Number of deaths from a specified cause during specified time period}}{\text{Total deaths during the same period}} \times 100$$

(continued)

EXHIBIT 3.1

Calculations Used in Health Impact Assessment

Number needed to treat (NNT) is the number of patients needed to receive a treatment to prevent one bad outcome. The NNT calculated should be rounded up to the next highest number. Before the NNT can be calculated, the absolute risk reduction (ARR) must be identified.

$$\text{ARR} = \text{Incidence in exposed} - \text{Incidence in nonexposed}$$
$$\text{NNT} = 1/\text{ARR}$$

The NNT can also be calculated in randomized trials using mortality rates:

$$\text{NNT} = 1/(\text{Mortality rate in untreated group} - \text{Mortality rate in treated group})$$

Disease impact number (DIN) is the number of those with the disease in question among whom one event will be prevented by the intervention.

$$\cfrac{1}{\left(\text{ARR} \times \begin{array}{l}\text{Proportion of people with the disease} \\ \text{who are exposed to the intervention}\end{array} \right)}$$

Population impact number (PIN) is the number of those in the whole population among whom one event will be prevented by the intervention.

$$\cfrac{1}{\left(\text{ARR} \times \begin{array}{c}\text{Proportion of people with} \\ \text{the disease who are exposed} \\ \text{to the intervention}\end{array} \times \begin{array}{c}\text{Proportion of the total} \\ \text{population with the disease} \\ \text{of interest}\end{array} \right)}$$

Years of potential life lost (YPLL) is used for setting heath priorities. Predetermined standard age at death in the United States is 75 years.

$$\text{YPLL (75)} = 75 - \text{Age at death from a specific cause}$$

Add the years of life lost for each individual for specific cause of death = YPLL

Calculations Used in Screening Programs

Sensitivity is the ability of a screening test to identify accurately those persons with the disease.

$$\text{Sensitivity} = \text{TP}/(\text{TP} + \text{FN})$$

Specificity reflects the extent to which it excludes the persons who do not have the disease.

$$\text{Specificity} = \text{TN}/(\text{TN} + \text{FP})$$

(continued)

EXHIBIT 3.1

	DISEASE	NO DISEASE
+ Test	True positive (TP)	False positive (FP)
− Test	False negative (FN)	True negative (TN)

Source: Adapted from Fulton, J. S., Lyon, B. L., & Goudreau, K. A., (2014). *Foundations of clinical nurse specialist practice* (2nd ed.). New York, NY: Springer Publishing Company.

Incidence and Prevalence

Incidence rates describe the occurrence of new events in a population over a period of time relative to the size of the population at risk. *Prevalence* rates describe the number of all cases of a specific disease or attribute in a population at a given point in time relative to the size of the population at risk. Incidence provides information about the rate at which new cases occur and is a measure of risk. For example, the formula for the incidence rate for HIV is:

$$\frac{\text{Total number of people who are diagnosed with HIV in a community during 2018}}{\text{Population in that community at midyear of 2018}} \times 1,000 = \text{Rate per } 1,000$$

Incidence rates provide us with a direct measure of how often new cases occur within a particular population and provide some basis on which to assess risk. By comparing incidence rates among population groups that vary in one or more risk factors, the APRN can begin to get some idea of the association between risk factors and disease. If, in the earlier example of breastfeeding, the APRN discovers breastfeeding rates are significantly different among different ethnic groups, the characteristics of the groups can be compared and the causes for this disparity can be hypothesized and tested.

Period prevalence measures the number of cases of disease during a specific period of time and is a measure of burden. The formula for the period prevalence rate for HIV in 2018 is:

$$\frac{\text{Total number of people who are HIV positive in a community during 2018}}{\text{Population in that community at midyear of 2018}} \times 1,000 = \text{Rate per } 1,000$$

In the formula given here, all newly diagnosed cases for the year plus existing cases are included. *Point prevalence* is defined as the number of cases of disease at a specific point in time divided by the number of people at risk at that specific point in time multiplied by a constant multiplier. An example of the use of point prevalence would be the information gathered from a survey in which an investigator asks questions such as who has diabetes, hypertension, epilepsy, or any other disease or event at that specific point in time. Prevalence, whether point or period, cannot give us an estimate of the risk of disease; it can only tell us about the burden of disease for a specified period of time. Prevalence is useful when comparing rates between populations but should be interpreted with caution. Diseases that are chronic will have a higher prevalence because at any given time, those with chronic disease will always have that disease. This can make it challenging to interpret prevalence rates as they do not tell us the risk of developing disease but they can be helpful when trying to determine resource needs for chronic diseases. With diseases that are short in duration, prevalence may not capture the true burden of disease for that population. Additionally, it is important to note that unidentified cases are not captured in either prevalence rates or incidence rates. Rates can only estimate the burden of disease, but they are the best way to draw comparisons using a common denominator.

An example of how prevalence rates are used in the literature is as follows:

The CDC (2018c) reported that the prevalence of obesity was 39.8% for U.S. adults in 2015–2016. Hispanics (47.0%) and non-Hispanic Blacks (46.8%) had the highest age-adjusted prevalence of obesity, followed by non-Hispanic Whites (37.9%) and non-Hispanic Asians (12.7%). The prevalence of obesity was 35.7% among young adults aged 20 to 39 years, 42.8% among middle-aged adults aged 40 to 59 years, and 41.0% among older adults aged 60 and over.

Information on the prevalence of adult obesity in the United States has led to increased attention to factors that cause obesity (especially in children). This has led to the development of new programs aimed at primary and secondary prevention.

Mortality Rates

Mortality rates, also known as death rates, can be useful when evaluating and comparing populations. As stated earlier, there are many factors that can affect the natural history of disease, and measuring mortality allows investigators to compare death rates among and within populations. The formula for mortality rate is:

$$\frac{\text{Number of deaths in a population during a specified time}}{\text{Average population estimate during the specified time}} \times \text{Constant multiplier}$$

Mortality rates can be specific or broad in definition and can include any qualifiers for time, age, or disease type. It is important to include those specifics in your denominator to ensure that the population value used is the best estimate of the population at risk. For example, to look at the number of deaths in 2018 due to breast cancer in women aged 18 to 40, the denominator should *only* include the midyear population of women aged 18 to 40 in 2018. It is also important to include those women who died during that year in the denominator. Again, it is impossible to know exactly how many women in that age group are at risk using a midyear population, but the key is to use similar sources of measurement so that comparisons can be made assuming similar sources are used to estimate the denominator.

Standardization of crude rates is an important consideration when comparing mortality rates among populations. Standardization is used to control the effects of age and other characteristics in order to make valid comparisons between groups. Age adjustment is an example of rate standardization and perhaps the most important one. No other factor has a larger effect on mortality than age. Consider the problem of comparing two communities with very different age distributions. One community has a much higher mortality rate for colon cancer than the other, leading investigators to consider a possible environmental hazard in that community, when in fact, that community's population is older, which could account for the higher mortality. Direct age adjustment or standardization allows a researcher to eliminate the age disparities between two populations by using a standardized population. This allows the researcher to compare mortality or death rates between groups by eliminating age differences between populations and comparing actual age-adjusted mortality rates to determine whether age truly plays a role in the crude unadjusted mortality rates.

There are two methods of age adjustment: direct, as mentioned earlier, and indirect. The direct method applies observed age-specific mortality or death rates to a standardized population. The indirect method applies the age-specific rates of a standardized population to the age distribution of an observed population and is used to determine whether one population has a greater mortality because of an occupational hazard or risk compared to the general population. (To learn how to perform age adjustment, refer to an advanced epidemiology text.)

The *case fatality rate* (CFR) is a measure of the severity of disease (such as infectious diseases) and can be helpful when designing programs to reduce the rate or disparity in the population. It should be noted that CFR is not a true rate as it has no explicit time implication but rather is a proportion of persons with disease who died from that disease after diagnosis. It is a measure of the probability of death among diagnosed cases. Its usefulness for chronic diseases is limited because the length of time from diagnosis to death can be long. CFR is also useful in determining when to use a screening test. Screening tests identify disease early so that an intervention or treatment can be initiated in the hopes of lessening the morbidity or mortality of that disease. Those diseases that are rapidly fatal may not necessarily be beneficial to screen unless the screening will allow for a cure or treatment to change the overall outcome or to prevent unnecessary spread of the disease. Screening is useful in identifying disease in asymptomatic individuals in whom further transmission of disease can be prevented or reduced, such as in HIV. CFRs, therefore, can be helpful for comparisons between study populations and can provide useful information that could help determine whether an intervention or treatment is working. The formula for CFR is as follows:

$$\text{Case fatality rate \%} = \frac{\text{Number of individuals with the specified disease after disease onset or diagnosis}}{\text{Number of cases of that specific disease}} \times 100$$

CFR is usually expressed as a percentage; so in this case, one would multiply this rate by a constant multiplier of 100 to obtain the percentage of disease that is fatal. It is important in all of these rates to include those who have died from the disease in the denominator. Removing those who have died from the denominator falsely increases the CFR, making the disease appear more fatal or severe (Gordis, 2014).

The *proportionate mortality ratio* is useful for determining the leading causes of death. The formula for proportionate mortality ratio is as follows:

$$\frac{\text{Number of deaths from a specified cause during specified time period}}{\text{Total deaths from all causes during the same specified time period}} \times 100$$

Again, this measure is usually reported as a percentage and reflects the burden of death due to a particular disease. This information is useful for policy makers who make decisions about the allocation of resources. (See Exhibit 3.1 for a list of these formulae.)

Survival and Prognosis

Mortality rates are very helpful when comparing groups and looking at disparities among populations. One cannot discuss mortality without having an understanding of survival and prognosis. Many diseases, particularly cancer, are studied over time, with attention placed on survival. Ideally, survival should be measured from the onset of disease until death, but the true onset of disease is generally unknown. Survival rates are usually calculated at various intervals from diagnosis or initiation of treatment. Prognosis is calculated using collected data to estimate the risk of dying or surviving after diagnosis or treatment begins. As mentioned earlier, CFRs give a good estimate of prognosis or severity of disease. However, they are best suited for acute diseases in which death occurs relatively soon after diagnosis. Survival analysis is better suited for chronic diseases or those diseases that take time to progress.

Survival time is generally calculated from the time of diagnosis or from the start of treatment. This can vary from patient to patient, as some patients may seek care immediately after symptoms present or may wait months to seek care. Some patients are diagnosed prior to symptom presentation after they screened positive on a screening test. Some may obtain a diagnosis immediately, whereas others may have poor access to care, and diagnosis is delayed by weeks to months or even years. Once a diagnosis is made, treatment may or may not occur immediately. Additionally, some patients may die before diagnosis or treatment. Because these individuals are not represented in survival analysis, this can lead to a falsely increased survival time. With that said, one can see how difficult it is to establish a true survival time after diagnosis. However, we can estimate survival if we use a common denominator and consistent criteria for measurement.

Before we discuss how to calculate and interpret survival data, we must touch on two important concepts, *lead time bias* and *overdiagnosis bias*. Lead time bias is a phenomenon whereby a patient is diagnosed earlier by screening and appears to have increased survival due to screening but rather dies at the same time he or she would regardless of screening. In other words, the time from which a patient is diagnosed earlier from screening is the lead time, and the bias is the error that occurs as a result of concluding that screening leads to a longer survival after diagnosis. As can be seen in the following timeline (Figure 3.1), the survival time is longer when screening is implemented, but the ultimate time of death is unchanged. Although this is not true for all screening tests, it is important to recognize the phenomenon of lead time bias as it can affect the conclusions that are made regarding survival, which ultimately can affect a patient's perceived prognosis.

Overdiagnosis bias occurs as a result of making a diagnosis from screening for a disease or cancer that would not have manifested clinically or has a slow progression, such that the person dies from another etiology. This type of bias has the potential to increase undue stress in individuals and can also falsely increase survival times, especially for diseases with slow progression. In both these types of biases, there is no difference in overall mortality in those screened versus those who were not screened. With that said, considerations must also be made for those screening tests in which a false-negative test reassures a patient who may not seek care and ultimately develops cancer and potentially has decreased survival due to delay in diagnosis. All of these biases need to be taken into consideration when interpreting survival data.

Prognosis is calculated using survival rates. There are two methods of conducting survival analysis and estimating prognosis that are discussed. The first is the *actuarial*

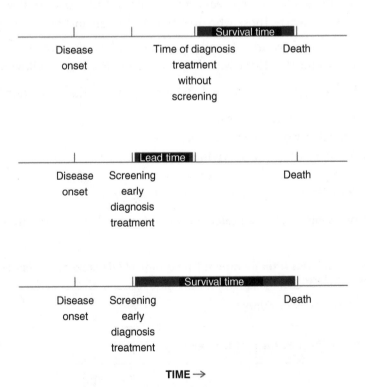

TIME →

FIGURE 3.1 Timeline illustrating lead time bias.

method, which measures the likelihood of surviving after each year of treatment (or a predetermined interval). This is calculated as follows: the probability of surviving 2 years if one survived 1 year, or the probability of surviving 3 years if one survived 2 years, and so on. Prognosis is most commonly described in the literature as the probability of surviving 1, 2, 3, or more years. Generally, survival is calculated as a probability P1, P2, P3, and so on. The survival after 1 year is designated as P1; if patients survived 1 year after treatment, those who survived to 2 years = P2; if patients survived 2 years after treatment, those who survived to 3 years = P3; and so on. To calculate P1, divide the number of survivors over the number of patients with the disease at the start of the study or treatment. It is important to note that those who are lost to follow-up (also known as withdrawals) or who are no longer studied must be removed from the denominator. When a study ends or is terminated, those patients are no longer followed and must be taken into consideration in your analysis, and this is called *censorship*. For simplicity, the following examples will assume no losses to follow-up, but it is important to recognize that those who are lost to follow-up or those who are censored must be taken into account in your calculations. Of note, in a more advanced epidemiology textbook, you will find that those who are lost to follow-up will be subtracted out of the denominator and multiplied by 1/2 to account for the chance they were at risk for half the interval. Again, for the purposes of this text, we will use a hypothetical example in which no patients are lost to follow-up. By definition, here is how to calculate P1, P2, and so on:

- P1 = (Number alive after 1 year of treatment)/(Number who started treatment)
- P2 = (Number alive after 2 years of treatment)/(Number who survived first year of treatment – Those who dropped out or were lost to follow-up)
- P3 = (Number alive after 3 years of treatment)/(Number who survived second year of treatment – Those who dropped out or were lost to follow-up)

To calculate the probability of surviving 1, 2, 3, or more years, the calculation is as follows:

P1 = probability of surviving 1 year
P1 × P2 = probability of surviving 2 years
P1 × P2 × P3 = probability of surviving 3 years
P1 × P2 × P3 × P4 = probability of surviving 4 years
P1 × P2 × P3 × P4 × P5 = probability of surviving 5 years

Using data from Table 3.1, we can calculate and interpret these probabilities.

TABLE 3.1 **Survival Rates After Treatment (Hypothetical Life Table of 100 Patients With No Patients Lost to Follow-Up)**

	NUMBER SURVIVED				
	AFTER 1 YEAR	AT 2 YEARS	AT 3 YEARS	AT 4 YEARS	AT 5 YEARS
Cohort (N = 100)	88	76	55	47	33

In this example:

P1 = 88/100 = 0.88

P2 = 76/88 = 0.86

P3 = 55/76 = 0.72

P4 = 47/55 = 0.85

P5 = 33/47 = 0.70

Probability of surviving 1 year = 0.88

Probability of surviving 2 years = 0.88 × 0.86 = 0.76

Probability of surviving 3 years = 0.88 × 0.86 × 0.72 = 0.54

Probability of surviving 4 years = 0.88 × 0.86 × 0.72 × 0.85 = 0.46

Probability of surviving 5 years = 0.88 × 0.86 × 0.72 × 0.85 × 0.70 = 0.32

It is important to distinguish between the probability of surviving 5 years and the probability of surviving 5 years given that someone survived 4 years. Generally, the longer someone survives after treatment, the more likely that person will make it to the next year. Overall survival after 5 years is always a smaller number as the probability of surviving each year is multiplied against each year (Gordis, 2014).

Note that the actuarial method can be used to look at outcomes other than survival or death as it can estimate probabilities of an outcome or event occurring such as a treatment side effect (e.g., vomiting, headache) or recurrence of disease. Another important consideration is survival over time. When looking at survival rates measured over years, it is important that an APRN take into account the improvements and advances in treatments over time. APRNs should consider comparing survival rates for earlier treatment regimens with those for newer regimens, as this can affect the validity of the overall survival if not taken into consideration. In addition, certain confounders (e.g., age, gender, ethnicity, socioeconomic status) may contribute to differences in survival rates and should be examined when performing a survival analysis (see Chapter 4, "Epidemiological Methods and Measurements in Population-Based Nursing Practice," for more on confounding). Recognition of these differences is a critical step for the evaluation of potential health disparities and is a perfect opportunity for an APRN to develop strategies to address the underlying issue causing those disparities.

In the literature, survival analysis using the actuarial method is plotted on a curve in which the x-axis represents time and the y-axis represents the number of survivors at each time interval. This is called a *survival curve* and represents the pattern of survival over predetermined time intervals. Using the data from the earlier example, the probabilities are plotted in a standardized survival curve (Figure 3.2).

The second type of survival analysis is the *Kaplan–Meier method*. This method is commonly used in medicine and is well suited for analyses of small and large populations, as well as comparisons between treatments or interventions. Although beyond the scope of this book, statistical analyses can be performed to compare treatments or interventions

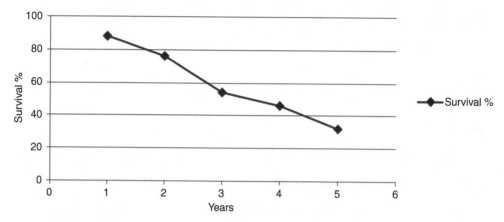

FIGURE 3.2 Hypothetical example of a survival curve using data from the earlier example.

using tests of significance (log-rank test) and logistic regression (proportional hazard models [Cox models]). As with any comparison trial, it is important to take into consideration the characteristics of those patients who are lost to follow-up because if they occur more frequently in one treatment group compared to another, this can affect the results. For example, if the majority of patients lost to follow-up are receiving treatment A and most of them can be characterized as impoverished with poor access to care, then this could skew the results of the remaining patients receiving treatment A. Thus, minimizing loss to follow-up or censored patients and/or maintaining similar losses with similar characteristics in each group is paramount to reducing bias and improving the strength of the study conclusions. This reiterates the importance of randomization, which will be discussed more thoroughly in Chapter 4, Epidemiological Methods and Measurements in Population-Based Nursing Practice.

Kaplan–Meier curves are used to plot survival, and these plots represent a stepwise pattern of survival in which the increments of time are not standardized (e.g., 1 year, 5 years), but rather each step represents an event (e.g., time to death or an outcome of interest). Kaplan–Meier curves are seen more commonly in the literature and are a better estimate of survival as they also take into consideration patients who are lost to follow-up or are censored. These curves also allow for comparisons between different treatment regimens (Figure 3.3).

Kaplan–Meier curves are different from traditional survival curves in that they do not slope downward after each event but rather maintain a horizontal line until the next event (e.g., death) occurs, and then a downward vertical line is drawn until the new cumulative survival is reached and the steps are continued until the study is completed. At the time in which no deaths are occurring (also known as the death-free period), the cumulative survival is maintained; however, hatch marks can be seen in these plots, which represent those lost to follow-up or censored during that interval (Jekel, Katz, Elmore, & Wild, 2007).

The importance of having the knowledge and skills to interpret and calculate survival data cannot be understated. APRNs can use survival data or outcome data in various ways. Most importantly, the evidence obtained from survival or outcome data can help

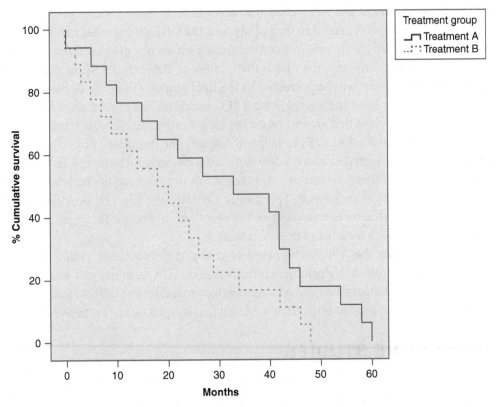

FIGURE 3.3 Hypothetical example of a Kaplan–Meier curve—comparison of treatment A to treatment B.

APRNs to design and justify interventions to improve the quality of life for diseases such as cancer. Comparisons to other groups can be made by addressing outcomes of interest to determine whether certain interventions make a difference in the quality of life and ultimately impact the survival of those involved.

Health Impact Assessment

As mentioned previously, rates can be used to describe the distribution of disease and other health-related states and events, but sometimes the APRN may be more concerned with knowing how data can be used to describe the relevancy of clinical practice. *Health impact assessment* (HIA) is the assessment of the potential health effects, positive or negative, of a particular intervention on a population. HIAs can evaluate population-directed programs or interventions before they are implemented and can provide recommendations on how those programs can potentially affect the health of a population irrespective of whether positive or negative. Certain calculations can be performed to determine the efficacy of a treatment or intervention. The number needed to treat (NNT), the disease impact number (DIN), and the population impact number (PIN) are formulae that are used in HIAs. NNT is the number of patients needed to receive a treatment to prevent one bad outcome, and the lower the NNT, the better for assessing superiority of treatments. However, the NNT takes into account only those patients being treated rather than all those with disease in the population. The DIN, on the other hand, uses the number of those with the disease in question among whom one event will be prevented by the intervention. Similarly, the PIN is the number of those in the whole population among whom one event will be prevented by the intervention (Heller & Dobson, 2000). Another calculation commonly used is the YPLL, which measures premature mortality, and the productive years that are lost related to early death (Merrill, 2017). Information on years of potential life lost (YPLL) helps to magnify the importance of primary prevention measures designed to address diseases such as obesity and other risk factors such as smoking. Each of these measurements is helpful in determining the benefits or risks of new interventions or treatments. Specifically, the DIN and the PIN provide a better population-based estimate of treatment or intervention impacts on the population as a whole. (See Exhibit 3.1 for a list of these formulae.)

It is important for the APRN who is involved in population-based evaluation to be aware of these concepts. More extensive information on HIA formulae and standardization can be found in most advanced epidemiology texts and on the CDC's *Health Impact Assessment Resources* page at https://www.cdc.gov/healthyplaces/hiaresources.htm.

DESCRIPTIVE STUDIES

Descriptive epidemiology is used to describe the distribution of disease and other health-related states and events in terms of personal characteristics, geographical distribution, and time. There are four types of descriptive studies: case reports, case series, cross-sectional studies, and correlation or ecologic studies. The data used in descriptive studies are often readily available and can be retrieved from such sources as hospital records, census data, or vital statistics records.

Case Reports and Case Series

Case reports are succinct written accounts of generally rare or unusual cases in which the treatment or management of the disease or condition is worth reporting. These are usually published to assist healthcare providers in the management of rare, unresearched, or undocumented cases. A case series is merely a report of a series of patients with similar diseases or conditions that describes their management or treatment in order to identify new strategies that may be helpful to treat patients with similar conditions. They also lead to future studies and can be helpful for APRNs as they can use these cases to build a case for future research of treatments or interventions that have not yet been rigorously studied.

Correlation Studies

Correlation studies are also referred to as ecologic studies and are used to conduct studies of aggregate or population characteristics. In ecologic studies, rates are calculated for characteristics that describe populations and are used to compare frequencies between different groups at the same time or the same group at different times. They are useful for identifying long-term trends, seasonal patterns, and event-related clusters. Because data are collected on populations instead of individuals, an event cannot be linked to an exposure in individuals, and the investigator cannot control for the effect of other variables. These types of studies lead to more rigorous studies that can control for variables of interest and look at individual data to determine whether an association truly exists. Correlational studies can only report that a correlation exists and cannot show an association exists as they compare population or aggregate data. An example of a correlation study would be one that shows a correlation between high fat content and breast cancer. Countries with a high fat content correlate to countries with higher rates of breast cancer. Without knowing individual data, one cannot determine whether women with breast cancer actually also have a high fat consumption (Gordis, 2014).

A study by Pillai, Maleku, and Wei (2013) provides an example of a correlational study. The authors used data from 143 countries to study the relationship between female literacy and maternal mortality. Their analysis reveals a significant negative relationship between female literacy rates and maternal mortality. Populations with a higher prevalence of literacy have lower maternal mortality rates and populations with a lower prevalence of literacy have higher maternal mortality rates. The authors point out limitations to their study, most importantly the difficulty of controlling for known correlates with maternal mortality (such as access to healthcare services) due to a scarcity of cross-national data. These data show that a correlation exists between the variables, but not necessarily a causal one. There are many possible explanations for the relationship, including (but not exclusively) demographic and economic differences among the countries. Correlation studies must be interpreted with caution, but important information can be obtained from the trends that could identify disparities and lead to further studies and hypothesis testing.

Cross-Sectional Studies

In *cross-sectional* studies, also known as prevalence studies, both exposures and outcomes are collected simultaneously. These studies provide a "snapshot" at one point in time and thus exclude people who have died or who chose not to participate, which can introduce bias. Temporal relationships are difficult to determine in these studies as only prevalence can be determined and the risk of developing disease cannot be estimated. Many cross-sectional studies are surveys that sample a population and its various characteristics. They can be inexpensive and can provide timely descriptive data about a group under study, but again, they do not tell us about causality or the true risk of developing a certain outcome such as disease.

Spoelstra, Given, von Eye, and Given (2010) conducted a cross-sectional study to determine whether individuals with a history of cancer fall at a higher rate than those without cancer. They also examined whether or not the occurrence of falls in the elderly was influenced by individual characteristics. The study population consisted of 7,448 community-dwelling elderly who were 65 years or older living in one state in the Midwestern United States. The analysis of the data revealed that having cancer was not a predictor of falls in this study. Further analysis revealed that predictors of falls in this population included race, sex, activities of daily living, incontinence, depression, and pain. Although cancer was not found to be a predictor of falls, the authors did find a high frequency of falls in that study population. The findings led the authors to conclude that it is important to develop a predictive model for fall risk in the community-dwelling elderly.

This study serves to illustrate both the advantages and disadvantages of cross-sectional studies. The study was carried out at one point in time using an existing data set (the minimum data set). One limitation of the study was that it missed people whose falls were not reported. Another limitation the authors cited was that they could not determine whether a specific cancer diagnosis, stage, or treatment was a risk factor for falls. Finally, they were unable to determine whether or not comorbidities may have placed individuals at a higher risk for falls. The inability to control for or identify the significance of potentially important variables is a disadvantage of using a cross-sectional study design. With that said, a cross-sectional study is a fairly quick method to obtain descriptive data and can be useful in identifying prevalence rates for specified populations.

ANALYTIC EPIDEMIOLOGY

Analytic epidemiology looks at the origins and causal factors of diseases and other health-related events. Analytic designs are often carried out to test hypotheses formulated from a descriptive study. The goal of analytic epidemiology is to identify factors that increase or decrease risk. Risk is the probability that an event will occur. For example, a patient who is obese might ask, "What is the likelihood that I will develop diabetes if I do not lose weight?"

Although descriptive studies allow a basis for comparison and can provide the APRN with data to identify potential risk factors and differences among groups, study designs, such as a prospective cohort, need to be carried out in order to determine whether there is an association between an exposure and a disease and to determine the strength of that association. To do this, the APRN can compare exposed and nonexposed groups and follow them over time to see who develops an outcome (such as a specific disease) and who does not. Comparison is an essential component of population studies. Case–control studies can also allow for comparisons by retrospectively looking back in time to see what exposure or risk factors are associated with being a case or a control. Comparisons can also be made by following a group using treatment A compared to treatment B or treatment A can be compared to no treatment at all. There are multiple study designs, but we will focus only on the most common study designs and discuss the advantages and disadvantages that each one poses in practice.

Cohort Studies

Cohort designs can be either prospective or retrospective. In a prospective cohort design, the investigator begins with a defined population and then follows a group of individuals who were either exposed or nonexposed to a factor of interest and then follows both groups to compare the incidence of an outcome or disease. In a cohort study, one can look at multiple outcomes that develop from an exposure. In a retrospective cohort design, exposure is ascertained from past records and outcome is ascertained at the time

TABLE 3.2   **Calculation of RR and Attributable Risk in a Cohort Study**

	DISEASE	NO DISEASE	TOTALS	
Exposure	a	b	a + b	Incidence in the exposed (Inc exp) = a/a + b
No Exposure	c	d	c + d	Incidence in the nonexposed (Inc nonexp) = c/c + d
Relative risk (RR) = Inc exp/Inc nonexp				
Attributable risk (AR) = Inc exp − Inc nonexp				
AR proportion in the exposed population = $\dfrac{\text{Inc exp} - \text{Inc nonexp}}{\text{Inc exp}}$				
AR proportion in the total population = $\dfrac{\text{Incidence in total population} - \text{Inc nonexp}}{\text{Incidence in total population}}$				

the study begins. If an association exists between the exposure and the outcome, then the incidence rate in the exposed group will be greater than that in the nonexposed group. The ratio of these is the *relative risk* (RR), which is the incidence rate in the exposed group divided by the incidence rate in the nonexposed group. RR is a measure of the strength of an association between an exposure and an outcome or disease (Table 3.2).

If the RR = 1 (the numerator equals the denominator), then the risk to the two groups is equal. If the RR >1 (the numerator is greater than the denominator), then the risk in the exposed group is greater than the risk in the nonexposed group and can be considered a positive association. If the RR <1 (the denominator is greater than the numerator), then the risk in the exposed group is less than the risk in the nonexposed group and can be considered protective. An example of a protective association may be the association between exercise and heart disease. Exercise can actually reduce the risk of heart disease and has an RR <1. Thus, it is considered a protective exposure.

Attributable risk (AR), absolute risk, or risk difference is the amount of risk that can be attributed to an exposure. For example, it is well known that smoking can cause lung cancer, but lung cancer can also occur in nonsmokers. The amount of disease that is associated with risks/exposures other than smoking is called the *background risk*. In order to calculate the risk attributable to a particular exposure, subtract the incidence of disease (lung cancer) in the exposed group (smokers) minus the incidence of disease (lung cancer) in the nonexposed group (background risk). This value is considered the AR due to exposure (see Table 3.2). If an APRN wants to know how much risk of disease can be reduced by removing a risk factor, one can calculate the ARR, which is synonymous with the AR. The relative risk reduction (RRR) is calculated the same as the AR proportion. This can be confusing as these terms are interchanged in medicine and epidemiology, but it is important to recognize and understand how these terms are used and interpreted. An example of RRR would be described as: What percentage of motor vehicle deaths could be reduced if we could eliminate texting while driving? This RRR percentage is what is commonly reported in the news and can be very helpful for policy makers and for justification of funding. The AR can also be calculated as a proportion of the total population. For example, to determine the amount of lung cancer attributable to smoking in the total population (AR proportion), one would have to know the incidence in the total population (to review how to calculate the incidence in the total population, refer to an advanced epidemiology textbook). APRNs should be familiar with how to calculate and interpret RR and AR, as these values are reported commonly in the literature and reports such as the *MMWR*.

Cohort studies are best carried out when the investigator has good evidence that links an exposure to an outcome, when the time interval between exposure and the outcome is short, and when the outcome occurs relatively often. One of the major problems with cohort studies is that they can be time-consuming and expensive, especially if the cohort needs to be followed for a prolonged length of time. Diseases that are rare or that take many years to develop may be better suited for a case–control study as it can be difficult to follow participants for many years, especially if the outcome of interest is rare. The longer the time period, the more likely participants will be lost to follow-up, and multiple exposures can potentially confound the relationship.

A cohort study was carried out in Norway to ascertain characteristics that would predict the risk of fibromyalgia (FM). The authors examined the association among leisure time, physical exercise, body mass index (BMI), and risk of FM (Mork, Vasseljen, & Nilsen, 2010). A longitudinal study followed 15,900 women without FM or physical impairment at baseline for 11 years. At the end of the study period, there were 380 reported cases of FM, and RRs were calculated for each of the study variables (exposures). Women who reported the highest exercise level had an RR of 0.77 (95% confidence interval [CI], 0.55–1.07). In looking at exercise, the authors controlled for the potential confounding factor of BMI. Overweight or obese women (BMI > 25.0 kg/m^2) had a 60% to 70% higher risk of FM compared with women of normal weight (BMI = 18.5 to 24.9 kg/m^2). In their study, overweight or obese women who exercised more than 1 hour/week had an RR of 1.72 (95% CI, 1.07–2.76), compared with normal-weight women with a similar activity level. The risk for overweight or obese women who were inactive (RR, 2.09; 95% CI, 1.36–3.21) or exercised less than 1 hour/week (RR, 2.19; 95% CI, 1.39–3.46) showed a positive association between risk of developing FM and low levels of exercise. The authors concluded that being overweight or obese was associated with an increased risk of FM, especially among women who also reported low levels of physical exercise. On the basis of these findings, they recommended that community-based measures aimed at reducing the incidence of FM should emphasize maintaining a normal weight and regular exercise.

Case–Control Studies

In a *case–control* study, the APRN must first identify a group of individuals with the outcome of interest (cases). A second group is identified without the outcome of interest (controls). The proportion of those cases that have a history of exposures is then compared to the proportion of the cases that were not exposed, and the proportion of the controls that were exposed is compared to the proportion of the controls that

TABLE 3.3 **Calculation of OR in a Case–Control Study**

	CASES	CONTROLS
Exposure history	a	b
No exposure history	c	d
Totals	a + c	b + d
	Proportion of cases exposed = a/a + c	Proportion of controls exposed = b/b + d
OR = ad/bc		

were not exposed. The measure of the effect of exposure is expressed as an odds ratio (OR), which is the ratio of the odds of having been exposed if you are a case to the odds of having been exposed if you are not a case. If the exposure is not related to the disease or outcome, the OR = 1. If the exposure is related to the disease or outcome, the OR >1, and if the OR <1, the exposure is considered protective. To calculate the OR, construct a 2 × 2 table in which the columns represent the cases and controls and the rows represent the exposed and nonexposed populations. It is important to set up the table correctly. If it is not set up correctly, it will affect the interpretation and conclusions. Once the table is complete, multiply the cross products to obtain the result (see Table 3.3).

In a case–control study, if there is an association between an exposure and disease, the history of exposure should be higher in persons who have the disease (cases) compared to those who do not have disease (controls). It is important to keep in mind that the OR is not a calculation of risk and cannot predict which exposures/risk factors will develop into a case or disease. The fact that a person is obese may put that person at risk for diabetes, but it does not mean that that person will get diabetes. In case–control studies, one cannot calculate RR; therefore, we cannot conclude that if you are obese you will develop diabetes, but rather, if your OR is greater than 1, you could conclude that those with diabetes (outcome) are more likely to be obese (risk factor/exposure).

Selection of cases and controls is an important step in case–control studies. Definite criteria should be used so that there is no ambiguity about how to distinguish between a case and a control. Exposure is not always all or nothing. Controls should resemble the cases as closely as possible except for the exposure to the factor under study. If the cases are drawn from a particular clinic, then ideally the controls should be drawn from the same clinic population. Matching is one method that can be used to select a sample so that potential confounders are distributed equally between the cases and controls. For example, if an APRN plans to evaluate an intervention to reduce burden among caregivers of dependent elderly in the home, it would be important to recognize the characteristics of the population studied prior to implementing the intervention. It is known that men and women have differing characteristics that affect their role as caregiver (Amankwaa, 2017). By matching for gender in the study, the APRN can eliminate this potentially confounding factor (gender). The problem with matching is that the investigator is not always aware of all of the potential confounding factors. It can be difficult to match each subject in a study, and in some cases, investigators can overmatch. When an investigator overmatches, one loses the ability to look at the matched variables as risk factors.

In case–control studies, the investigator begins with cases and controls and goes back retrospectively to look for exposures. In cohort studies, the investigator begins with exposed and nonexposed individuals and follows individuals over time to see who develops or does not develop an outcome or disease. Case–control studies allow the APRN to look at cases and the probability of having an exposure or risk factor. Cohort studies allow an APRN to follow a cohort over time to determine whether being exposed to a risk factor impacts the likelihood of developing a disease or diseases, or improves outcomes (as in an intervention). If associations are found, further studies are necessary to determine causal links and to prevent ecologic fallacy. When examining the results of case–control and cohort studies, it is important for the APRN to consider whether or not all other explanations for an identified association have been eliminated. No single epidemiological study can satisfy all criteria for causality. The APRN needs to look at the accumulation of evidence, as well as the strength of individual studies.

Randomized Controlled Trials

Randomized controlled trials (RCTs) or clinical trials are useful for evaluating treatments (including technology) and for assessing new ways of organizing and delivering health services. In population-based studies, the issue is often health promotion and disease prevention rather than treatment of an existing disease. Interventions can also be studied in RCTs, with the target involving defined populations rather than individuals and often involving educational, program, or policy interventions. When carefully designed, RCTs can provide the strongest evidence for evaluating treatments and interventions.

The basic design of an RCT is to assign subjects randomly to either receive the new treatment/intervention or not receive the new treatment/intervention. Inclusion and exclusion criteria for the participants must be precise and written in advance to eliminate any errors within the study or any future comparison studies. As with cohort studies, RCTs can compare more than two groups. Analysis is carried out to compare outcomes between the randomized groups. As mentioned earlier, comparisons can be made between different interventions, different treatments, or to a control group that has received no intervention or treatment.

There are many examples of how RCTs have been used to evaluate the effectiveness of interventions in specific groups of people. For example, they have been used to evaluate the effectiveness of the Orem self-care model on pain relief in people with rheumatoid arthritis (Saeedifar, Memarian, Fatahi, & Ghelichkhani, 2018), and the use of a community-based skill building intervention to improve heart failure management in community dwelling adults (Dickson, Melkus, Dorsen, Katz, & Riegel, 2015), as well as to test the impact of a nurse-delivered intervention to reduce intimate partner violence (Gupta et al., 2017). These studies illustrate how useful the randomized trial design is for testing a new intervention. RCTs are an excellent vehicle to provide evidence to enhance practice.

Sample Size

Sample selection and sample size determination are critical steps in the research process. Sample size determination is necessary to identify the minimum number of subjects needed to enroll in a study to identify true differences and associations between groups and thus has implications for the investigators as they need to allocate ample resources based on sample size to carry out the study. Power analysis is used to determine sample size. There are several factors that influence the size of the sample: variance, significance, power, and effect size.

Variance

Variance is the variation about the mean. For example, if you are looking at a continuous variable such as blood pressure, the variance away from the mean is defined as s^2. Variance (s^2) is the square of the standard deviation (s). The standard deviation takes into account all blood pressure measurements and essentially sums the difference of each blood pressure measurement away from the mean (see a statistic textbook for more details). If you do not have data with which to calculate the standard deviation, you can review the literature or look at a pilot data set to determine this number. A study that has very little variance (i.e., most of the values fall close to the mean) would require a smaller sample size than a study in which the blood pressure measurements have a very large range and a wider sigmoid curve.

Significance and Power

Significance is the probability that an observed difference or relationship exists and usually is defined as a p-value ($p < 0.05$). The smaller the p-value (e.g., $p < 0.01$), the larger the required sample size. *Power* ($1 - \beta$) is the capacity of the study to detect differences or relationships that actually exist in the population or the capacity to correctly reject a null hypothesis, that is, prevent a type II error. The larger the power required, the less likelihood of committing a type II error. Most studies use a power of 80% or 0.80, or, if a more rigorous power is necessary (e.g., 90%), a larger sample size is required.

Effect Size

Effect size is the actual difference between groups and treatments that you hope to see in your study. One way to identify effect size is to review previous studies; another method is to conduct a pilot study. For example, if you are designing an educational intervention and want to see a 20% improvement of knowledge after the intervention, 20% is your effect size. If you want to see a smaller change in knowledge (e.g., 10%), then a larger sample will be required to detect a smaller effect or difference. In summary, effect sizes occur along a range of values. For example, if you want to see a 5% change in results of an outcome, you will need many more participants than if you want to see a 30% change.

Understanding what goes into power analysis is an important step in designing a study. Power analysis can be calculated using computer programs. There are many free software programs available on the Internet to assist with power analysis. Typing "sample size calculation" in a search engine such as Yahoo or Google will lead an APRN to many sites.

Screening

Screening is a tool used to detect disease in groups of asymptomatic individuals with the goal of reducing and/or preventing morbidity and mortality. Screening tests can be applied to groups of individuals or to high-risk populations. There are multiple examples of screening tests, including the Pap smear, the tuberculosis skin test (PPD test), the mammogram, and so on.

Determining whether a screening test is appropriate requires the APRN to address several aspects of the disease of interest. Screening is neither available nor appropriate for all diseases. In order for a screening program to be effective, certain criteria should be met. The target population needs to be identifiable and accessible and the disease should affect a sufficient number of people to make screening cost-effective. The preclinical period should be sufficient to allow treatment before symptoms appear so that early diagnosis and treatment make a difference in terms of outcome.

Finally, it is necessary for the screening test to be sensitive enough to detect most cases of the disease and to be specific enough to limit the number of false-positive tests. Screening tests should also be relatively inexpensive, easy to administer, and have minimal side effects.

The validity of a screening test refers to its ability to accurately identify those who have the disease. Sensitivity and specificity are measures of a screening test's validity. Sensitivity is a measure of a screening test's ability to accurately identify disease when it is present. Specificity is a measure of a screening test's ability to correctly identify a person without disease with a negative test. The positive predictive value (PPV) is a measure of the probability of a positive test result when the disease is present. The negative predictive value (NPV) of a test is a measure of the probability that the disease is absent when there is a negative test (see Table 3.4).

Directing screening tests toward high-risk populations has many advantages. By screening populations with a higher disease prevalence, we can actually increase the PPV of that test. Screening low-prevalence populations can lead to more false positives, which can be costly and harmful to patients. Thus, selection of the disease to be tested and the patient population to be screened are both important to consider when designing a new test.

The APRN can evaluate the success of screening programs by looking at a variety of outcomes. For example, some of the outcomes that can be followed include

TABLE 3.4   Computing Sensitivity, Specificity, and Predictive Values in Screening Tests

	DISEASE	NO DISEASE	TOTALS	
+ Test	a	b	a + b	PPV = a/a + b
– Test	c	d	c + d	NPV = d/c + d
Totals	a + c	b + d		
	Sensitivity = a/a + c	Specificity = d/b + d		

the reduction in overall mortality in screened individuals, a reduction in the CFR in screened individuals, an increase in the percentage of cases detected at earlier stages, a reduction in complications, and improvement of quality of life in screened individuals.

In 2018, the U.S. Preventive Services Task Force (USPSTF) released their final recommendations for cervical cancer screening (USPSTF, 2018). The complete recommendations can be found on the USPSTF web site (www.uspreventiveservicestaskforce.org/Page/Name/us-preventive-services-task-force-issues-new-cervical-cancer-screening-recommendations). One of the recommendations for cervical cancer screening is that women aged 21 to 65 should get a Pap smear every 3 years. A second recommendation is that women aged 30 to 65 who wish to be screened less frequently can choose a combination Pap smear and human papillomavirus (HPV) testing every 5 years. The Task Force does not recommend cervical cancer screening using HPV testing in women younger than age 30. This is because evidence indicates that the expected harms (such as false positives) in this age group outweigh the potential benefits.

According to the Task Force, "since the implementation of widespread cervical cancer screening, there has been a dramatic reduction in cervical cancer deaths in the United States" (USPSTF, P4). For this reason, the Task Force urges healthcare providers to encourage women to be screened for cervical cancer, especially those who have never been screened, or who have not been screened within the past 5 years. These guidelines provide an example of how evidence on the specificity and sensitivity of a screening test can be used to create more evidence-based clinical guidelines. Therefore, screening tests need to be tailored to the disease under investigation, and many factors need to be taken into consideration; for example, How many false negatives can be missed? How many false positives are acceptable? Can screening and early detection really make a difference in the outcome of the disease? Understanding these factors and balancing them with targeted screening in high-risk populations are important considerations in screening implementation. The USPSTF provides screening guidelines on a variety of disease states with recommendations (e.g., colorectal, prostate, and breast cancers). APRNs can visit their website located at https://www.uspreventiveservicestaskforce.org for the latest recommendations.

SUMMARY

The natural history of disease refers to the progression of a disease from its preclinical state to its clinical state, and knowledge of these stages provides a framework for understanding approaches to the prevention and control of disease. Primary prevention refers to the process of altering susceptibility or reducing exposure to susceptible individuals and includes general health promotion and specific measures designed to prevent disease prior to a person getting a disease. Primary prevention measures are generally carried out during the stage of susceptibility. With secondary prevention, it is sometimes possible to either cure a disease at a very early stage or slow its progression to prevent complications and limit disability. Secondary prevention measures are carried out during the preclinical or presymptomatic stage of disease. Tertiary prevention takes place during the middle or later stages of a disease (the clinical stage of disease) and refers to measures taken to alleviate disability and restore effective functioning.

The dynamic nature of disease calls for a sophisticated model for explaining causation. When designing interventions for populations, the APRN needs to keep in mind that disease develops as the result of many antecedent factors and not as a result of a single, isolated cause.

Descriptive epidemiology is used to describe the distribution of disease and other health-related states and events in terms of personal characteristics, geographical distribution, and time. It also helps APRNs design studies and measure mortality and prognosis. Analytic epidemiology looks at the origins and causal factors of diseases and other health-related events. Epidemiologic methods can be used to identify populations at risk and to evaluate interventions provided to patient populations. Population-based evaluation and planning depend on understanding the many and varied factors that influence health and disease. APRNs can use their understanding of epidemiological methods in concert with their clinical expertise to develop policies and implement and evaluate new programs and interventions to improve population outcomes.

EXERCISES AND DISCUSSION QUESTIONS

Exercise 3.1 In 2018, there were 105 new cases of type 2 diabetes reported in Smithville, a city of 500,000. This brought the total number of active cases of type 2 diabetes in Smithville to 3,075. During this time, there were 105 deaths attributable to the disease.

    a.   What was the incidence rate per 100,000 for type 2 diabetes in 2018?

    b.   What was the prevalence rate of type 2 diabetes per 100,000 in 2018?

    c.   What was the cause-specific death rate of type 2 diabetes in 2018?

Exercise 3.2 A city contains 100,000 people (45,000 males and 55,000 females), and 1,000 people die per year (600 males and 400 females). There were 50 cases (40 males and 10 females) of lung cancer per year, of whom 45 died (36 males and 9 females).

    Using this information compute:

    a.   The crude mortality rate per 1,000

    b.   The sex-specific mortality rate per 1,000

    c.   The cause-specific mortality rate per 1,000 for lung cancer

    d.   The case fatality rate for lung cancer

    e.   The proportionate mortality ratio for lung cancer

Exercise 3.3 A new rapid blood test was created to test for HPV in a rural clinic. The following is a 2 × 2 chart which describes the results of the test. Answer questions a to g using the 2 × 2 chart.

	HPV	NO HPV	TOTALS
Positive (+) test	95	37	132
Negative (−) test	39	278	317
Totals	134	315	449

a. What is the sensitivity of this test?

b. What is the specificity of this test?

c. What is the positive predictive value?

d. What is the negative predictive value?

e. Describe in words the sensitivity of this test.

f. Describe in words the negative predictive value.

g. What is the disease prevalence in this population?

Exercise 3.4 An epidemiologic study is conducted to learn about the relationship between celiac disease and colon cancer. Suppose there are 77 cases of colon cancer in 68,000 person-years in persons with celiac disease and 54 cases of colon cancer in 215,000 person-years in those without celiac disease. (The overall rate in both groups combined = 131 cases in 283,000 person-years overall.) Use this information to answer questions a to c.

a. Calculate the rate of colon cancer in the celiac group (R_1), in the no celiac group (R_0), and overall (R). Express all rates "per 100,000 person-years."

R1 =
R0 =
R =

b. Calculate and *interpret* the relative risk of colon cancer associated with celiac disease.

c. Calculate and *interpret* the attributable risk of colon cancer associated with celiac disease.

Exercise 3.5

a. What is the fundamental difference between a case–control study and a cohort study?

b. What are the advantages and the disadvantages of a cross-sectional study?

c. What are the characteristics of a correlational study?

d. You read about a new protocol (HTN T) that was used successfully to improve blood pressure control in an urban clinic population. A major feature of HTN T is the use of technology (such as text messaging) to communicate with patients. You work in a rural clinic and currently use protocol HTN 1. You wonder if HTN T would improve blood pressure control in your clinic population. Explain how you could use a randomized clinical trial to evaluate whether HTN T improves blood pressure control in your clinic population.

Exercise 3.6 You are reviewing the survival statistics from your hospital using a new treatment (treatment A) compared to the old treatment (treatment B) for breast cancer. The following table lists the number of survivors after each year of treatment for both treatments A and B. Answer the following questions using the table. Assume no patients were lost to follow-up.

TREATMENT A	NUMBER SURVIVED				
	AT 1 YEAR	AT 2 YEARS	AT 3 YEARS	AT 4 YEARS	AT 5 YEARS
Cohort (N = 1,229)	1,102	987	835	725	633

TREATMENT B	NUMBER SURVIVED				
	AT 1 YEAR	AT 2 YEARS	AT 3 YEARS	AT 4 YEARS	AT 5 YEARS
Cohort (N = 1,179)	1,084	886	755	602	544

- Calculate the survival rates for treatments A and B for each year after treatment: P1, P2, P3, P4, and P5.

- Calculate the probability of surviving for 1, 2, 3, 4, and 5 years cumulatively for each of the treatments.

- Your administrator would like to know how the treatments compared to each other. You are asked for the following information:

  – What is the likelihood of surviving 5 years if you made it to 4 years of treatment for each of the treatments?

  – How does treatment A compare to treatment B for each year of survival after treatment?

  – Which treatment has the best 5-year survival rate?

- Plot the survival curve for both treatments on the same graph.

- Why might there be differences between these two treatments?

- What are some potential confounders that may contribute to one treatment working better than the other?

■ Explain the advantages and disadvantages of screening tests.

■ What are the limitations to performing survival analysis?

■ How might patients lost to follow-up affect the validity of survival analysis?

■ What are the differences between the actuarial method of survival analysis and the Kaplan–Meier method?

Exercise 3.7

■ Perform a search to determine the incidence, prevalence, and survival rates for one of the following cancers in your state (lung cancer, breast cancer, colon cancer, prostate cancer, cervical cancer)

   – Perform a search and describe the screening recommendations for the cancer you selected.

   – Describe the advantages and disadvantages of cancer screening for the cancer you selected.

   – How does the incidence, prevalence, and survival rates in your state compared to the national rates.

   – What are potential confounders for the cancer you selected?

   – What disparities in cancer incidence, mortality, and survival were you able to determine from your search?

3.8 What factor has the single biggest impact on mortality?

REFERENCES

American Association of Colleges of Nursing. (2006). *The essentials of doctoral education for advanced practice nursing.* Washington, DC: Author. Retrieved from https://www.aacnnursing.org/DNP/DNP-Essentials

Amankwaa, B. (2017). Informal caregiver stress. *ABNF Journal, 28*(4), 92–95.

Centers for Disease Control and Prevention. (2011). Decrease in smoking prevalence—Minnesota, 1999–2010. *Morbidity and Mortality Weekly Report, 60*(5), 138–141. Retrieved from http://www.ncbi.nlm.nih.gov/pubmed/21307824

Centers for Disease Control and Prevention. (2018a). *Fast facts: Smoking and tobacco use.* Retrieved from http://www.cdc.gov/tobacco/data_statistics/fact_sheets/fast_facts/index.htm#use

Centers for Disease Control and Prevention. (2018b). *Morbidity and Mortality Weekly Report.* Retrieved from http://www.cdc.gov/mmwr/about.html

Centers for Disease Control and Prevention. (2018c). Overweight and obesity. Retrieved from https://www.cdc.gov/obesity/data/adult.html

Dickson, V. V., Melkus, G. D., Dorsen, C., Katz, S., & Riegel, B. (2015). Improving heart failure self-care through a community-based skill-building intervention: A study protocol. *Journal of Cardiovascular Nursing, 30*(4), S14–S24. doi:10.1097/jcn.0000000000000161

Fulton, J. S., Lyon, B. L., & Goudreau, K. A., (2014). *Foundations of clinical nurse specialist practice* (2nd ed.). New York, NY: Springer Publishing Company.

Gordis, L. (2014). *Epidemiology* (5th ed.). Canada: Elsevier Saunders.

Gupta, J., Falb, K. L., Ponta, O., Xuan, Z., Campos, P. A., Gomez, A. A., . . . Olavarrieta, C. D. (2017). A nurse-delivered, clinic-based intervention to address intimate partner violence among low-income women in Mexico City: Findings from a cluster randomized controlled trial. *BMC Medicine, 15*(1), 128. doi:10.1186/s12916-017-0880-y

Harkness, G. (1995). *Epidemiology in nursing practice.* New York, NY: Mosby.

Heller, R. F., & Dobson, A. J. (2000). Disease impact number and population impact number: Population perspectives to measures of risk and benefit. *British Medical Journal, 321*(7266), 950–953. doi:10.1136/bmj.321.7266.950

Heller, R. F., & Page, J. (2002). A population perspective to evidence-based medicine: "Evidence for population health." *Journal of Epidemiology and Community Health, 56,* 45–47. doi:10.1136/jech.56.1.45

Jekel, J. F., Katz, D. L., Elmore, J. G., & Wild, D. M. J. (2007). *Epidemiology, biostatistics, and preventive medicine* (3rd ed.). Philadelphia, PA: Saunders Elsevier.

Merrill, R. M. (2017). *Introduction to epidemiology* (7th ed.). Burlington, MA: Jones & Bartlett Learning.

Minnesota Department of Health. (2018). The positive health impacts of raising tobacco taxes in Minnesota. Retrieved from http://www.health.state.mn.us/divs/hpcd/tpc/topics/taxes.html

Mork, P. J., Vasseljen, O., & Nilsen, T. I. L. (2010). Association between physical exercise, body mass index, and risk of fibromyalgia: Longitudinal data from the Norwegian Nord-Trøndelag Health Study. *Arthritis Care & Research, 62,* 611–617. doi:10.1002/acr.20118

National Heart, Lung, and Blood Institute and Boston University. (2018). *The Framingham study.* Retrieved from https://www.framinghamheartstudy.org/fhs-about/history

Park, S., Xu, F., Town, M., & Blanck, H. (2016). Prevalence of sugar-sweetened beverage intake among adults—23 states and the District of Columbia, 2013. Retrieved from https://www.cdc.gov/mmwr/volumes/65/wr/mm6507a1.htm?s_cid=mm6507a1_w

Pillai, V. K., Maleku, A., & Wei, F. H. (2013). Maternal mortality and female literacy rates in developing countries during 1970–2000: A latent growth curve analysis. *International Journal of Population Research, 2013,* 1–11. doi:10.1155/2013/163292

Saeedifar, E. S., Memarian, R., Fatahi, S., & Ghelichkhani, F. (2018). Use of the Orem self-care model on pain relief in women with rheumatoid arthritis: A randomized trial. *Electron Physician, 10*(6), 6884–6891. doi:10.19082/6884

Spoelstra, S., Given, B., von Eye, A., & Given, C. (2010). Falls in the community-dwelling elderly with a history of cancer. *Cancer Nursing, 33*(2), 149–155. doi:10.1097/NCC.0b013e3181bbbe8a

U.S. Preventive Services Task Force. (2018). U.S. Preventive Services Task Force issues new cervical cancer screening recommendations. Retrieved from https://www.uspreventiveservicestaskforce.org/Page/Name/us-preventive-services-task-force-issues-new-cervical-cancer-screening-recommendations

INTERNET RESOURCES

CDC, Health Impact Assessment: www.cdc.gov/healthyplaces/hia.htm

Morbidity and Mortality Weekly Report: www.cdc.gov/mmwr

U.S. Preventive Services Task Force: https://www.uspreventiveservicestaskforce.org

U.S. Preventive Services Task Force (USPSTF), U.S. Preventive Services Task Force Issues New Cervical Cancer Screening Recommendations: https://www.uspreventiveservicestaskforce.org/Page/Name/us-preventive-services-task-force-issues-new-cervical-cancer-screening-recommendations

CHAPTER 4

EPIDEMIOLOGICAL METHODS AND MEASUREMENTS IN POPULATION-BASED NURSING PRACTICE: PART II

PATTY A. VITALE | ANN L. CUPP CURLEY

INTRODUCTION

In order to provide leadership in evidence-based practice, advanced practice registered nurses (APRNs) require skills in the analytic methods that are used to identify population trends and evaluate outcomes and systems of care (American Association of Colleges of Nursing [AACN], 2006). APRNs need to be able to carry out studies with strong designs and solid methodology, taking into account the factors that can affect study results. This chapter discusses the complexities of data collection and the strengths and weaknesses of study designs used in population research. Critical components of data analysis are discussed, including bias, causality, confounding, and interaction.

ERRORS IN MEASUREMENT

A dilemma that may occur with population research is the difficulty of controlling for variables that are not being studied but that may have an impact on the results. Finding a statistical association between an intervention and an outcome or an exposure and a particular disease is meaningful only if variables are correctly controlled, tested, and measured. The purpose of a well-designed study is to properly identify the impact of the variable (or variables) under study and to avoid bias and/or design flaws caused by another, unmeasured variable.

Statistics are used to analyze population characteristics by inference from sampling (Statistics, 2002, p. 1695). They help us translate and understand data. Before we can begin to understand a measured difference between groups, we have to identify the variation. But statistical analysis cannot overcome problems caused by a flawed study. When a researcher draws the wrong conclusion because of a problem with the research methodology, the result is a type I or type II error, also referred to as *errors of inference*. A *type I error* occurs when a null hypothesis is rejected when in fact it is true. A *type II error* occurs when one fails to reject a null hypothesis when in fact it is false. Take, for example, an APRN who carries out a study to determine whether a particular intervention improves medication compliance in hypertensive patients. To keep the example simple, the intervention will simply be referred to as "Intervention A." A null hypothesis proposes no difference or relationship between interventions or treatments. In this case, the null hypothesis is: There is no difference in medication compliance between hypertensive patients who receive Intervention A and those who receive no intervention. Let us assume that the APRN completes the study and carries out the statistical analysis of the data. The following conclusions are possible:

1. There is no significant difference in medication compliance between the two groups.

2. There is a significant difference in medication compliance between the two groups.

Now let us assume that the correct conclusion is number 1, but the APRN concludes that there is a difference in medication compliance between the two groups (rejects the null hypothesis when it is true). The APRN has committed a type I error. If the correct conclusion is number 2, but the APRN concludes that there is no difference in medication compliance between the two groups (fails to reject the null hypothesis when it is false), then a type II error has occurred (Table 4.1).

When using data or working with data sets, it is critical to understand that mistakes can occur where measurements are involved. There are two basic forms of error of measurement: *random error* (also known as nondifferential error) and *systematic error* (also known as bias). Random errors occur as the result of the usual, everyday variations that are expected and that can be anticipated during certain situations. The result is a fluctuation in the measurement of a variable around a true value. Systematic errors occur not as the result of chance but because of inherent inaccuracies in measurement. They are typically constant or proportional to the true value. Systematic error is generally considered the more critical of the two. It can be the result of either a weak study design or a deliberate distortion of the truth.

TABLE 4.1 Type I and Type II Errors

	RELATIONSHIP DOES NOT EXIST	RELATIONSHIP EXISTS
Conclude Relationship Does Not Exist (Fail to Reject Null Hypothesis)	Correct Decision	Type II Error (β)
Conclude Relationship Exists (Reject Null Hypothesis)	Type I Error (α)	Correct Decision Power (1 − β)

Random Error

Random error measurements tend to be either too high or too low in about equal amounts because of random factors. Although all errors in measurement are serious, random errors are considered to be less serious than bias because they are less likely to distort findings. Random errors do, however, reduce the statistical power of a study and can occur because of unpredictable changes in an instrument used for collecting data or because of changes in the environment. For example, if one of three rooms being used to interview subjects became overheated occasionally during data collection, making the subjects uncomfortable, it could affect some of their responses. This effect in their responses is an example of a random error of measurement.

Systematic Error

There are several types of systematic error or bias and all of them can impact the validity of study results. Bias can occur in many ways and is commonly broken down into two categories: selection and information bias. Such things as how the study design is selected, how subjects are selected, how information is collected, how the study is carried out (the conduct), or how the study is interpreted by investigators are all forms of potential bias. These problems can result in a deviation from the truth, which can lead to false conclusions.

Selection Bias

Selection bias occurs when the selected subjects in a sample are not representative of the population of interest or representative of the comparison group, and as a result, this selection of subjects can make it appear (falsely) that there is or is not an association between an exposure and an outcome. Selection bias is not simply an error in the selection of subjects for a study, but rather the systematic error that occurs with "selecting a study group or groups within the study" (Gordis, 2014, p. 263). Nonprobability sampling (nonrandom sampling) is strongly associated with selection bias. In nonprobability sampling, members of a target population do not share equal chances of being selected for the study or intervention/treatment group. This can occur with studies using convenience samples or volunteers. People who volunteer to participate in a study may have characteristics that are different from people who do not volunteer, and this can impact the outcome of the results and is simply referred to as *volunteer bias*. Similarly, people who do not respond to surveys may possess characteristics different from those who do respond to surveys. Thus, it is important to characterize nonresponders as much as possible, as the characteristics of responders may be very different from those of nonresponders and can lead to errors in survey interpretation. The best way to avoid this type of bias is to keep it at a minimum unless the characteristics of nonresponders can be identified and addressed. Another form of selection bias is *exclusion bias*, and this can occur when one applies different eligibility criteria to the cases and controls (Gordis, 2014). *Withdrawal bias* can occur when people of certain characteristics drop out of a group at a different rate than they do in another group or are lost to follow-up at a different rate. This can also lead to systematic error in the interpretation of data. APRNs must be aware of these types of error early in their study design. All of these types of systematic error can have an impact on how data are interpreted; therefore, minimizing these types of error through careful assessment of subject selection and eligibility criteria, and monitoring of characteristics in the populations of interest are critical for successful research and program implementation. Finally, probability sampling methods (random sampling) can be used to ensure that all members of a target population have an equal chance of being selected into a study, thereby eliminating the chance of selection bias (Merrill, 2017; Shorten & Moorley, 2014).

Information Bias

Information bias deals with how information or data are collected for a study. This includes the source of data that are collected, such as hospital records, outpatient charts, or national databases. Many of these types of data are not collected for research purposes, so they may be incomplete, inaccurate, or contain information that is misleading. This can complicate data analysis as the information abstracted from these sources may be incorrect and can lead to invalid conclusions. *Measurement bias* is a form of information bias and occurs during data collection. It can be caused by an error in collecting information for an exposure or an outcome. Calibration errors can occur when using instruments to measure outcomes. This type of bias can also occur when an instrument is not sensitive enough to measure small differences between groups or when interventions are not applied equally (e.g., blood pressure measurements taken using the wrong cuff size). Information bias also includes how the data are recorded and classified. This can lead to *misclassification bias*, in which a control may be recorded as a case or a case is classified as having an exposure or exposures that he or she did not actually have. Misclassification bias can be subdivided into differential and nondifferential. For example, *differential misclassification* occurs when a case is misclassified into exposure groups more often than controls. In this case, this type of bias usually leads to the appearance of a greater association between exposure and the cases than one would find if this bias was not present (Gordis, 2014). In *nondifferential misclassification,* the misclassification occurs as a result of the data-collection methods such that a case is entered as a control or vice versa. In this situation, the association between exposure and outcome may be "diluted," and one may conclude there is not an association when one really exists (Gordis, 2014). Another example of misclassification bias occurs when members of a control group are exposed to an intervention. This results in *contamination bias.* An example would be a nurse who floats from the floor where hourly rounding is being carried out to a control floor where no rounding is supposed to occur, but the nurse carries out hourly rounding on the control floor. In this case, contamination bias minimizes the true differences that would have been seen between groups. However, these cases should not be reassigned; in fact, any unexpected or unplanned crossover that occurs should be analyzed in the original group to which it was assigned by the investigator. This is known as the *intent-to-treat principle.* For example, patients who are assigned to one group or another and crossover intentionally or accidentally to the other group should be analyzed according to their original assignment. *Intent to treat* simply means that you assign patients to the original group you intended to treat them in from the start of the study regardless of the treatment they received.

If information is obtained from interviews, there can be bias introduced based on how the questions are asked or there may be variance between interviewers in how the questions are prompted to the subject. *Recall bias* happens when subjects are asked to remember or recall events from the past. For example, people who experience a traumatic event in their lives may recall events of that day more accurately and with more detail than someone asked to recall events from a day without significance. *Reporting bias* occurs when a subject may not report a certain exposure as he or she may be embarrassed or not want to disclose certain personal information, or the subject may report certain things to gain approval from the investigator (Gordis, 2014). The effects of bias can impact a study in two ways. It can make it appear that there is a significant effect when one does not exist (type I error), or there is an effect but the results suggest there is no effect (type II error; see Table 4.1).

Finally, an APRN needs to be aware of both *publication bias* and *citation bias* (additional types of *information bias*), particularly when carrying out systematic reviews or meta-analyses. Publication bias refers to the tendency of peer-reviewed journals to publish a higher percentage of studies with significant results than those studies with non-significant or negative statistical results. Citation bias refers to the practice of selective citation of articles based on their results.

Publication bias has been identified and studied for decades (Joober, Schmitz, Annable, & Boksa, 2012; Mlinarić, Horvat, & Šupak Smolčić, 2017; Song et al., 2009). Song et al. (2009) completed a meta-analysis to determine the odds of publication by study results. Although they identified many problems that were inherent in studying publication bias (e.g., they pointed out that studies of publication bias may be as vulnerable as other studies to selective publication), they concluded that "[t]here is consistent empirical evidence that the publication of a study that exhibits significant or 'important' results is more likely to occur than the publication of a study that does not show such results" (p. 11).

Duyx, Urlings, Swaen, Bouter, and Zeegers (2017) conducted a meta-analysis of citation bias. They found that articles that report statistically significant results are cited more often than articles that report nonsignificant results. They also found that this occurs more often in the biomedical sciences than the natural sciences. As has been found in studies on publication bias, these authors warn that citation bias can lead to an over representation of positive results and unfounded beliefs.

There are several issues related to these two types of information bias. They can give readers a false impression about the impact of an intervention, they can lead to costly and futile research, they can distort the literature on a topic, and can be unethical. People who participate in research studies (subjects) are often told that their participation will lead to a greater understanding of a problem. There is a breach of faith when the results of these studies are not published and shared in the scientific community (Joober et al., 2012; Siddiqi, 2011). The publication and citation of both categories of research is ethical and provides a more balanced and objective view of current evidence.

In summary, bias must be recognized and addressed early in the study design. Ultimately, bias should be avoided when possible, but if it is recognized, it should be acknowledged in the interpretation of results and addressed in the study discussion.

CONFOUNDING

Confounding occurs when it appears that a true association exists between an exposure and an outcome, but in reality, this association is confounded by another variable or exposure. An interesting study by Matsumoto, Ishikawa, and Kajii (2010) raised questions about the potential confounding effect of weather on differences found among communities in Japan. They investigated the rural–urban gap in stroke incidence and mortality by conducting a cohort study that included 4,849 men and 7,529 women in 12 communities. On average, subjects were followed for 10.7 years. Information on geographic characteristics (such as population density and altitude), demographic characteristics (including risk factors for stroke), and weather information (such as rainfall and temperature) were obtained and analyzed using logistic regression. The researchers discovered a significant association between living in a rural community and stroke, independent of risk factors. However, further analyses revealed that the actual link may be between the weather and stroke. They proposed that the difference seen in the incidence of stroke in these communities may be related not to living in a rural versus an urban community, but by the weather differences between communities. Low temperatures are known to cause an increase in coagulation factors and plasma lipids, and therefore, differences in weather could have an impact on the incidence of stroke. They cite the small number of communities as a limitation of the study, and for this reason they did not generalize their findings. But they did raise an important point: It is important to be aware of the many variables (e.g., biological, environmental) that may confound a relationship in population studies (Matsumoto et al., 2010).

Identification of confounding or other causes of spurious associations are important in population studies. A confounder is a variable that is linked to both a causative factor or an exposure and the outcome. There are many examples of confounders, such as age, gender, and socioeconomic status. Confounding occurs when a study is performed, and it appears from the study results that an association exists between an exposure and an outcome, when, in fact, the association is actually between the confounder and the outcome. Another example of confounding might occur if an APRN carried out a study to determine whether there is a relationship between age and medication compliance without controlling for income. Younger, working patients might be more compliant not because of the age factor, but because they have the resources to buy their medications. If confounding is ignored, there can be long-term implications as the APRN may implement interventions for medication compliance with education programs aimed at older patients without considering problems related to income. The intervention would ultimately not succeed because the relationship is false or not causal due to confounding. By definition, confounders must be known risk factors for the outcome and must not be affected by the exposure or the outcome (Gordis, 2014). Confounding, although difficult to avoid, must be recognized and accounted for in studies.

There are some techniques that an APRN can use to reduce the effects of confounding variables. Random assignment to treatment and nontreatment groups can reduce confounding by ensuring each group has similar shared characteristics that otherwise might lead to spurious associations. In the earlier example, if you were concerned about the socioeconomic status and education level, you may stratify early on for those characteristics and randomly assign from each of those groups so that they are equally represented in your intervention and nonintervention groups. When random assignment is not possible, the matching of cases and controls for possible confounding variables can improve equal representation of subjects and can minimize the effect of confounding. Investigators can match groups or individuals. Group matching allows groups with similar characteristics of interest to be matched to each other. Each group should share a similar proportion of the characteristics of interest. Usually, cases should be selected first, and the control group should be selected with similar proportions of the characteristics of interest (Gordis, 2014).

In individual matching, each individual case is matched to a control with similar characteristics of interest. This is referred to as matched pairs. One has to be careful not to match cases and controls for too many characteristics, as it can be difficult to find a control or the control may be too similar to the case and true differences may not be able to be demonstrated in the analysis phase. Using strict inclusion and exclusion criteria also can be helpful and should be applied similarly for comparison groups. There are limitations to the latter two methods.

Although it is possible to match for known confounding variables, there may be other unknown confounding variables that cannot be controlled for and, if not recognized, can impact study conclusions. If the study groups are matched for gender, then gender cannot be evaluated in the final analysis. Additionally, if the study is matched for too many variables, this can also limit the study as all of the matched variables cannot be studied, and this may limit the ability to make valid conclusions. There is a similar problem with inclusion and exclusion criteria as both criteria should be applied the same to each of the study groups. The method for analyzing data can also help reduce problems related to confounding.

Multivariable regression, for example, can measure the effects of multiple confounding variables. This method is useful only when the variables are recognized and acknowledged. Recognition of confounders requires a basic understanding of the relationship between an exposure and a disease or an outcome, and can also be identified by performing a stratified analysis first. Once confounders are determined, then these variables can be added in and removed from the model one at a time. Interaction needs to be assessed, and the exposure–disease relationship is determined. These inferential methods estimate the contribution of each variable to the outcome while holding all other variables constant in the model. The objective is to include a set of variables that are theoretically or actually correlated with both the intervention and the outcome to reduce the bias of treatment effect. Therefore, the goal of regression analysis is to identify causal relationships by recognizing the confounders to ensure found relationships are real and not spurious (Kellar & Kelvin, 2013; Starks, Diehr, & Curtis, 2009).

INTERACTION

Whenever two or more factors or exposures are being studied simultaneously, the possibility of *interaction* exists. Interaction occurs when one factor impacts another such that one sees a greater or lesser effect than would be expected by one factor alone. *Synergism* occurs when the combined effect of two or more factors is greater than the sum of the individual effects of each factor. And, conversely, the opposite or negative impact can be seen with *antagonism* of factors. One example of synergism is seen with the interaction of exercise and diet. The combination of these two factors can actually reduce the risk of heart disease more than each factor alone. Synergistic models can have an additive effect in which the effect of one factor or exposure is added to another or can have a multiplicative effect in which the effect of one factor multiples the effect of another factor. For example, epidemiologists identified an interactive effect between cigarettes and alcohol; these two factors together have a multiplicative effect on the risk of developing digestive cancers (Sjödahl et al., 2007). There are many synergistic effects that can be found in clinical practice, especially as they pertain to drugs. First-generation antihistamines, such as chlorpheniramine, have a synergistic effect on opioids such as codeine. Patients are warned not to take them in combination as the sedative effects are more significant when taken together. APRNs who carry out investigations need to be aware of the potential interactions when examining the effects of multiple exposures on an outcome. A discussion on how to determine whether a model is multiplicative or additive can be found in more detail in an advanced epidemiology textbook, but a basic understanding is necessary for interpreting the different outcomes that can occur from multiple exposures.

There are clearly many sources of error that can occur while conducting a study. The informed APRN needs to identify and acknowledge these types of errors and work to minimize them. Therefore, it is essential that APRNs recognize when errors occur and how they can impact a study, and should be familiar with measures that can be taken to avoid or minimize errors.

RANDOMIZATION

Randomized controlled trials (RCTs) are considered inherently strong because of their rigorous design. Random selection of a sample and random assignment to groups are objective methods that can be used to prevent bias and produce comparable groups. Random assignment helps to minimize bias by ensuring that every subject has an equal chance of being selected and that results are more likely to be attributed to the intervention being tested and not to some other extraneous factor such as how subjects were assigned to the treatment or control group. It is impossible to know all of the characteristics that could influence results. The random assignment of subjects to different treatment groups helps to ensure that study groups are similar in the characteristics that might affect results (e.g., age, gender, ethnicity, and general health).

Blinding

Another problem encountered in research occurs when investigators or subjects themselves have an effect on study results. This can happen when a researcher's personal beliefs or expectations of subjects can influence his or her interpretation of the outcome. Sometimes observers can err in measuring data toward what is expected. If subjects know or believe that they are given a placebo or the nonexperimental treatment, it may cause them to exaggerate symptoms that they would dismiss if given the experimental treatment. These actions by both investigators and subjects are not necessarily intentional; they can occur subconsciously.

The best way to eliminate or minimize this type of bias is to use a *single-blind* or a *double-blind* study design. In a double-blind study, both the subjects and the investigators are blinded, that is, unaware of which group is receiving the experimental treatment or intervention. Sometimes it is impossible to blind the investigator because of the nature of the treatment, in which case a single-blind design, in which the subjects are unaware of which group they are in, can be used. If blinding cannot be used, measures need to be taken that ensure that study groups are followed with strict objectivity.

DATA COLLECTION

As mentioned earlier, how data are collected and analyzed can lead to bias when conducting a study. The training of investigators to ensure that data are collected uniformly from all subjects and the use of a strict methodology for data collection and analysis contribute to a strong study design. Objective criteria should be used for the collection of all data. Strict inclusion and exclusion criteria should be developed in writing so that there are no questions as to what criteria are to be applied to the study. Avoiding subjective criteria is important as it can lead to inconsistent application of criteria. For example, if you chose "ill appearance" as an exclusion criterion, it may be difficult to apply this criterion uniformly as each APRN may have different levels of experience making this assessment. Objective criteria, such as heart rate greater than 120 beats per minute, respiratory rate greater than 24 breaths per minute, or oxygen saturations less than 90%, are easy to apply uniformly. Of course, even those criteria can be incorrectly assessed by someone who is inexperienced; however, one can see that these types of data are more easily reproducible within and between studies. One way to assess reliability between raters in a study is by using the *kappa statistic*. This statistic tests how reliable different investigators or data collectors are in their assessment or interpretation of data beyond what one would expect by chance alone.

$$kappa = \frac{(\text{Percent agreement observed}) - \begin{array}{c}(\text{Percent agreement expected} \\ \text{by chance alone})\end{array}}{100\% - (\text{Percent agreement expected by chance alone})}$$

If you were to evaluate two observers without any training, you would expect them to agree a certain percentage of the time and that percentage represents the chance of agreement, usually around 50%. Using the kappa statistic, you can estimate how reliable this agreement is by subtracting out the percentage expected by chance alone. In general, any kappa below 0.60 indicates inadequate agreement among the raters and little confidence should be placed in the study results. These values, although not perfect, can give an investigator an assessment of how well her or his observers are agreeing with each other in their data interpretation (McHugh, 2012). The kappa statistic appears frequently in the literature, and the APRN should be familiar with its use and limitations.

One of the first steps in data analysis is to compare the demographic information of each of the groups studied to ensure that they are matched for important characteristics and that they represent the population of interest. Frequencies of data can be generated and compared for similarities and differences. This should be done early on so that any imbalance between groups is addressed before it becomes a problem in the analysis stage. This reiterates the importance of generating strict inclusion and exclusion criteria that can be followed with minimal error.

CAUSALITY

Ernst Mach, an Austrian professor of physics and mathematics and a philosopher, argued that all knowledge is based on sensation and that all scientific measurements are dependent on the observer's perception. He proposed that "in nature there is no cause and effect" (Huttemann, 2013, p. 102). This is a relevant quote to begin a discussion of causality, because causality is a complex issue faced by all investigators. A single clinical disease can have many different "causes," and one cause can have several clinical consequences. Causality becomes even more complex when we begin to look at chronic diseases. Chronic diseases can have multiple etiologies. Cardiac disease, for example, has multiple causes such as genetic predisposition, obesity, smoking, lack of exercise, poor diet, or any combination of these factors.

A useful definition of causation for population research is that an increase in the causal factor or exposure causes an increase in the outcome of interest (e.g., disease). With that said, if an association is found between an exposure and an outcome, then the next question is: Is it causal? There are many theories of causation, some of which have been addressed in Chapter 3, Epidemiological Methods and Measurements in Population-Based Nursing Practice: Part I, but no one theory can explain entirely the complex interactions of an exposure with the development of disease or an outcome.

There are multiple criteria that can help determine causality. No one criterion in and of itself determines causality, but each one may help strengthen the argument for or against causality. One important criterion is the determination of a statistical *strength of association*. Statistics are used to test hypotheses: Is an exposure or risk factor present significantly more often in a population with the disease than without? If a new intervention is put into place, is there a significant improvement in the targeted outcome? The strength of association is measured by such things as relative risk and attributable risk. Another criterion is the confirmation of a *temporal relationship*: The suspected exposure or risk factor needs to occur before the disease or outcome. For example, a person needs to smoke before he or she develops lung cancer in order to attribute lung cancer to smoking as a potential causal agent. To show a causal relationship requires the elimination of all known *alternative explanations* and an experienced investigator will seek out other potential explanations to explain why such a relationship may not exist (Katz, Elmore, Wild, & Lucan, 2013).

Two additional important considerations are scientific plausibility and the ability to replicate findings. *Scientific plausibility* refers to coherence with our current body of knowledge as it relates to the phenomenon under study. That is, do the results make sense based on what we know about the phenomenon? For example, is it biologically plausible that exposure to cigarette smoke (e.g., benzene, nicotine, tar) could convert normal cells into cancer cells? Additionally, the ability to *replicate findings* in different studies and in different populations provides strong evidence that a causal association exists. Other criteria for causation include the *dose–response* relationship. For example, with increasing exposure (e.g., smoking), one can see increasing risk of disease (e.g., lung cancer). Similarly, if one has a *cessation of exposure*, one would expect a cessation or reduction of disease. Finally, another criterion worth mentioning is consistency with other knowledge. This criterion takes into consideration knowledge of other known factors (e.g., environmental changes, product sales, behavioral changes) that may indicate a causal relationship. For example, if a law is passed that prohibits smoking in public places, it may result in fewer cases of smoking-related diseases reported in area hospitals. These criteria, in concert with a strong study design and methodology, can assist an APRN in determining the likelihood of causality when an association is found between an exposure and an outcome (Gordis, 2014).

Causes can be both direct and indirect. An example of a direct cause would be an infectious agent that causes a disease. Pertussis (whooping cough, a bacterial infection) is caused by *Bordetella pertussis*. The disease is a direct cause of the organism. Toxic shock syndrome is an example of an indirect cause. Although the staphylococcal organism and its toxins are the direct cause of the syndrome, the indirect cause (and the first factor that was identified) is tampons.

Even the infectious disease process is not simple. Both the host and the environment can have an impact on the infectious disease process. Characteristics of the host (e.g., age, previous exposures, general health, and immune status) can influence the development of the disease. Environmental conditions also play a role. A good example is influenza, which is most prevalent during certain times of the year. Infectious disease departments document these seasonal trends during the year, and they are available for healthcare providers to review. Such information can assist in antibiotic selection, hospital staffing, and educational campaigns to ensure immunizations or prevention programs are put into place. Awareness of seasonal fluctuations in certain diseases, trends in drug resistance, or changes in the community that affect the overall management of a patient are important in an APRN's practice. By following these trends, the APRN can better assess the needs of the community and ensure that appropriate resources are available to address the fluctuations that occur naturally in all communities.

SCIENTIFIC MISCONDUCT (FRAUD)

Scientific misconduct includes (but is not limited to) gift authorship, data fabrication and falsification, plagiarism, and conflict of interest. It can have an impact on researchers, patients, and populations (Karcz & Papadakos, 2011). No one wants to believe that there are investigators who commit fraud by deliberately distorting research findings, but it does happen. Unfortunately, in some cases, the fraud is intentional; in other cases it occurs via a series of missteps from methodology to analysis. As mentioned earlier, multiple forms of bias or confounding can be introduced into a study, and these, if ignored, can lead to spurious results. Intentionally ignoring these issues, especially without addressing them as a limitation, can be fraudulent. Acceptance for publication in a prominent peer-reviewed journal and/or evidence that the protocol was approved by an institutional review board (IRB) does not ensure the accuracy and/or ethical conduct of that research.

Perhaps one of the most infamous cases of fraud involved a well-respected peer-reviewed journal. In 1998, *The Lancet* published an article written by Andrew Wakefield and 12 others that implied a link between the measles–mumps–rubella (MMR) vaccine and autism and Crohn's disease. Although epidemiologists pointed out several study weaknesses, including a small number of cases, no controls, and reliance on parental recall, it received wide notice in the popular press. It was 7 years before a journalist uncovered the fact that Wakefield altered facts to support his claim and exploited the MMR scare for financial gain. *The Lancet* retracted the paper in 2010 (Godlee, Smith, & Marcovitch, 2011). A series of articles in the *British Medical Journal* (Deer, 2011) revealed how Wakefield and his associates distorted data for financial gain. Before this article was retracted, it caused widespread fear among parents and accelerated an antivaccine movement that many blame for the resurgence of infectious diseases among children.

In 2006, a writer for *The New York Times* (Interlandi, 2006) wrote an article that described a case of fraud that involved a formerly tenured professor at the University of Vermont. Dr. Eric Poehlman was tried in a federal court and found guilty. He was sentenced to 1 year and 1 day in jail for fraudulent actions that spanned 10 years. His misconduct included using fraudulent data in lectures and in published papers, and using these data to obtain millions of dollars in federal grants from the National Institutes of Health (NIH). He pleaded guilty to fabricating data on obesity, menopause, and aging. Interlandi's article, which includes a very detailed account of Dr. Poehlman's actions and his downfall, documents how a "committed cheater can elude detection for years by playing on the trust—and self-interest—of his or her junior colleagues" (p. 3).

It is safe to say that the majority of researchers carry out their research with scrupulous attention to detail and with integrity, but APRNs need to be aware that instances such as those mentioned do happen. As stated in Chapter 3, Epidemiological Methods and Measurements in Population-Based Nursing Practice: Part I, it is important that when an APRN is making decisions related to population-based evaluation, the decisions need to be based on a sound methodological framework that includes ethical considerations of the effect of the research on the population as a whole. It is also important that APRNs are aware that fraud occurs in research and that they should be vigilant not only in how they carry out research but also in how they critically review the results of studies by other investigators.

STUDY DESIGNS

There is no perfect study design; however, there are strategies that can be used to decrease the threat of bias and increase the likelihood that hypotheses are answered accurately.

The awareness that bias and confounding can cause a threat to the validity of study results is important and may be unavoidable; however, recognizing these limitations and addressing them within your study is even more critical. The design of high-quality and transparent studies creates a good foundation for evidence-based practice. Table 4.2 outlines the strengths and weaknesses of study designs used in population research.

Randomized Controlled Trials

When carefully designed, RCTs can provide the strongest evidence for the effectiveness of a treatment or intervention. Subjects are randomly assigned to either the intervention group (which will receive the experimental treatment or intervention) or the control group (which will receive the nonexperimental treatment or no intervention). Inclusion and exclusion criteria for the participants must be precise and spelled out in advance.

RCTs are considered strong designs because of their ability to minimize bias; however, if the randomization is not executed in a truly random manner, then the design can be flawed, or if the data are not reported consistently, then errors can lead to invalid conclusions.

TABLE 4.2 **Strengths and Weaknesses of Study Designs**

TYPE OF STUDY	STRENGTHS	WEAKNESSES
Randomized controlled trials	■ Lower likelihood of confounding variables ■ Minimize bias in treatment assignment ■ Able to control intervention or treatment	■ Labor intensive ■ Costly ■ Lengthy ■ Sometimes impractical or unethical to conduct
Cohort designs	■ Able to identify confounding and address in the study ■ Able to control exposure ■ Able to calculate relative risk and incidence rates ■ Can study multiple outcomes	■ Labor intensive ■ Costly ■ Lengthy
Case-control	■ Inexpensive ■ Shorter time to completion ■ Able to study variables with long latency or impact periods ■ Provides a means to compare groups ■ Able to calculate odds ratios ■ Able to study rare or fatal diseases ■ Can study multiple exposures	■ Risk of bias and confounding variables ■ Sometimes unable to measure or determine exposure ■ Selection bias ■ Measurement error ■ Recall bias ■ Cannot assess risk
Cross-sectional	■ Able to calculate prevalence of population studied ■ Assesses exposures and outcomes at one time ■ Provides a snapshot of study population ■ Inexpensive	■ Risk of confounding variables ■ Selection bias ■ Cannot control for or identify the significance of potentially important variables ■ Cannot assess risk

Consolidated Standards of Reporting Trials (CONSORT) is a method that has been developed to improve the quality and reporting of RCTs. It offers a standard way for authors to prepare reports of trial findings, facilitate their complete and transparent reporting, and aid their critical appraisal and interpretation (CONSORT, 2018). The CONSORT checklist items focus on reporting how the trial was designed, analyzed, and interpreted; the flow diagram displays the progress of all participants through the trial (CONSORT, 2018). The CONSORT guidelines are endorsed by many professional journals and editorial organizations. They are part of an effort to improve the quality and reporting of research that is conducted to make better clinical decisions. Both the CONSORT checklist and the CONSORT flow diagram can be accessed at www.consort-statement.org.

RCTs are believed to provide the most reliable scientific evidence, but they can be expensive, time-consuming, and sometimes difficult to conduct for ethical reasons. There are general guidelines that APRNs can follow when conducting a study to provide a framework for a quality design. They are as follows:

- Formulate an answerable research question (see Chapter 5, Applying Evidence at the Population Level).

- Complete an extensive review of the literature to determine what is currently known about the problem and to provide a sound theoretical background (see Chapter 5, Applying Evidence at the Population Level).

- Select a study design that will best answer the research question.

- Choose a study design that is feasible in terms of both time and money.

- Once a design is chosen, plan every step of the research process before beginning the study (e.g., determination of inclusion and exclusion criteria, selection of primary and secondary outcomes of interest).

- Ensure that comparison groups are as similar as possible; stratify for possible confounders early on to avoid making false conclusions.

- Determine sufficient sample size to ensure the study has adequate power for result interpretation.

- Use objective criteria for the collection of all data.

- Train all investigators to ensure that data are collected uniformly.

- Choose the appropriate methods for data analysis.

- Provide sufficient and clear details of the study in papers and presentations to allow others to understand how the study was carried out and to allow them to assess for possible biases (e.g., provide an audit trail).

Cohort Studies

Cohort designs can be either prospective or retrospective. In a prospective cohort design, the investigator selects a group of individuals who were exposed to a factor of interest and compares it to a group of nonexposed individuals and follows both groups to determine the incidence of an outcome (e.g., disease). This type of design should be carried out when the APRN has good evidence (a sound theoretical base) that links an exposure to an outcome. A well-designed, prospective cohort study has the potential to provide better evidence than a poorly designed RCT. One of the major problems with cohort studies is that they can be time-consuming and expensive if the cohort needs to be followed for a prolonged period of time, and the longer the time period involved, the more likely that participants can and will be lost to follow-up. This potential loss of subjects can result in withdrawal bias, particularly when people with certain characteristics drop out of one group at a different rate than that of another group or are lost to follow-up at different rates. Both of these occurrences can lead to spurious results or results that are difficult to generalize. For example, subjects who participate for the duration of a study may be healthier than those who drop out, leading to potential characteristic differences between groups that may affect the final analysis. These types of differences can falsely dilute observed differences between groups or falsely strengthen results and should be avoided when possible.

When conducting a cohort study, investigators should provide detailed information on the following: subjects' data that are lost or incomplete, subjects' rates of withdrawal or loss to follow-up, characteristics of subjects that are lost to follow-up or who have withdrawn from the study, and, when possible, reasons for the dropouts. They should also include detailed descriptions of the groups that are included in the analysis of outcomes (e.g., age, gender, family history, and severity of disease).

Des Jarlais, Lyles, Crepaz, and the TREND Group (2004) first presented the Transparent Reporting of Evaluations with Nonrandomized Designs (TREND) in the *American Journal of Public Health*. These guidelines provide a framework for the design and reporting of nonrandomized studies in order to facilitate research synthesis. The TREND checklist has 22 steps and was designed for use as an evaluation tool of nonrandomized behavioral or public health intervention studies. The TREND statement and checklist are available through the Centers for Disease Control and Prevention website, www.cdc.gov/trendstatement. These types of studies should include a defined intervention and research design that provides for an assessment of the efficacy or effectiveness of the intervention. The TREND guidelines provide APRNs with a comprehensive checklist for designing studies and writing research reports.

Case-Control Studies

In a *case-control* study, the investigator first identifies a group of individuals with the attribute of interest (cases), and a second group is identified without the attribute of interest (controls). Cases and controls can be matched individually or as a group for variables that might cause confounding (e.g., age, gender, and ethnicity), or they can be unmatched. If unmatched, then each group should have similar characteristics. As mentioned earlier, matching can be on an individual level or group level. In Chapter 3, Epidemiological Methods and Measurements in Population-Based Nursing Practice: Part I, we defined the odds ratio (OR) in case-control studies as the odds of being an exposed case compared to the odds of being an exposed control (ad/bc). This is the calculation for an unmatched study. However, when we calculate the OR for a matched

TABLE 4.3A 2 × 2 Table for Calculating Odds Ratio in an Unmatched Case-Control Study

	CASES	CONTROLS
Exposed	a	b
Nonexposed	c	d
OR = ad/bc (unmatched pairs)		

TABLE 4.3B 2 × 2 Table for Calculating Odds Ratio in a Matched Pairs Case-Control Study

	EXPOSED CONTROLS	NONEXPOSED CONTROLS
Exposed Cases	a	b
Nonexposed Cases	c	d
OR = b/c (matched pairs)		

pairs study (e.g., matching of individual pairs for a variety of characteristics), we need to take into consideration only those situations in which cases have different exposures. We are not interested in comparing cases with controls if both are exposed (as in "a") or both are unexposed (as in "d"). Therefore the OR for a matched case-control study is calculated as b/c. Also, of note in a matched case-control study, the 2 X 2 table is set up differently as individual cases are matched to individual controls (Tables 4.3A and B).

Case-control studies tend to be inexpensive and relatively quick to complete, but they have several weaknesses. Because subjects in the groups are not randomly assigned, associations found in the analysis may be the result of exposure to another, unknown variable. To decrease the likelihood of bias, definite criteria should be used so that there is no ambiguity about how to distinguish between a case and a control. Controls should resemble the cases as closely as possible except for exposure to the factor under study. If the cases are drawn from a medical surgical unit in an acute care hospital, then ideally the controls should be drawn from the same population. Matching, as previously described, is one method that can be used so that potential confounders are distributed equally between the cases and controls. A problem with case-control studies is that data are usually abstracted from medical records that are not designed for collection of research material; so data obtained from medical records may be limited and may not provide adequate or accurate information on exposures. For example, data collected from medical records may be incomplete (e.g., missing diagnoses), may use old diagnostic criteria, or may be coded or entered incorrectly. Additionally, if abstracting data from interviews, biases, such as recall bias or reporting bias, may play a role in how data are recorded and ultimately can affect the interpretation and final conclusions of a study.

DATABASES

Databases have become ubiquitous in the healthcare field, and their use is growing. Many of the larger and better known databases are discussed throughout this text. There is a good reason for their frequent mention. Nurses in all fields and in all positions enter data electronically into databases of some kind. Managers use databases to assess the level of satisfaction of their patient population and nursing staff. Direct care nurses use data to assess the performance of their units on important patient care indicators (such as falls) and record patient information into electronic health records that may be linked with larger databases or registries. Departments dedicated to quality improvement track infection rates, readmission rates, and other identified indicators of quality of care. Health departments track infectious diseases as well as other indicators linked to population health.

Some databases are for a single site (e.g., one acute care hospital or one community), but it is becoming increasingly common for databases to be linked or for databases to include information at the state, regional, and national level (e.g., trauma registries that log all incoming trauma data from all trauma centers in the state). State and federal regulatory agencies, such as the Agency for Healthcare Research and Quality (AHRQ) and the Centers for Medicare & Medicaid Services (CMS), are requiring healthcare providers to report specific patient safety indicators. Some of these data, such as those compiled by CMS, are being posted for public view. Other organizations, such as the American Nurses Credentialing Center (ANCC), are requiring data entry for accreditation by programs, such as Magnet®, and setting performance standards using benchmarks.

Databases are being developed to meet the needs of specific populations. One such database was developed for quality-improvement and service planning for palliative care and hospice facilities in North Carolina. The system was developed and implemented over a 2-year period and grew from one community-based site to four. The patient data are entered at the point of care (e.g., hospital, nursing home, and hospice). The information captured by the database has strengthened the ability of providers to identify areas for improvement in quality of care and the service needs of the palliative care population (Bull et al., 2010).

Nursing care data that are captured using technology can be aggregated, analyzed, and benchmarked. The information can provide APRNs with a clear picture of the population that they serve and help to guide decisions for the provision of services. Patrician, Loan, McCarthy, Brosch, and Davey (2010) described the creation of the nurse-sensitive indicators for the military nursing outcomes database (MilNOD). The information gleaned from this database allows military nurse leaders to track nursing and patient quality indicators and to target areas for managerial and clinical performance improvement. For more information on MilNOD go to https://www.usuhs.edu/node/3370/.

There are many issues that the APRN needs to be aware of when using or developing databases. Databases require a high level of technological expertise to create, maintain, and use. Trained technicians and specialized equipment are required. Unanticipated technology-related problems can occur. In North Carolina, the mountains created a barrier for wireless communication of data and another system had to be installed to be able to communicate among sites. MilNOD designers identified the need to focus on a standardized approach for data collection. To minimize bias in their data set, the designers also created standardized definitions and specific and detailed protocols to ensure data are entered accurately and consistently.

Roberts and Sewell (2011) have outlined important requirements for the development and use of databases. Among the important points that they make is that nurses must understand the basics of entering data into databases and how data must be structured. Computer systems must be able to communicate with each other. This includes systems located within one site as well as systems in other sites if it is a multisite system. They also emphasize the need to be consistent in how data are coded.

Successful databases are created collaboratively. Members of the healthcare team who will be entering and using the data need to work together with technicians who understand systems. And the creation of a workable database is just a beginning. Once the data are entered, they need to be analyzed and checked for accuracy (*data editing*). Posting data that are summarized and benchmarked using graphs and trend lines on shared drives that are accessible to direct care nurses as well as nurse leaders brings the information to people who directly impact care and helps nurses to identify areas for improvement. Nurses at all levels should be involved in data management and analysis.

SUMMARY

APRNs need to carry out studies with strong methodology and designs and understand the factors that can influence study results. One problem with population research is that it is difficult to identify and control for variables that are not part of the study but that may have an effect on the results. When a researcher analyzes data in a study and draws the wrong conclusion, the result is a type I or type II error, also referred to as errors of inference. A type I error occurs when a null hypothesis is rejected when in fact it is true. A type II error occurs when a null hypothesis is not rejected when in fact it is false. There are two kinds of error of measurement—random error and systematic error, and it is essential that APRNs are aware how these errors can occur, how they can impact a study, and what measures can be taken to avoid or minimize them. RCTs are considered the gold standard in population research and offer the best protection for preventing bias, but they are not always feasible. Well-designed cohort and case-control studies are acceptable alternatives when RCTs are not an option.

Databases are increasingly used in healthcare. Aggregated data provide valuable information about population groups that can be used to direct care and establish evidence for clinical guidelines. APRNs should work closely with technology experts in the planning, implementation, and use of databases in order to maximize their ability to analyze data in an accurate and systematic manner. Strong methodology and data collection with a sound research design are the foundation for an excellent study/intervention that ultimately can contribute to evidence-based practice.

EXERCISES AND DISCUSSION QUESTIONS

Exercise 4.1 An APRN carries out a study to determine if a new media campaign (Intervention M) improved vaccination rates in her community.

- What is the null hypothesis?

The APRN carries out the study and concludes that "Vaccination rates did not improve significantly following implementation of Intervention M." In fact, vaccination rates *did* improve significantly following implementation of Intervention M.

- What type of error has the APRN committed?

Exercise 4.2 In a small pilot study, 10 women with liver cancer and 10 women with no apparent disease were contacted and asked whether they had hepatitis B. Each woman with cancer was matched by age, ethnicity, weight, and parity to a woman without cancer. The results are shown below.

PAIR NUMBER	LIVER CANCER	NO LIVER CANCER
1	HEPATITIS B	HEPATITIS B
2	HEPATITIS B	NO HEPATITIS B
3	HEPATITIS B	NO HEPATITIS B
4	NO HEPATITIS B	NO HEPATITIS B
5	NO HEPATITIS B	NO HEPATITIS B
6	HEPATITIS B	HEPATITIS B
7	HEPATITIS B	NO HEPATITIS B
8	NO HEPATITIS B	HEPATITIS B
9	HEPATITIS B	NO HEPATITIS B
10	NO HEPATITIS B	NO HEPATITIS B

- a. Construct the 2 x 2 table for **matched** pairs.
- b. Calculate the estimated odds ratio for a matched-paired analysis.
- c. Interpret this statistic.
- d. What is the purpose of matching cases and controls?

Exercise 4.3 You are working in a health center at a large university and are concerned about an increase in the incidence of antibiotic-resistant gonorrhea in the student population that you serve. Before you launch an educational campaign aimed at both your staff and the university community, you need to establish the severity of the problem.

- Identify a database at the local, state, or national level that can help you obtain the necessary information.

- How can you determine the incidence and prevalence of gonorrhea in your community?

- What are some of the potential errors that can occur in the reporting of gonorrhea to a local, state, or national database?

■ How might this effect your interpretation of the data?

■ What are some of the barriers to reporting in your community?

You determine from your investigation that there is a significant problem in your community.

■ Describe how you would address the increasing rate of gonorrhea in the population that you serve.

■ What type of study design would you use to evaluate the effectiveness of your intervention?

■ What are potential confounders?

Exercise 4.4 You are a manager on a medical unit in a community hospital. You are concerned about a recent increase in falls with injury on your unit. You have not had any recent changes in staffing or patient mix and acuity.

■ How might you assess this situation?

■ Where might you find the data in your hospital to support your concern?

■ What type of study could you perform to identify the cause(s) for the increase in falls with injury?

■ How will you select your population of study?

■ How will you select a control group or comparison group?

■ What are potential errors in measurement that you may encounter?

REFERENCES

American Association of Colleges of Nursing. (2006). *The essentials of doctoral education for advanced practice nursing.* Retrieved from http://www.aacn.nche.edu/publications/position/DNPEssentials.pdf

Bull, J., Zafar, Y., Wheeler, J., Harker, M., Gblokpor, A., Hanson, L., . . . Abernethy, A. (2010). Establishing a regional, multisite database for quality improvement and service planning in community-based palliative care and hospice. *Journal of Palliative Medicine, 13*(8), 1013–1020. doi:10.1089/jpm.2010.0017

CONSORT. (2018). *Transparent reporting of trials.* Retrieved from http://www.consort-statement.org

Deer, B. (2011). How the case against the MMR vaccine was fixed. *British Medical Journal, 342,* 77–82. doi:10.1136/bmj.c5347

Des Jarlais, D., Lyles, C., Crepaz, N., & the TREND Group. (2004). Improving the reporting quality of nonrandomized evaluations of behavioral and public health interventions: The TREND statement. *American Journal of Public Health, 94*(3), 361–366. doi:10.2105/AJPH.94.3.361

Duyx, B., Urlings, M. J. E., Swaen, G. M. H., Bouter, L. M., & Zeegers, M. P. (2017). Scientific citations favor positive results: A systematic review and meta-analysis. *Journal of Clinical Epidemiology, 88,* 92–101. doi:10.1016/j.jclinepi.2017.06.002

Godlee, F., Smith, J., & Marcovitch, H. (2011). Wakefield's article linking MMR vaccine and autism was fraudulent [Editorial]. *British Medical Journal, 342,* 64–66. doi:10.1136/bmj.c7452

Gordis, L. (2014). *Epidemiology* (5th ed.). Canada: Elsevier Saunders.

Huttemann, A. (2013). A disposition-based process-theory of causation. In S. Mumford & M. Tugby (Eds.), *Metaphysics and science* (pp. 101–122). Oxford, UK: Oxford University Press.

Interlandi, J. (2006, October 22). An unwelcome discovery. *The New York Times.* Retrieved from http://www.nytimes.com/2006/10/22/magazine/22sciencefraud.html

Joober, R., Schmitz, N., Annable, L., & Boksa, P. (2012). Publication bias: What are the challenges and can they be overcome? *Journal of Psychiatry & Neuroscience, 37*(3), 149–152. doi:10.1503/jpn.120065

Karcz, M., & Papadakos, P. J. (2011). The consequences of fraud and deceit in medical research. *Canadian Journal of Respiratory Therapy, 47*(1), 18–27.

Katz, D., Elmore, J. G., Wild, D. M. G., & Lucan, S. C. (2013). *Jekel's epidemiology, biostatistics, preventive medicine, and public health* (4th ed.). Canada: Elsevier Saunders.

Kellar, S. P., & Kelvin, E. A. (2013). *Munro's statistical methods for health care research* (6th ed.). Philadelphia, PA: Wolters Kluwer/Lippincott Williams & Wilkins.

Matsumoto, M., Ishikawa, S., & Kajii, E. (2010). Rurality of communities and incidence of stroke: A confounding effect of weather conditions? *Rural and Remote Health, 10,* 1493. Retrieved from http://www.rrh.org.au

McHugh, M. (2012). Interrater reliability: The kappa statistic. *Biochemia Medica, 22*(3), 276–282. doi:10.11613/BM.2012.031

Merrill, R. M. (2017). *Introduction to Epidemiology* (7th ed.) Burlington, MA: Jones and Bartlett Learning.

Mlinarić, A., Horvat, M., & Šupak Smolčić, V. (2017). Dealing with the positive publication bias: Why you should really publish your negative results. *Biochemia Medica, 27*(3), 030201. doi:10.11613/BM.2017.030201

Patrician, P., Loan, L., McCarthy, M., Brosch, L., & Davey, K. (2010). Towards evidence-based management: Creating an informative database of nursing-sensitive indicators. *Journal of Nursing Scholarship, 42*(4), 358–366. doi:10.1111/j.1547-5069.2010.01364.x

Roberts, A., & Sewell, J. (2011). Data aggregation: A case study. *CIN: Computers, Informatics, Nursing, 29*(1), 3–7. doi:10.1097/NCN.0b013e3181fb5c0c

Shorten, A., & Moorley, C. (2014). Selecting the sample. *Evidence-Based Nursing, 17*(2), 32–33. doi:10.1136/eb-2014-101747

Siddiqi, N. (2011). Publication bias in epidemiological studies. *Central European Journal of Public Health, 19*(2), 118–120. Retrieved from http://web.b.ebscohost.com/ehost/detail/detail?vid=14&sid=12f13f7c-adf3-40ee-8c3c-ed3d6d69996a%40sessionmgr115&hid=116&bdata=JnNpdGU9ZWhvc3QtbGl2ZQ%3d%3d#db=rzh&AN=2011210575

Sjödahl, K., Lu, Y., Nilsen, T., Ye, W., Hveem, K., Vatten, L., & Lagergren, J. (2007). Smoking and alcohol drinking in relation to risk of gastric cancer: A population-based, prospective cohort study. *International Journal of Cancer, 120*(1), 128–132. doi:10.1002/ijc.22157

Song, F., Parekh-Bhurke, S., Hooper, L., Loke, Y., Ryder, J., Sutton, A., . . . Harvey, I. (2009). Extent of publication bias in different categories of research cohorts: A meta-analysis of empirical studies. *BMC Medical Research Methodology, 9,* 79. Retrieved from http://web.ebscohost.com/ehost/pdfviewer/pdfviewer?hid=110&sid=01961f3d-cd2e-4770-86af-bc7107e2f85e%40sessionmgr113&vid=4

Starks, H., Diehr, P., & Curtis, J. R. (2009). The challenge of selection bias and confounding in palliative care research. *Journal of Palliative Medicine, 12*(2), 181–187. doi:10.1089/jpm.2009.9672

Statistics. (2002). *The American heritage dictionary of the English language* (4th ed., p. 1695). Boston, MA: Houghton Mifflin.

INTERNET RESOURCES

CDC, Transparent Reporting of Evaluations with Nonrandomized Designs (TREND): https://www.cdc.gov/trendstatement

CONSORT, Transparent Reporting of Trials: http://www.consort-statement.org

Uniformed Services University, Military Nursing Outcomes Database (MilNOD): https://www.usuhs.edu/node/3370

CHAPTER 5

APPLYING EVIDENCE AT THE POPULATION LEVEL

VERA KUNTE | ANN L. CUPP CURLEY

INTRODUCTION

Nurses in advanced practice have an obligation to improve the health of the populations that they serve by providing evidence-based care. The American Association of Colleges of Nursing (AACN) has outlined eight essentials that represent the core competencies for the education of doctorally prepared advanced practice registered nurses (APRNs). The first essential "Scientific Underpinnings for Practice" and the third essential "Clinical Scholarship and Analytical Methods for Evidence-Based Practice" stress the integration of evidence-based practice into advanced nursing practice (AACN, 2006). APRNs are educated at the graduate level in research and critical appraisal, and possess both scientific knowledge and clinical expertise. These specialized abilities prepare the APRN to demonstrate the importance of evidence-based practice to others and to facilitate the incorporation of such evidence into practice (Buck, Chucta, Francis, Vermillion, & Weber, 2017).

In this chapter, the APRN will learn how to gather, appraise, and synthesize information in order to design interventions that are based on evidence to improve population health. Nurses need a sound knowledge of research methodology to support an evidence-based practice. They also require a wide array of knowledge gleaned from the sciences and the ability to translate that knowledge quickly and effectively to benefit patients (Fencl & Mathews, 2017). The goal of this chapter is to summarize the skills required for evidence-based practice and to provide specific examples of how APRNs use these skills to improve population outcomes.

Evidence is defined as facts or observations that support a conclusion or assertion. Melnyk and Fineout-Overholt (2015) define *evidence-based practice* as

> a paradigm and life-long problem solving approach to clinical decision-making that involves the conscientious use of the best available evidence (including a systematic search for and critical appraisal of the most relevant evidence to answer a clinical question) with one's own clinical expertise and patient values and preferences to improve outcomes for individuals, groups, communities and systems. (p. 604)

A related concept is "best practices," which refers to providing high quality care based on evidence to achieve optimal outcomes (Nelson, 2014). Nurses require several skills to become practitioners of evidence-based care and to improve clinical outcomes. They must be able to identify clinical problems, recognize patient safety issues, compose clinical questions that provide a clear direction for study, conduct a search of the literature, appraise and synthesize the available evidence, and successfully integrate new knowledge into practice. The APRN plays an important role in this complex process of incorporating evidence-based practice into policies and standards of care to improve population outcomes. In population-based care, there is additional complexity in determining the values and needs of diverse groups of people. Making decisions related to population-based health requires consideration of the effects of the intervention on the population as a whole. Balancing the overall needs of groups of people with the rights of individuals requires careful and thoughtful consideration. A sound evidence-based practice provides a foundation to better assess and meet those needs based on current evidence.

ASKING THE CLINICAL QUESTION

There are many situations that drive clinical questions. Clinical practice and observation, as well as information obtained by reading the professional literature, can lead nurses to ask questions such as "Why is this happening?," "Would this approach to care work in my clinical practice?," or "What can we do to improve this outcome?" An APRN who reads an article about an innovation in practice that leads to an improvement in a population outcome might wonder whether such an intervention would work in another setting. The observation that the readmission rates for a particular diagnosis are increasing, or that rates for a particular disease are higher in one population than in another, or that patient satisfaction scores for a particular group of patients are lower can all lead to a search of the literature for evidence to change and improve outcomes. It may also lead to further research to improve outcomes or the implementation of new interventions to change outcomes. But before the search can begin, it is important that clinical questions are defined clearly and in a way that can be effectively answered and applied to practice.

Clinical questions should be written in a format that provides a clear direction for examination. PICO is a popular framework used to develop clinical questions. The acronym stands for population studied (P), intervention (I), comparison (C), and outcome (O). Sometimes, practitioners use PICOT, in which the "T" stands for "time frame."

When framing a qualitative question, the PICo approach is preferred. The letters in PICo refer to population (P), phenomena of interest (I), and context (C). An outcome is not needed in a qualitative synthesis (o) (Aromataris & Munn, 2017). As you formulate your PICO question, it is helpful to describe the type of question you are asking to better define your research method. Is this an intervention, diagnosis, etiology, or prognosis type of question? (Lansing Community College Library, 2018, Table 5.1).

Once the type of question you wish to ask is identified, the next step is to clearly describe the patient population to be studied. This is essential, as the background literature search must be relevant to the targeted population. Think of how best to describe the population that you are interested in learning more about. What are its most important characteristics? For example, an APRN who works in long-term care (LTC) may observe that the nursing staff, especially the nursing assistants, working in LTC facilities lack knowledge and training in end-of-life (EOL) care. This APRN also notes that many of the elderly patients in LTC do not have advanced directives and have high rates of hospital admissions and emergency department (ED) transfers at EOL. To accurately define the population, an APRN needs to identify any important characteristics of the group that is to be addressed or examined in the proposed study or intervention. Using the same example, since many elderly patients reside in LTC facilities and since nursing staff in this setting are observed to be unprepared in EOL care, the APRN decides to target this particular population for study. Therefore, the population to be studied would be described as follows:

■ *Population:* Nursing staff working in LTC facilities.

The second step is to determine the intervention or process you want to study. As mentioned earlier, defining the method of study early on can help develop the PICO question more fully. In this particular example, the APRN is aware that nursing staff in LTC facilities receive very little training in EOL care. Since the nursing assistants are the ones that provide most of the care in LTC facilities and often form close bonds with the residents, the APRN decides to include them in the population "nursing staff." In the professional literature there are many studies demonstrating the success of staff EOL education programs in other settings (Braun & Zir, 2005; Ersek, Grant, & Kraybill, 2005). The APRN decides to provide an educational program on EOL care for the nursing staff in LTC facilities. When older adults are asked about and provided with information about advance directives, they are more likely to complete advance directives (Ko, Lee, & Hong, 2016). The APRN postulates that by improving the EOL knowledge of the nursing staff in LTC facilities, the nursing staff will be better able to help the residents make informed EOL decisions.

■ *Intervention:* An education program on end of life communication.

In this particular example, the APRN plans to compare nursing staff EOL knowledge and LTC resident EOL decision making before and after an education program.

■ *Comparison:* Nursing staff EOL knowledge and resident EOL decision making before and after an education program (education vs. no education).

TABLE 5.1 PICOT Questions > Types of Evidence > Databases

Type of Clinical Question	Primary Research	Synthesized Research (Secondary Literature)	Other Evidence (Secondary Literature)
	Use CINAHL and MEDLINE to find: • Randomized controlled trials (RCT) • Controlled trials • Case-control studies • Cohort studies • Descriptive studies • Qualitative studies • Instrument development research	Use Cochrane Collection Plus, CINAHLPLUS, and Medline to find: • Systematic reviews • Meta-analyses	Use CINAHLPLUS, Medline, Joanna Briggs Institute, nursing, healthcare, and government organizations to find: • Clinical practice guidelines Use published clinical articles (not research based), peer institution practices, expert clinician practices to find: • Expert opinion
Therapy "What is the best treatment or intervention?"	RCT, controlled trials	Systematic reviews	Clinical practice guidelines
Prevention "How can I prevent this problem?"	RCT, controlled trials	Systematic reviews	Clinical practice guidelines

(continued)

TABLE 5.1 PICOT Questions > Types of Evidence > Databases (*continued*)

PICOT Question	Types of Evidence		Evidence Pyramid: Look for the highest level of evidence appropriate for your clinical question.
Diagnosis/Assessment "What is the best way to assess or best diagnostic test for this patient?"	Instrument development research		**Level 1:** Systematic reviews and meta-analysis of RCTs; evidence-based clinical practice guidelines
Causation "What causes this problem?"	Cohort, case control, descriptive, or qualitative studies	Systematic reviews	**Level 2:** One or more RCTs
Prognosis "What are the long-term effects of this problem?"	Cohort or descriptive studies	Systematic reviews	**Level 3:** Controlled trials (no randomization)
Meaning "What is the meaning of this experience for patients?"	Qualitative studies	Systematic reviews	**Level 4:** Case-control or cohort study
			Level 5: Systematic review of descriptive and qualitative studies
			Level 6: Single descriptive or qualitative study
			Level 7: Expert opinion

Evidence Pyramid: Level I, Level II, Level III, Level IV, Level V, Level VI, Level VII

RCT, randomized controlled trials.

Source: Used with permission of Lansing Community College Library. (2019). What is PICOT? Retrieved from http://libguides.lcc.edu/c.php?g=167860&p=6198388

The last step is the outcome: What does the APRN want to see improved? What does the APRN expect to accomplish? The objective in this case was to increase the EOL knowledge of nursing staff in LTC facilities and to increase the EOL decision-making capacity of the residents.

■ *Outcome:* Staff EOL knowledge based on a test administered before and after the education program. Rates of LTC resident advance directives and hospital transfers at EOL before and after an education program.

Using these steps, the APRN can now compose the final PICO question: Will a 3-week EOL education program: (a) increase the EOL knowledge of LTC facility nursing staff, (b) increase the rate of resident advance directives, and (c) decrease the rate of resident hospital transfers at EOL (Kunte, Johansen, & Isenberg-Cohen, 2017). Development of the PICO question provides the APRN with a better understanding of the clinical problem, allows for specific measures to be introduced, and provides the foundation for a well-designed study. The next step is to perform a thorough and comprehensive literature review.

THE LITERATURE REVIEW

The literature search should further define and clarify the clinical problem; summarize the current state of knowledge on the subject; identify relationships, contradictions, gaps, and inconsistencies in the literature; and finally, suggest the next step in solving the problem (American Psychological Association [APA], 2009). The search of the literature can be conducted by the APRN or the APRN can engage the assistance of a research librarian if available. Librarians are educated to find and access information and are excellent resources for assisting with literature reviews. Navigating databases in order to find relevant information can be a complex process. The searcher needs to use the correct terms, search the correct databases, and use a well-designed and systematic search strategy. The searcher should also document each step of the process in order to provide an audit trail and avoid duplication of work. An audit trail provides transparency to the breadth and depth of the strategies used to find the evidence and allows others to follow the decision-making process (Amankwaa, 2016). In the absence of a librarian, there are steps that the APRN can take to increase the likelihood of a successful search.

In order to find the most relevant literature to inform decision-making, the searcher should use key terms from the PICO question (i.e., population studied, intervention, comparison, and outcomes of interest). The first step is to search each key term separately and then to take steps to refine the search. The APRN should use at least two databases for the literature search. Access to some databases requires a subscription, while others are free. The Cochrane Collaboration is an international organization that provides up-to-date systematic reviews (currently more than 7,500). It can be accessed through the Cochrane Collaboration website (www.cochrane.org) that requires a subscription in many countries, including the United States (with the exception of Wyoming). For a complete list of countries with free access, go to the Cochrane page at www.cochranelibrary.com/help/access. Some of the content is free. For example, access to summaries or older versions of the reviews can be accessed without a subscription, but for access to full systematic reviews, a paid subscription is required (The Cochrane Collaboration, 2018). PubMed is a free resource. It includes MEDLINE and is the U.S. National Library of Medicine (NLM) journal literature search system. It includes more than 28 million citations for biomedical literature from MEDLINE, journals, and online books, and includes citations from full-text content (NLM, 2018). A free tutorial on how to use PubMed is available at www.nlm.nih.gov/bsd/pubmed _tutorial/ml001.html.

The Joanna Briggs Institute (JBI) and the Cumulative Index to Nursing and Allied Health Literature (CINAHL) are excellent databases that both require a subscription. The JBI includes The JBI Library of Systematic Reviews, which is an international, not-for-profit, membership-based organization located within the University of Adelaide, Australia (JBI, 2018). Students receive a discounted subscription rate to the JBI. JBI can be accessed at joannabriggs.org. CINAHL is a comprehensive resource for nursing and allied health literature. It is owned and operated by EBSCO Publishing, which currently offers access to five different versions (CINAHL, CINAHL Plus, CINAHL with Full Text, CINAHL Plus with Full Text, and CINAHL Complete). The main differences among them are the variety of added content; CINAHL is the basic database (EBSCO Publishing, 2018).

Searches of a single keyword can result in a very large number of articles. For example, a CINAHL search for full-text articles using the keyword "end of life" yielded a list of 17,202 articles. Including more than one concept in the search is more likely to provide relevant and useful articles. *Boolean logic* is the term used to describe certain logical operations that are used to combine search terms in many databases. Using the Boolean connector AND narrows a search by combining terms; it will retrieve documents that use the two keywords. Combining words with a Boolean connector such as AND (e.g., *nursing home AND end of life*) can narrow the search. In CINHAL, using *nursing home AND end of life* reduced the number to 584 articles. Using OR, on the other hand, broadens a search to include results that contain either of the words that are typed in the search. OR is a good tool to use when there are several common spellings or synonyms of a word. An example in this case would be *nursing home OR LTC facility*. Using NOT will narrow a search by excluding certain search terms. NOT retrieves documents that contain one but not the other of the search terms entered and is appropriate to use when a word is used in different contexts. An example would be *nursing home NOT rehabilitation facility*. Parentheses indicate relationships between search terms. When they are used, the computer will process the search terms in a specified order and also combine them in the correct manner. For example, (*nursing home OR LTC facility*) *AND end of life* combines these terms to get the most relevant results. A search conducted in the full-text database of CINAHL using these words and connectors yielded 608 articles.

There are other methods that can be used to make searches more relevant and useful. Specifying limits, such as English language only, peer-reviewed journals only, randomized controlled trials only, and a date range can narrow a search and increase the relevance of the information retrieved. Keep in mind that the more limits that are placed on the search, the fewer the results. A search using (*nursing home OR LTC facility*) AND end of life, full text only, English only, limited to articles published in the past 5 years yielded 232 articles. However, it is recommended that the initial search should be broad and explored before restricting the search limits, as this could lead to information bias. For this PICO question, the following keywords were used both alone and in combinations: *end of life, end of life training program, advance directive, hospital transfer, nursing staff, nursing assistants, nursing home, LTC facility, and nursing home resident*

A search of electronic databases does not complete the search for the most current known evidence about a topic. A hand search of current and relevant journals may reveal information that has not yet been entered into an electronic database. Studies can also appear in publications other than journals such as books, and in noncommercial "grey" literature like government reports, conference proceedings, monographs, working papers, and unpublished doctoral dissertations (Riesenberg & Justice, 2014). Projects and reports that are completed by specialized organizations, such as foundations and professional membership groups, may appear only on websites. Internet searching can help locate such resources and can scan organizational websites of professional and specialized organizations such as the National Hospice and Palliative Care Association, the American Public Health Association, the American Nurses Association, and the Robert Wood Johnson Foundation. The APRN should also consider contacting experts who may know of important findings and recent discoveries in a particular field. A technique known as snowballing (citation tracking using the citation databases such as Science Citation Index, Social Sciences Citation Index, and Arts and Humanities Citation Index) might also be helpful (Wright, Golder, & Rodriguez-Lopez, 2014). After reviewing the literature, many references that may not have been discovered in an Internet search can be found by simply reviewing the references of collected literature.

Finally, really simple syndication (RSS) feeds provide a convenient way for subscribers to obtain constantly updated information (see also Chapter 6, Using Information Systems to Improve Population Outcomes). These function as a new version of a database. Rather than searching individual websites, nurses can browse content, summaries of content, headlines, and/or links to information quickly and in one place from an aggregator that automatically downloads the new data to the user. Sites such as PubMed allow subscribers to customize the information for which they want alerts. For those who want to do the searching, instant RSS search (http://ctrlq.org/rss/) provides a venue to find feeds for news, websites, podcasts, and more.

During the literature search, APRNs should keep in mind the difference between primary and secondary sources. Primary sources are those materials or documents created during the time under study and directly experienced by the writer. For example, an original article written by researchers that summarizes the methods and findings of a study carried out by them is an example of a primary source. Other examples of primary sources are letters, diaries, and speeches. Secondary sources interpret and analyze primary sources. An example is a news article announcing a new scientific discovery. A key here is that secondary sources generally analyze and interpret the findings in primary sources and this can lead to bias. It is always advisable to use primary sources when seeking evidence for a change in practice.

ASSESSING THE EVIDENCE

Once a list of articles is obtained, the next step is to assess and synthesize the evidence. Appraising evidence for its usefulness can be a challenge. While reviewing the evidence, the APRN needs to ask some fundamental questions that address the relevance of information such as "How confident am I that the relationships and knowledge in this particular study will apply to the situation in question?" (Wakefield, 2014). To determine whether the evidence discovered is enough to drive a practice change, it is important to ask "Is the evidence strong enough to use the results?" "Are the findings applicable to my setting?," "If I adopt the practice, what will be the impact on the target population?" (Melnyk, 2016). It is also essential to examine the "efficacy" (evidence of an effect under ideal conditions, such as double-blind, randomized controlled trials [RCTs]) and "effectiveness" (evidence of what actually works in practice) of the findings and of the study. In summary, during the process of determining which studies to include in a synthesis, the APRN needs to ask not only "Does this intervention work?" and "For whom does this intervention work?," but also "When, why, and how does it work?"

Since all published evidence is not completed with equal rigor, the value of published articles varies on a continuum from the lowest to the highest value. A search can potentially find an enormous number of articles, but not all articles may be useful. Because there is often a limited amount of time that is available to assess and synthesize the evidence, it is helpful to have a method that provides guidance as to which articles might be the most valid and useful. After conducting an extensive search of sources, the APRN must establish criteria for inclusion and exclusion of studies (Wakefield, 2015)

A systematic review is a comprehensive summary of the best available evidence on a particular topic at the time the review was written (Polit & Beck, 2017). There are several organizations that provide guidelines and resources for the conduct of systematic reviews. Many of these help healthcare professionals keep pace with the professional literature by maintaining a database of completed systematic reviews. Information on some sources is listed in Table 5.2. These reviews are completed using strict inclusion and exclusion criteria, and aim to include as much of the research that is relevant to the clinical question being asked as possible. The overall objective of an appraisal is to assess the general strength of the evidence in relation to the particular issue being studied. The Evidence for Policy and Practice Information and Coordinating Centre at the Institute of Education, University of London (2018), describes in detail, the method used for conducting a comprehensive systematic review on its website (see Table 5.2).

To begin the appraisal, it is helpful to use a table to summarize and group the information according to key areas. Table 5.3 is an example of a tool that can be used to

TABLE 5.2 Online Resources for Evidence-Based Practice

ORGANIZATION	DESCRIPTION	WEB LINK
The Cochrane Collaboration	The Cochrane Collaboration is an independent, not-for-profit organization	www.cochrane.org
	Systematic reviews are published in The Cochrane Library—summaries and abstracts are free of charge; a subscription is required for full use of the library resources	
	Publishes the *Cochrane Handbook for Systematic Reviews* community.cochrane.org/book_pdf/764	
The Joanna Briggs Institute (JBI), Australia	JBI is a professional, peer-review organization	connect.jbiconnectplus.org
	The JBI Library of Systematic Reviews is a refereed library that publishes systematic reviews of literature; subscription is required; student rates are available	
Centre for Reviews and Dissemination (CRD), University of York, UK	The CRD is part of the National Institute for Health Research (NIHR)	www.york.ac.uk/inst/crd
	The CRD makes available systematic reviews on health and public health questions	
	Access is available to archived records of DARE, NHS EED (production ceased in 2015), and HTA (production halted in 2018) databases and guidelines for undertaking systematic reviews	
The Evidence for Policy and Practice Information and Co-ordinating Centre (EPPI-Centre) at the Institute of Education, University of London	The EPPI-Centre is part of the Social Science Research Unit at the Institute of Education, University of London	eppi.ioe.ac.uk/cms
	Provides the main findings, technical summary, or full technical reports of individual EPPI-Centre Systematic Reviews	
	Available online: Methods for a Systematic Review www.betterevaluation.org/sites/default/files/Methods.pdf	
U.S. National Library of Medicine (NLM)	PubMed (which includes MEDLINE) is the NLM literature search system; it includes more than 20 million citations for biomedical literature from MEDLINE, journals, and online books and includes citations from full-text content	www.nlm.nih.gov
	PubMed Central (PMC) is a web-based repository of biomedical journal literature providing free, unrestricted access to more than 1.5 million full-text articles	
	Publishes and provides the following: systematic reviews, meta-analyses, reviews of clinical trials, evidence-based medicine, consensus development conferences, and guidelines	

DARE, database of abstracts of reviews of effects; HTA, health technology assessment; NHS EED, national health service economic evaluation database guide.

document the critical elements of the evidence such as the design of the study, the study population, and the outcomes. It provides the APRN with a standardized method for evaluating the important points gleaned from the literature search; it can also serve as an audit trail, so others can judge the rigor and quality of the review.

TABLE 5.3 **Example of Literature Review and Synthesis for Evidence-Based Practice Tool**

CLINICAL QUESTION:							
TITLE OF ARTICLE	AUTHORS WITH CREDENTIALS	QUESTION	STUDY DESIGN	LEVEL OF EVIDENCE	DESCRIPTION OF SAMPLE	MEASURES	RESULTS

An important step in the research review process is the organization and grading of the evidence. A hierarchical level-of-evidence approach is a useful way to rank evidence according to its strength and helps to remove subjectivity from the assessment. The design of the study used by investigators to minimize bias determines the strength of the evidence. Most hierarchies classify the best evidence (studies that provide the most reliable evidence) at the top of the list and those with the least reliable evidence at the bottom of the list. By first rating the strength, and then critiquing individual studies, the practitioner can "ensure that the evidence is credible and appropriate for inclusion into practice" (Peterson et al., 2014, p. 59).

Levels of evidence are graded based on scientific merit. An example of some of the groups that have established hierarchies of evidence are the American Academy of Pediatrics, the Oncology Nursing Association, the Oxford Centre for Evidence-Based Medicine, the Cochrane Institute, and the Joanna Briggs Institute.

The AACN's evidence-leveling system (most recently revised in 2012) shown in Table 5.4, is an example of this type of system and is a useful tool in the appraisal of research evidence. As with most hierarchical systems, the AACN system classifies the levels of evidence in descending order, with the highest level of evidence placed in Level A and the lowest in Level M.

The evidence-leveling system of the Centre for Reviews and Dissemination (CRD) at the University of York includes study designs like case-control and cohort studies that are used in population research (Exhibit 5.1). Similar to the AACN system, it classifies the levels of evidence in a descending order, with well-designed RCTs at the top and case studies at the bottom.

TABLE 5.4 American Association of Colleges of Nursing's Evidence-Leveling System: 2012 Revisions to 2008 Hierarchy

CATEGORY	LEVEL	DESCRIPTION
Experimental Evidence	A	Meta-analysis or metasynthesis of multiple controlled studies with results that consistently support a specific action, intervention, or treatment (systematic review of a randomized controlled trial)
	B	Evidence from well-designed controlled studies, both randomized and nonrandomized, with results that consistently support a specific action, intervention, or treatment
	C	Evidence from qualitative, integrative reviews, or systematic reviews of qualitative, descriptive, or correlational studies or randomized controlled trials with inconsistent results
Recommendations	D	Evidence from peer-reviewed professional organizational standards, with clinical studies to support recommendations
	E	Theory-based evidence from expert opinion or multiple case reports
	M	Manufacturer's recommendation only

Source: Peterson, M. H., Barnason, S., Donnelly, B., Hill, K., Miley, H., Riggs, L., & Whiteman, K. (2014). Choosing the best evidence to guide clinical practice: application of AACN levels of evidence. *Critical Care Nurse, 34*(2), 58–68. doi:10.4037/ccn2014411

EXHIBIT 5.1

HIERARCHY OF STUDY DESIGNS USED TO ASSESS THE EFFECTS OF INTERVENTIONS

Centre for Reviews and Dissemination, University of York, UK

This list is not exhaustive, but covers the main study designs.

Randomized controlled trials

The simplest form of RCTs is known as the parallel group trial, which randomizes eligible participants to two or more groups, treats according to assignment, and compares the groups with respect to outcomes of interest. Participants are allocated to groups using both randomization (allocation involves the play of chance) and concealment (ensures that the intervention that will be allocated cannot be known in advance). There are different types of randomized study designs:

Randomized crossover trials

All participants receive all the interventions; for example, in a two-arm crossover trial, one group receives intervention A before intervention B, and the other group receives intervention B before intervention A. It is the sequence of interventions that is randomized.

(continued)

EXHIBIT 5.1

Cluster randomized trials
A cluster randomized trial is a trial in which clusters of people, rather than single individuals, are randomized to different interventions. For example, whole clinics or geographical locations may be randomized to receive particular interventions, rather than individuals.

Quasi-experimental studies
The main distinction between randomized and quasi-experimental studies is the way in which participants are allocated to the intervention and control groups; quasi-experimental studies do not use random assignment to create the comparison groups.

Nonrandomized controlled studies
Individuals are allocated to a concurrent comparison group, using methods other than randomization. The lack of concealed randomized allocation increases the risk of selection bias.

Before-and-after study
Comparison of outcomes in study participants before and after the introduction of an intervention. The before-and-after comparisons may be in the same sample of participants or in different samples.

Interrupted time series
Interrupted time series designs are multiple observations over time that are "interrupted," usually by an intervention or treatment.

Observational studies
A study in which natural variation in interventions or exposure among participants (i.e., not allocated by an investigator) is investigated to explore the effect of the interventions or exposure on health outcomes.

Cohort study
A defined group of participants is followed over time and comparison is made between those who did and did not receive an intervention.

Case-control study
Groups from the same population with (cases) and without (controls) a specific outcome of interest are compared to evaluate the association between exposure to an intervention and the outcome.

Case series
Description of a number of cases of an intervention and the outcome (without comparison with a control group). These are not comparative studies.

Source: From Centre for Reviews and Dissemination. (2008). *Systematic reviews: CRD's guidance for undertaking reviews in healthcare [Internet].* York: University of York. Retrieved from http://www.york.ac.uk/inst/crd/index_guidance.htm. Used with permission from Centre for Reviews and Dissemination, University of York, UK.

The inclusion of different study designs in a systematic review can provide valuable insight as it has a direct impact on the complexity of the information. For example, although qualitative studies are not classified as high levels of evidence, they can still provide an APRN with important information to better understand observed phenomena. The findings of qualitative studies offer answers to different types of questions and help to describe complex human interactions. A classic example is Beck's (1993) qualitative study that used grounded theory to explore the phenomenon of postpartum depression. Because it was a qualitative study, the results were not generalized to the population of all women with postpartum depression. Instead, Beck's research offered the reader vivid descriptions of the women in her study, and an insight into how she derived the evocative theme of "teetering on the edge" to effectively illustrate the women's experience.

Validity

Once the APRN has completed evidence collection, each individual study needs to be appraised for the internal and external validity of the design. A hallmark of good research is that it is carried out by researchers who are aware of the existence of error and who design studies in such a way that errors are minimized. Table 5.3 is a useful tool to facilitate the appraisal of evidence by providing a method to organize the individual aspects or components of the study. The APRN uses this information to examine the soundness of the design, conduct an analysis of the study (internal validity), and to determine how well the study results can be applied to other settings and populations (external validity) (Andrade, 2018).

When appraising the quality of a study, the APRN should attempt to assess how accurate the findings are and whether they are of relevance in the particular setting or population of interest. The appraisal should include the appropriateness of the study design to the research question, the risk of bias, the overall quality of the methods used to carry out the study, the outcome measure, the quality of the intervention, appropriateness of the analysis, the quality of the research report, and the generalizability of the results. When appraising a qualitative study, the APRN evaluates its credibility and trustworthiness by reviewing the methods of observation, data collection, reporting strategies and audit trails (Cope, 2014). The APRN may choose to perform an "integrative review" (Christmals & Gross, 2017) where qualitative evidence is synthesized with quantitative findings on a specific topic to generate a new perspective or interpretation. Holloway and Galvin (2017) assert that both methodologies are equally important, since qualitative and quantitative "researchers ask different questions" and "therefore generate different answers" (p. 24).

Nurses are often intimidated when faced with evaluating the data analysis section in a research article. An important fact to keep in mind is that statistical significance is not synonymous with proof and that sometimes overemphasis is placed on statistically significant findings. It is equally important to evaluate the clinical significance of the results and how they affect treatment outcomes. Researchers report a statistical significance when they are confident that the difference they found between groups is real and not likely to be caused by chance. When determining clinical significance, however, the treatment benefit or amount of meaningful clinical improvement in treated individuals is assessed (Jensen & Corralejo, 2017). If a statistically significant result is not clinically significant, it should not be used to guide clinical practice (Heavey, 2015, p. 27). The APRN should review the results section of a research report carefully to determine whether or not the method of analysis used by the researcher answers the research question(s) or hypothesis and provides enough information to support the interpretation of the results.

Transparency

Transparency is another important concept for consideration during the appraisal of research publications. Transparency in research is a reflection of both the accountability and the integrity of the investigator(s). Clarity about the research methods and techniques used ensures the rigor of the research study and the validity of its outcomes (McKechnie, Chabot, Dalmer, Julien, & Mabbott, 2016). It should be possible, for example, for the study and results to be replicated by others. There should also be a disclosure of relationships that have the potential to cause a conflict of interest. A conflict of interest may occur when a researcher's objectivity is impacted by economic (ownership of stocks or shares), commercial (payouts by companies), or personal interests (when a researcher's status may be impacted by the results of the research) (APA, 2009). For example, an investigator with ties to a company that is closely related to the area of research may stand to profit from steering the results in a particular direction. Even when investigators disclose their conflicts of interest, the APRN should critically review the research for potential bias.

Research Synthesis

The literature review not only provides a historical account of past work in the area of interest but also supports or refutes the necessity for ongoing study. The background for any study is founded on a thorough and comprehensive literature review. It serves as a justification for current research goals and introduces the reader to important past studies that have similar outcomes of comparison. Although not all studies will have an array of historical evidence in the literature, review of similar study designs or interventions can still provide a strong justification if the background is well researched.

The overall purpose of the example described earlier was to determine whether an EOL education program for nursing staff would improve staff EOL knowledge and improve EOL outcomes of the elderly residents living in LTC facilities. All persons, especially the elderly, should receive quality EOL care that meets national standards. Table 5.5 provides a portion of the research synthesis that was completed using the sample PICO question. The literature search demonstrated that more than one third of the residents in nursing homes did not have advance directives and received expensive, aggressive EOL care. Those residents that had advance directives were more likely to die in the nursing home, and have lower rates of hospitalizations at EOL. The review provided evidence that nursing staff play an important role in the decision-making process in LTC facilities, since they are familiar with the wishes of the residents. But several

TABLE 5.5 Tool Used to Assess Literature Review: Interventions, Purpose, Populations, and Outcomes

TITLE/AUTHOR	DESCRIPTION OF INTERVENTION	PURPOSE AND POPULATIONS	OUTCOMES ACHIEVED
1. Braun, K., & Zir A. (2005). Using an interactive approach to teach nursing home workers about end-of-life care. *Journal of Hospice & Palliative Nursing, 7*(5), 280–288.	Qualitative study using descriptive design with focus groups. Interactive education program primarily for nurse aides. Participants completed 8 1-hour modules.	To improve knowledge of nursing home staff on end-of-life care. 144 participants from 10 nursing homes attended the ACORN course (8 RNs, 6 social workers, 82 nurse aides, 4 activity aides)	Participants had high scores on posttests for all modules. They also had significantly improved scores on personal comfort with providing end-of-life care.
2. Ersek, M., Grant, M. M., & Kraybill, B. M. (2005). Enhancing end-of-life care in nursing homes: Palliative Care Educational Resource Team (PERT) program. *Journal of Palliative Medicine, 8*(3), 556–566.	Quasi-experimental design, with an adapted cohort analysis. Four day-long classes were conducted monthly. Some classes were separate and others were combined classes for the nurses and nurse aides. Separate pre-/posttests for aides and nurses, self-evaluation, and supervisor evaluation of staff knowledge.	To describe the development and evaluation of Palliative Care Educational Resource Team (PERT) program, designed to improve end of life abilities of nursing home staff; 61 nurse aides and 108 nurses from 44 nursing homes participated; 3 groups from 3 different areas	Participants demonstrated significant increases in EOL knowledge, and self-evaluation of EOL skills, Supervisors' evaluations of participants' EOL care also showed improvement scores.
3. Johnson, S., & Bott, M. J. (2016). Communication with residents and families in nursing homes at the end of life. *Journal Of Hospice And Palliative Nursing: JHPN: The Official Journal Of The Hospice And Palliative Nurses Association, 18*(2), 124–130.	Secondary analysis of data from a previously administered qualitative study. Three research questions were explored: (a) who should communicate with the resident/family about death and dying; (b) when communication should occur around death and dying; c) what differences exist in communication among nursing staff	A secondary analysis was conducted to determine perception of EOL communication between the resident/family and direct care staff in nursing homes; 2,932 direct care staff from 85 randomly selected Midwestern facilities participated	More than 90% of staff thought that physician or social worker should communicate about death and dying with residents/families. Only 53% thought that direct care staff should talk with patients. Staff was more likely to talk about EOL on admission or upon the resident's family's request.
4. Jones, A. L., Moss, A. J., & Harris-Kojetin, L. D. (2011). Use of advance directives in long-term care populations. *NCHS Data Brief,* (54), 1–8.	Analysis of data from two national surveys: 2004 National Nursing Home survey and 2007 National Home and Hospice Survey	To analyze the effects of the Patient Self-Determination Act on the rate of advance directives in patients in long-term care facilities. The 2004 NNHS and 2007 NHHCS are periodic cross-sectional surveys of nationally representative samples of U.S. long term care facilities	28% of home healthcare patients and 655 of nursing home residents have at least one advance directive. Recipients under 65 and Black care recipients are less likely to have advance directives.

(continued)

TABLE 5.5 Tool Used to Assess Literature Review: Interventions, Purpose, Populations, and Outcomes (*continued*)

TITLE/AUTHOR	DESCRIPTION OF INTERVENTION	PURPOSE AND POPULATIONS	OUTCOMES ACHIEVED
5. Ko, E., Lee, J., & Hong, Y. (2016). Willingness to complete advance directives among low-income older adults living in the USA. *Health & Social Care in the Community, 24*(6), 708–716.	This study was conducted as part of a larger study that explored advance care planning in low-income adults. A cross-sectional design was used. Face-to-face interviews were conducted with the participants. Questionnaires used were: EOL preference questionnaire, attitude towards advance decision-making questionnaire, and the Luben Support Network Scale. Willingness to complete an advance directive and availability of healthcare proxy were yes/no questions	To explore low-income older adults' willingness to complete advance directives, and the role of social support and other predictors that impact their willingness. It included 204 older adults living in two supportive housing facilities or members of a senior center. Participants were selected through random sampling methods. Inclusion criteria included age over 60 and mentally competent.	The majority of participants (72.1%) reported a willingness to complete advance directives. Self-rated health, attitudes toward advance decision-making and social support were some of the factors affecting their decisions.
6. Lange J. W., Shea J., Grossman S. C., Wallace M., & Ferrell B. R. (2009). Validation of the end-of-life nursing education consortium knowledge assessment test: An abbreviated version. *Journal of Hospice & Palliative Nursing, 11*(5), 284–290.	Questions from each of the nine domains with highest item-to-total correlations were selected from the original test.	To test the validity of a 50-item version of the original 109-item EOL knowledge assessment tool developed by end-of-life nursing education consortium; 141 graduate and undergraduate nursing students pretested the shorter version; 30 graduate students also completed the original version.	Scores on the 109-item and 50-item versions were highly correlated. Among graduate students pretest scores were well below the 80% target. This supports the need for end-of-life education. The shorter version is useful to assess baseline EOL knowledge
7. Mather, M., Jacobsen, L. A., & Pollard, K. M. (2015). Aging in the United States. *Population Bulletin, 70*(2).	Population Reference Bureau (PRB) analyzes data from the U.S. decennial census, American Community Survey, Current Population Survey, Vital Statistics, and other products of the federal statistical system. This bulletin provided statistics on the older adults living in the United States	The PRB collects and supplies statistics about the environment, and structure and health of populations.	There will be 2.3 million nursing home residents in 2030 if the share of Americans ages 65+ living in nursing homes remains at 2010 levels.

(continued)

TABLE 5.5 Tool Used to Assess Literature Review: Interventions, Purpose, Populations, and Outcomes (*continued*)

TITLE/AUTHOR	DESCRIPTION OF INTERVENTION	PURPOSE AND POPULATIONS	OUTCOMES ACHIEVED
8. Teno, J. M., Gozalo, P. L., Bynum, J. P. W., Leland, N. E., Miller, S. C., Morden, N. E., … Mor, V. (2013). Change in end-of-life care for Medicare beneficiaries: Site of death, place of care, and healthcare transitions in 2000, 2005, and 2009. *JAMA, 309*(5), 470–477.	Retrospective cohort study. A multivariable regression model was used to examine outcomes. Patients in the last 6 months of life were grouped according to diagnosis of cancer, chronic obstructive pulmonary disease, or dementia, and EOL experiences analyzed.	Study reviewed records of a 20% random sample of fee-for-service Medicare beneficiaries, aged 66 years and older, who died in 2000 (n = 207,202), 2005 (n = 29,819), and 2009 (n = 286,282) to describe changes in site of death, place of care, and explore healthcare transitions	Comparing 2000, 2005, and 2009 data showed a decrease in deaths in acute care hospitals and increase in hospice use at the time of death. However there were increases in intensive care unit (ICU) use in the last 30 days, and healthcare transitions at the end of life
9. Unroe, K. T., Cagle, J. G., Lane, K. A., Callahan, C. M., & Miller, S. C. (2015). Nursing home staff palliative care knowledge and practices: Results of a large survey of frontline workers. *Journal of Pain And Symptom Management, 50*(5), 622–629.	Palliative care survey (PCS) was offered to all employees who could attend. Completion was voluntary. Some completed a paper survey, others completed via Survey Monkey.	To compare palliative care knowledge and practices among nursing home staff and to examine relationships between facility characteristics and knowledge levels; 1,200 employees from 51 nursing homes in Indiana responded to the survey (71% response rate).	Nurse aides had significantly lower practice and knowledge scores compared to LPNs, RNs, and social workers. Although all groups had high levels of knowledge about physical symptoms, general EOL knowledge was low for all staff.

ACORN, appropriate care of residents in nursing homes.

Source: From Kunte, V., Johansen, M. L., & Isenberg-Cohen, S. (2017). Improving long-term care residents' outcomes by educating nursing staff on end-of-life communication. *Journal of Hospice & Palliative Nursing, 19*(6), 550–555. doi:10.1097/NJH.0000000000000386

studies also showed that nursing staff, especially nursing assistants, in LTC facilities have minimal knowledge of EOL care and are uncomfortable initiating these conversations with residents. Finally, a search for staff education revealed the evidence-based EOL Nursing Education Consortium (ELNEC) Geriatric program, which is specially designed to address the EOL care education needs of nurses and nursing assistants who care for older adults in a wide range of community settings. No studies were found that correlated nursing education with nursing home residents' EOL outcomes. The literature review identified a gap in knowledge, highlighted the significance of the problem and justified the need for the study.

This project was implemented at two LTC facilities, one in the inner city and the other located in the suburbs. The nurses and nursing assistants on select units at each facility were invited to participate in this project. Nursing staff at each site received three weekly 30-minute education sessions based on the curriculum of the ELNEC-Geriatric program.

To measure the nursing staff knowledge outcome, nurses completed a pre-/posttest based on the communication module of the ELNEC-Geriatric program, while the nursing assistants completed a pre-/posttest developed by the Hospice and Palliative Nurses Association (HPNA) for nursing assistants. At the end of the program, participants rated the level of their knowledge of EOL communication before and after the program and how much the information learned would change the way they communicated about EOL care.

To measure resident outcomes, data were collected on those residents present on the units at the time the project was initiated and again from the same resident cohort post implementation. Baseline information on the absence/presence of an advance directive and the number of transfers to the emergency department (ED)/hospital from each facility for these residents was collected for the 2 months prior to implementing the program, and for the 2 months following the completion of the education program.

The results in this study were consistent with other studies discovered during the literature review. Nursing staff that participated in this project demonstrated an improvement in EOL knowledge on the test and in a self-evaluation of their EOL skills. As in other studies, the gains made in the knowledge tests were higher for the nursing assistants as compared to the nurses, probably because they had a higher need for education on EOL issues.

An evaluation of the resident outcomes demonstrated a dramatic decrease of almost 44% in resident transfers to the hospital/ED in the postimplementation phase. During that same time, a very small increase (2%) in the number of advance directives was noted, all of which occurred at the suburban LTC facility. The results were disappointing, but not surprising, as there was a big difference in the rates of residents with advance directives at the two facilities. These findings are reflective of other documented research, where prior to the program less than 10% of the predominantly minority residents at the urban facility had an advance directive, while at the suburban facility over 75% of the predominantly White residents did.

The summation of this work from literature review, to research synthesis, to pilot project is an excellent example of how APRNs can use this approach to design interventions to improve population outcomes.

INTEGRATION OF EVIDENCE INTO PRACTICE

Often, time lags occur when applying new research findings to clinical practice. The time period between the discovery that an intervention works and the application of that new knowledge into actual practice can take up to 17 years (Miller, Drummond-Hayes, & Carey, 2015). In 1999, the American Society of Anesthesiology (ASA) published evidence-based guidelines for preoperative fasting in healthy patients undergoing elective procedures. Moving away from the accepted tradition of NPO after midnight, the ASA advocated fasting periods of 2 hours for clear liquids, 6 hours for a light meal (tea and toast) and 8 hours for heavier meals before elective surgery. Crenshaw and Winslow (2002) conducted a study to determine how well the ASA guidelines were being followed. They interviewed 155 patients in one hospital about their preoperative fasting, comparing preoperative fasting instructions, actual preoperative fasting, and ASA-recommended fasting durations for liquids and solids. They found that the majority of patients continued to receive instructions to remain NPO after midnight for both liquids and solids, whether they were scheduled for early or late surgery. They also discovered that, on average, the patients fasted from liquids and solids for 12 hours and 14 hours, respectively, with some patients fasting as long as 20 hours from liquids and 37 hours from solids. These fasts were significantly longer than those recommended by the ASA. Clearly, in this case, the authors discovered a significant lag time between the generation of new knowledge and the implementation of that knowledge into practice.

A follow-up study in 2004 sought to evaluate the effects of the implementation of a preoperative fasting policy and the education of healthcare practitioners on preoperative fasting practices at their facility. Unfortunately, the authors found that the traditional practice of allowing NPO after midnight persisted (Crenshaw & Winslow, 2008). The authors identified the difficulty of changing entrenched traditions as one reason that preoperative fasting in excess of evidence-based recommendations persisted.

Since the publication of the original preoperative fasting guidelines (ASA, 1999), the ASA has published two updates (ASA, 2011; ASA 2017) reiterating the adverse effects of prolonged fasting and maintaining the previously recommended fasting periods. Still, after all these years, many facilities cling to outdated protocols. Recent research shows that just 25% of hospitals report compliance with the ASA guidelines (Thampy, Issa, Schostak, & Soto, 2018) and that the average preoperative NPO time for patients still hovers around 14 hours (Chon, Ma, & Mun-Price, 2017).

Similarly, given the many advances in nursing research, many nurses still adhere to ineffective, outdated practices; often there is no evidence of benefit, and in some cases even evidence of potential harm. In a nationwide survey, 2,356 nurses responded to the 20 questions asked by the journal *Nursing* to assess their knowledge of evidence-based practices (Miller, Drummond-Hayes, & Carey, 2015). The authors discussed the nurses' responses to the questions in a report, titled "20 Questions: Evidence-based practice or sacred cow." The survey results demonstrated that nurses were familiar with widely accepted practices like recommendations for preventing ventilator-associated pneumonia (VAP), central line associated bloodstream infections (CLABSI) and catheter-associated urinary tract infections (CAUTI). However, questions about evidence-based practices related to gastric residual volumes, placement of feeding tubes, stopping and starting tube feedings, the use of the Trendelenberg position for patients in shock, and pre-operative fasting, elicited a high number of incorrect responses (Miller, Drummond-Hayes, & Carey, 2015). When the same questionnaire was used at a facility seeking to compare its nurses' knowledge of best practices, the investigators found that their results closely matched the responses on the national survey (Cavlovich, 2016). Both survey results corroborate the need for further education on evidence-based practices and for policy reviews and revisions.

In order to effect change, the APRN needs to understand why these time intervals exist between the development of new knowledge and the incorporation of that knowledge into practice. Many national and international studies have explored the reasons for nurses not keeping up to date in their practice. In a recent integrative review, Camargo et al. (2018) examined nurses' knowledge, attitudes, practices and barriers to integrating evidence in their nursing care. As reported in prior studies, the researchers found that although most nurses have positive attitudes about evidence-based practice, the challenges related to their lack of knowledge and critical appraisal skills, work overload, lack of resources, and resistance to change still persist. Higher competence in evidence-based practice was directly related to higher academic degrees; older nurses and those who graduated many years ago demonstrated lower competence (Camargo et al., 2018)

In their groundbreaking ethnographic study, Gabbay and le May (2004) found that primary care providers rarely accessed or used current evidence but instead relied on "mindlines" while making complex clinical decisions. The researchers define mindlines as "internalized guidelines that are formed primarily from interactions with colleagues and people perceived as opinion leaders." Mindlines arise from experience and an individual process of acquiring and sharing information with trusted professional sources leading to "day to day practice based on socially constituted knowledge" (p. 1015). Instead of viewing practitioner mindlines as barriers to be overcome, Gabbay and le May (2016) argue that a network of trusted opinion leaders who are well grounded in evidence-based practice are the key to transferring research evidence to clinical practice.

Tradition is a difficult barrier to overcome. Nurses need to question practices based on tradition and instead use evidence whenever possible to guide nursing practice. Besides education, nurses need mentors to improve their evidence retrieval skills and to promote evidence implementation into daily practice (Friesen, Brady, Milligan, & Christensen, 2017). Depending on the focus of their advanced degrees, APRNs are experts who can assume the roles of highly skilled practitioners and/or leaders and educators in their respective clinical fields. APRNs are uniquely situated to be trusted opinion leaders and mentors to help bring about practice change and influence patient outcomes. They can challenge clinical staff to identify and remove barriers to evidence-based practice. Because they receive advanced education in research, APRNs can guide staff nurses in developing PICO questions, searching and synthesizing the literature, and changing practice interventions to reflect current knowledge (Campo Guinea, Pumar-Méndez, Ara Lucea, & Cenizo Simón-Ricart, 2015).

Models of Evidence-Based Practice

Several models have been created to facilitate the implementation of evidence-based practice. They provide an organized approach to integrate evidence into practice and sustain the change. A practice model ensures that professional nursing practice is consistent and minimizes practice variations that often increase risk and create gaps in care. Some examples of the models in use are the Advancing Research and Clinical Practice through Close Collaboration (ARCC©) Model, the Johns Hopkins Nursing Evidence-Based Practice Model (JHNEBPM), the Chronic Care Model (CCM), and the Iowa Model of Evidence-Based Practice to Promote Quality of Care. The overriding characteristic of each is that it provides a structured method for incorporating best evidence into practice.

The focus of the ARCC model is to bring research experts together with direct care nurses to integrate research into practice. Developed by Bernadette Melnyk and the faculty of the School of Nursing at the University of Rochester in 1999, it was originally designed to bring academic communities together with acute and community-based healthcare organizations. The APRN as mentor plays a prominent role in the ARCC model, as one of its key components is educating and coaching nursing staff on evidence-based practice. Fineout-Overholt, Levin, and Melnyk (2004) conducted a study to test this model in two pediatric units at acute care facilities. The authors identified the following crucial factors for implementing evidence-based practice: administrative support, creation of a clear role for nurses that includes evidence-based practice, adequate infrastructure (such as computer resources and databases), evidence-based practice mentors to work directly with direct care nurses, time and money to carry out studies, and creation of an evidence-based practice culture. In this study, direct care nurses valued the importance of APRN mentorship in bringing about practice change as opposed to simply being told what to do. The authors stress that APRN mentors facilitate and sustain a culture of evidence-based practice by working closely with direct care nurses. Several studies support the ARCC model which has since been implemented in a number of healthcare organizations worldwide (Melnyk & Fineout-Overholt, 2015).

Similar to the ARCC model, the origin of the JHNEBPM is found in a successful partnership between academia and a healthcare institution. This model was developed in collaboration with the Johns Hopkins Hospital and the Johns Hopkins University School of Nursing. In this model, the three-step PET process (**p**ractice question, **e**vidence, and **t**ranslation), provides the framework to incorporate best evidence into clinical practice (Dang & Dearholt, 2018). The essential cornerstones of the model are practice, education, and research, and at its core, is evidence. The JHNEBPM encourages critical thinking and provides a framework to guide nurses as they seek and find the best available evidence to improve patient outcomes.

The CCM (Group Health Research Institute, 2014) employs a holistic approach to chronic disease management through the use of evidence-based practice. It summarizes the basic elements for improving care in health systems at the community, organization, practice, and patient levels. It has six components: the healthcare delivery system, community, patient self-management support, decision support, delivery system design, and clinical information system. The emphasis of this model is on health promotion. O'Toole et al. (2010) investigated its effectiveness in providing primary care to homeless veterans. A retrospective cohort design was used to compare veterans who received their primary care in a clinic that used the CCM to a matched cohort of veterans who received their primary care in "usual care" clinics. Veterans enrolled in the clinic using the CCM for delivery of primary care had fewer ED visits and greater improvements in blood pressure and low-density lipoproteins than did the control cohort. The authors cited the importance of the location of the clinic (the clinic was located in an urban Virginia hospital so that it was geographically convenient) and of tailoring interventions to the target population (the clinic addressed issues such as the need for housing and food). They concluded that how primary care is delivered and organized is important in chronic disease management. In another study, 3,519 veterans with multiple chronic conditions were surveyed using The Patient Assessment of Chronic Illness Care (PACIC), to examine their perception of chronic care received at the Veterans Administration following the CCM (Balbale, Etingen, Malhiot, Miskevics, & LaVela, 2016). The veterans' scores on the scale were high; they perceived their care to be well organized, reported that they were well informed about their condition, and appreciated being involved in making decisions about their care.

The Iowa Model of Evidence-Based Practice to Promote Quality of Care was "developed to serve as a guide for nurses and other healthcare providers to use research findings for improvement of patient care" (Titler et al., 2001, p. 498). Responding to the advances in healthcare and user feedback, the Iowa Model was revised in 2015 to streamline it and make it easy to use (Buckwalter et al., 2017). Important features of the model are decision points and feedback loops that are characteristic of the ongoing process of improving care through research. The model includes six steps, beginning with problem identification (step 1) and ending with dissemination of the results of the project both internally and externally to share lessons learned with other organizations (step 6). Case Study 5.1 illustrates how a clinic used this practice model to facilitate practice change and improve patient outcomes.

CASE STUDY 5.1

USE OF THE IOWA MODEL TO INCREASE BREASTFEEDING INITIATION RATES OF URBAN CLINIC MOTHERS

Trigger
Nurses working in a perinatal clinic determined that the rate of breastfeeding initiation for their patients was low, approximating 40%. The clinic provides prenatal and maternity services to an ethnically diverse, inner-city population in the northeastern United States.

Identify purpose, determine priority
Since the institution was designated "Baby Friendly," improving breastfeeding exclusivity rates was a top organizational priority.

(continued)

CASE STUDY 5.1

Form team, assemble, appraise, and synthesize the literature

A team was created that included a clinical nurse specialist (CNS), the case managers for the perinatal clinic, and a lactation nurse specialist. A literature review was carried out by the CNS and the lactation nurse and more than 30 articles were retrieved and appraised. The literature search revealed information on the benefits of breastfeeding, breastfeeding rates among inner-city populations, research on effective strategies for increasing rates, and culturally appropriate materials for teaching.

Included in the key findings:

- Breastfeeding can reduce the incidence of many disease states in childhood and throughout adulthood, such as diabetes, sudden infant death syndrome (SIDS), ear infections, allergies, asthma, and obesity (American Academy of Pediatrics, 1999; Chulada, Arbes, Dunson, & Zeldin, 2003).

- The opinions of healthcare providers regarding breastfeeding have enormous impact on urban women, their partners, and families (Philipp, Merewood, Gerendas, & Bauchner, 2004).

- Methods to increase the rates of breastfeeding have been unsuccessful for African Americans because these methods are not culturally sensitive.

This information was summarized, shared, and discussed with team members. The team created a plan to increase the breastfeeding rates of the clinic population.

Pilot change and carryout study

The clinic initiated education programs for clinic staff and community providers and increased lactation services. The clinic environment was changed to include sensitive pictures of ethnically diverse breastfeeding mothers, and improvements were made in bilingual educational brochures. Each clinic counselor was given a protocol book describing specific literature, videos, and discussion to be provided to patients at each trimester. The healthcare providers documented the education that was provided to each patient, and patients completed a postpartum questionnaire that was used to evaluate interventions and factors influencing feeding choice.

Determine whether the change is appropriate for adoption in practice

Five years after the initiation of the evidence-based change, breastfeeding initiation rates had increased to 70%. Analysis of the patient evaluations revealed that counseling and reading material were cited as the most influential factors in making the choice to breastfeed. Other important factors were the opinions of family and healthcare professionals.

The nurses determined that prenatal education interventions that address varied learning styles and delivered in defined segments may be effective in influencing the feeding decisions of new mothers. The educational programs must be culturally sensitive, and staff education is vital to ensure effective and accurate delivery of information.

(continued)

Continue to monitor structure, process, and outcome data

The team has continued to monitor lactation rates and to review new information on lactation education as it has become available. Educational materials are updated on a regular basis. Eight years after the start of the initiative, their breastfeeding rates placed the hospital among the top 10 in the state. The clinic and its associated hospital achieved Baby-Friendly Designation in 2012, the second in the state. In order to achieve this goal, the clinic needed to demonstrate that they have integrated the "10 Steps to Successful Breastfeeding" (n. d.) into their practice for healthy newborns.

Disseminate Results

The department CNS and the lactation consultant presented the results of this project internally as podium and/or poster presentations at hospital-based events and conferences and published in hospital newsletters. Results were also disseminated externally via poster presentations at other local and regional institutions.

Source: Adapted from Procaccini, D., & Mahony, J. (2014). *Survey of educational interventions to increase the breastfeeding initiation rates of urban clinic mothers.* Unpublished manuscript.

Ultimately, APRNs need to determine which practice model will best suit their needs. Schaffer, Sandau, and Diedrick (2013) conducted an extensive literature review of practice models. They examined the key factors (characteristics) and usefulness of several. They concluded that in selecting a practice model, nurses should consider "how the model facilitates EBP projects, provides guidelines for evidence critique, guides the process for implementing practice change, and can be used across practice areas" (p. 1206). Their guidelines can be used to help APRNs select a practice model.

SUMMARY

The use of research evidence to guide practice can lead to the implementation of interventions that will improve population outcomes, but this is a complex process. The ability to identify clinical problems and issues, ask clinical questions in a format that allows for study, conduct a search of the literature, appraise and synthesize the available evidence, and successfully integrate new knowledge into practice requires specialized skills and knowledge. This process can be challenging and time-consuming. Researchers have identified many barriers to evidence-based practice, including the lack of belief by practicing nurses that research can make a real difference. APRNs are uniquely positioned to influence nursing care through their roles as leaders, educators, and clinical experts. This chapter described some of the basic skills needed to integrate and synthesize information in order to design interventions that are based on evidence to improve population health. APRNs need to use their specialized knowledge and advanced practice roles to identify the barriers to evidence-based practice and build the capacity to implement change. They also require the ability to engage individuals, teams, and organizations in the process. By adopting a culture of evidence-based practice in the work environment, APRNs have the opportunity to facilitate change that can lead to improved quality of care and enhanced population outcomes.

EXERCISES AND DISCUSSION QUESTIONS

Exercise 5.1 Describe in your own words a clinical problem you would like to examine.

- Explain why you think it is important to address this problem

Exercise 5.2 Write a clinical question using the PICO format.

Exercise 5.3 Carry out a literature review for the PICO question you wrote in Exercise 5.2.

- Establish criteria for inclusion and exclusion of studies.

- Synthesize and appraise the information using Table 5.3.

Exercise 5.4 Which practice model would you use to implement an evidence-based change in your practice area?

- Provide a rationale for your choice of model.

- Describe how you would apply the model to address your PICO question.

REFERENCES

Amankwaa, L. (2016). Creating protocols for trustworthiness in qualitative research. *Journal of Cultural Diversity, 23*(3), 121–127. Retrieved from http://search.ebscohost.com/login.aspx?direct=true&db=mnh&AN=29694754&site=ehost-live

American Academy of Pediatrics. (1999). 10 Steps to supporting a parents' choice to breastfeed their baby. In *AAP Task Force on Breastfeeding* (pp. 1–5). Washington, DC: Author.

American Association of Colleges of Nursing. (2006). *The essentials of doctoral education for advanced practice nursing.* Retrieved from https://www.aacnnursing.org/DNP/DNP-Essentials

American Psychological Association. (2009). *Publication manual of the American psychological association* (6th ed.). Washington, DC: Author.

American Society of Anesthesiologists. (1999). Practice guidelines for preoperative fasting and the use of pharmacologic agents to reduce the risk of pulmonary aspiration: Application to healthy patients undergoing elective procedures. *Anesthesiology. 90*, 896–905. doi:10.1097/00000542-199903000-00034

American Society of Anesthesiologists. (2011). Practice guidelines for preoperative fasting and the use of pharmacologic agents to reduce the risk of pulmonary aspiration: Application to healthy patients undergoing elective procedures, An updated report by the American Society of Anesthesiologists Committee on Standards and Practice Parameters. *Anesthesiology. 114*, 495–511. doi:10.1097/ALN.0b013e3181fcbfd9

American Society of Anesthesiologists. (2017). Practice guidelines for preoperative fasting and the use of pharmacologic agents to reduce the risk of pulmonary aspiration: Application to healthy patients undergoing elective procedures, An updated report by the American Society of Anesthesiologists Task Force on Preoperative Fasting and the Use of Pharmacologic Agents to Reduce the Risk of Pulmonary Aspiration. *Anesthesiology. 126*, 376–393. doi:10.1097/ALN.0000000000001452

Andrade, C. (2018). Internal, external, and ecological validity in research design, conduct, and evaluation. *Indian Journal of Psychological Medicine, 40*(5), 498–499. doi:10.4103/IJPSYM.IJPSYM_334_18

Aromataris, E., & Munn, Z. (Eds). (2017). *Joanna Briggs Institute Reviewer's Manual*. The Joanna Briggs Institute. Retrieved from https://reviewersmanual.joannabriggs.org

Balbale, S. N., Etingen, B., Malhiot, A., Miskevics, S., & LaVela, S. L. (2016). Perceptions of chronic illness among veterans with multiple chronic conditions. *Military Medicine, 181*(5), 439–444. doi:10.7205/MILMED-D-15-00207

Beck, C. T. (1993). Teetering on the edge: A substantive theory of post partum depression. *Nursing Research, 42*(1), 42–48. doi:10.1097/00006199-199301000-00008

Braun, K., & Zir, A. (2005). Using an interactive approach to teach nursing home workers about end-of-life care. *Journal of Hospice & Palliative Nursing, 7*(5), 280–288. doi:10.1097/00129191-200509000-00015

Buck, J. S., Chucta, S., Francis D. A., Vermillion, B. K., & Weber, M. L. (2017). Integrating the evidence-based practice competencies into the role of advanced practice nurses. In B. M. Melnyk, L. Gallagher-Ford, & E. Fineout-Overholt (Eds.), *Implementing the evidence-based practice competencies in healthcare: A practical guide for improving quality, safety, & outcomes* (pp. 205–224). Indianapolis, IN: Sigma Theta Tau International.

Buckwalter, K. C., Cullen, L., Hanrahan, K., Kleiber, C., McCarthy, A. M., Rakel, B., . . . Tucker, S. (2017). Iowa Model of Evidence-Based Practice: Revisions and validation. *Worldviews on Evidence-Based Nursing, 14*(3), 175–182. doi:10.1111/wvn.12223

Camargo, F. C., Iwamoto, H. H., Galvão, C. M., Pereira, G. de A., Andrade, R. B., & Masso, G. C. (2018). Competences and barriers for the evidence-based practice in nursing: An integrative review. *Revista Brasileira De Enfermagem, 71*(4), 2030–2038. doi:10.1590/0034-7167-2016-0617

Campo Guinea, N., Pumar-Méndez, M. J., Ara Lucea, P., & Cenizo Simón-Ricart, A. (2015). Impact of advanced nursing practice on staff development and evidence-based practice. *Revista De Enfermeria (Barcelona, Spain), 38*(7–8), 32–37. Retrieved from http://search.ebscohost.com/login.aspx?direct=true&db=mnh&AN=26448998&site=ehost-live

Cavlovich, D. (2016). The sacred cow project: Is your practice "udderly" out of date? *Nursing, 46*(11), 18–20. doi:10.1097/01.NURSE.0000502767.81097.d1

Centre for Reviews and Dissemination. (2008). Systematic reviews: CRD's guidance for undertaking reviews in health care [Internet]. York, UK: University of York. Retrieved from http://www.york.ac.uk/inst/crd/index_guidance.htm

Chon, T., Ma, A., & Mun-Price, C. (2017). Perioperative fasting and the patient experience. *Cureus, 9*(5), e1272. doi:10.7759/cureus.1272

Christmals, C. D., & Gross, J. J. (2017). An integrative literature review framework for postgraduate nursing research reviews. *European Journal of Research in Medical Sciences, 5*(1), 7–15.

Chulada, P. C., Arbes, S. J., Dunson, D., & Zeldin, D. C. (2003). Breast-feeding and the prevalence of asthma and wheeze in children: Analyses the Third National Health and Nutrition Examination Survey, 1988–1994. *Journal of Allergy and Clinical Immunology, 111*(2), 328–236. doi:10.1067/mai.2003.127

Cochrane Collaboration. (2018). *About us*. Retrieved from http://www.cochrane.org/about-us

Cope, D. G. (2014). Methods and meanings: Credibility and trustworthiness of qualitative research. *Oncology Nursing Forum, 41*(1), 89–91. doi:10.1188/14.ONF.89-91

Crenshaw, J. T., & Winslow, E. H. (2002). Preoperative fasting: Old habits die hard. *American Journal of Nursing, 102*(5), 36–44. doi:10.1097/00000446-200205000-00033

Crenshaw, J. T., & Winslow, E. H. (2008). Preoperative fasting duration and medication instruction: Are we improving? *Association of Operating Room Nurses Journal, 88*(6), 963–976. doi:10.1016/j.aorn.2008.07.017

Dang, D., & Dearholt, S. (Eds). (2018*). Johns Hopkins Nursing Evidence-Based Practice Model and guidelines* (3rd ed.). Indianapolis, IN: Sigma Theta Tau International.

EBSCO Publishing. (2018). *CINAHL databases*. Retrieved from http://www.ebscohost.com/nursing/products/cinahl-databases

Ersek, M., Grant, M. M., & Kraybill, B. M. (2005). Enhancing end-of-life care in nursing homes: Palliative Care Educational Resource Team (PERT) program. *Journal of Palliative Medicine, 8*(3), 556–566. doi:10.1089/jpm.2005.8.556

Evidence for Policy and Practice Information Coordinating Centre. (2018). *EPPI-Centre methods for conducting systematic reviews*. Retrieved from https://www.betterevaluation.org/sites/default/files/Methods.pdf

Fencl, J. L., & Matthews, C. (2017). Translating evidence into practice: How advanced practice RNs can guide nurses in challenging established practice to arrive at best practice. *AORN Journal, 106*(5), 378–392. doi:10.1016/j.aorn.2017.09.002

Fineout-Overholt, E., Levin, R. F., & Melnyk, B. (2004). Strategies for advancing evidence-based practice in clinical settings. *Journal of the New York Nurses' Association, 35*(2), 8–32.

Friesen, M. A., Brady, J. M., Milligan, R., & Christensen, P. (2017). Findings from a pilot study: Bringing evidence-based practice to the bedside. *Worldviews on Evidence-Based Nursing, 14*(1), 22–34. doi:10.1111/wvn.12195

Gabbay, J., & le May, A. (2004). Evidence based guidelines or collectively constructed "mindlines?" Ethnographic study of knowledge management in primary care. *British Medical Journal, 329*, 1013–1017. doi:10.1136/bmj.329.7473.1013

Gabbay, J., & le May, A. (2016). Mindlines: Making sense of evidence in practice. *The British Journal of General Practice: The Journal of the Royal College of General Practitioners, 66*(649), 402–403. doi:10.3399/bjgp16X686221

Group Health Research Institute. (2014). *The chronic care model.* Retrieved from http://www.improving-chroniccare.org/index.php?p=Model_Elements&s=18

Heavey, E. (2015). Differentiating statistical significance and clinical significance. *American Nurse Today, 10*(5), 26–28. Retrieved from http://search.ebscohost.com/login.aspx?direct=true&db=ccm&AN=103258353&site=ehost-live

Holloway, I., & Galvin, K. (2017). *Qualitative Research in Nursing and Healthcare* (4th ed.). Ames, IA: John Wiley and Sons, Inc.

Jensen, S. A., & Corralejo, S. M. (2017). Measurement issues: Large effect sizes do not mean most people get better–Clinical significance and the importance of individual results. *Child & Adolescent Mental Health, 22*(3), 163–166. doi:10.1111/camh.12203

Ko, E., Lee, J., & Hong, Y. (2016). Willingness to complete advance directives among low-income older adults living in the USA. *Health & Social Care in the Community, 24*(6), 708–716. doi:10.1111/hsc.12248

Kunte, V., Johansen, M. L., & Isenberg-Cohen, S. (2017). Improving long-term care residents' outcomes by educating nursing staff on end-of-life communication. *Journal of Hospice & Palliative Nursing, 19*(6), 550–555. doi:10.1097/NJH.0000000000000386

Lansing Community College Library. (2019). *What is PICOT?* Retrieved from http://libguides.lcc.edu/c.php?g=167860&p=6198388

McKechnie, L., Chabot, R., Dalmer, N., Julien, H. & Mabbott, C. (2016). Writing and reading the results: the reporting of research rigour tactics in information behaviour research as evident in the published proceedings of the biennial ISIC conferences, 1996–2014. *Information Research, 21*(4). Retrieved from http://www.informationr.net/ir/21-4/isic/isic1604.html

Melnyk, B. M. (2016). Level of evidence plus critical appraisal of its quality yields confidence to implement evidence-based practice changes. *Worldviews on Evidence-Based Nursing, 13*(5), 337–339. doi:10.1111/wvn.12181

Melnyk, B. M., & Fineout-Overholt, E. (2015). *Evidence-based practice in nursing and healthcare: A guide to best practice* (3rd ed.). Philadelphia, PA: Wolters Kluwer Health/Lippincott Williams & Wilkins.

Miller, J., Drummond-Hayes, D., & Carey, K. W. (2015). 20 questions: Evidence-based practice or sacred cow? *Nursing, 45*(8), 46–55. doi:10.1097/01.NURSE.0000469234.84277.95

Nelson, A. M. (2014). Best practice in nursing: A concept analysis. *International Journal of Nursing Studies, 51*(11), 1507–1516. doi:10.1016/j.ijnurstu.2014.05.003

O'Toole, T., Buckel, L., Bourgault, C., Redihan, S., Jiang, L., & Friedman, P. (2010). Applying the chronic care model to homeless veterans: Effect of a population approach to primary care on utilization and clinical outcomes. *American Journal of Public Health, 100*(12), 2493–2499. doi:10.2105/AJPH.2009.179416

Peterson, M. H., Barnason, S., Donnelly, B., Hill, K., Miley, H., Riggs, L., & Whiteman, K. (2014). Choosing the best evidence to guide clinical practice: Application of AACN levels of evidence. *Critical Care Nurse, 34*(2), 58–68. doi:10.4037/ccn2014411

Philipp, B. L., Merewood, A., Gerendas, E. J., & Bauchner, H. (2004). Breastfeeding information in pediatric textbooks needs improvement. *Journal of Human Lactation, 20*(2), 206–210. doi:10.1177/0890334404263921

Polit, D., & Beck, C. T. (2017). *Nursing research: Generating and assessing evidence for nursing practice* (10th ed.). Philadelphia, PA: Wolters Kluwer Health/Lippincott Williams & Wilkins.

Procaccini, D., & Mahony, J. (2014). *Survey of educational interventions to increase the breastfeeding initiation rates of urban clinic mothers.* Unpublished manuscript.

Riesenberg, L. A., & Justice, E. M. (2014). Conducting a successful systematic review of the literature, part 2. *Nursing, 44*(6), 23–26. doi:10.1097/01.NURSE.0000446641.02995.6a

Schaffer, M. A., Sandau, K. E., & Diedrick, L. (2013). Evidence-based practice models for organizational change: Overview and practical applications. *Journal of Advanced Nursing, 69*(5), 1197–1209. doi:10.1111/j.1365-2648.2012.06122.x

Thampy, M. S., Issa, H. A., Schostak, M. L., & Soto, R. G. (2018, October). To eat or not to eat: Examining adherence to ASA NPO guidelines among Michigan hospitals. Poster presented at *Anesthesiology, 2018*, Orlando, FL.

The Joanna Briggs Institute. (2018). *About us*. Retrieved from http://joannabriggs.org/about.html

Titler, M., Kleiber, C., Steelman, V., Rakel, B., Budreau, G., Everett, C., . . . Goode C. J. (2001). The Iowa Model of evidence-based practice to promote quality care. *Critical Care Nursing Clinics of North America, 13*(4), 497–509. doi:10.1016/S0899-5885(18)30017-0

U.S. National Library of Medicine. (2018). *About the National Library of Medicine*. Retrieved from http://www.nlm.nih.gov/about/index.html

Wakefield, A. (2014). Searching and critiquing the research literature. *Nursing Standard, 28*(39), 49–57. doi:10.7748/ns.28.39.49.e8867

Wakefield, A. (2015). Synthesizing the literature as part of a literature review. *Nursing Standard, 29*(29), 44–51. doi:10.7748/ns.29.29.44.e8957

Wright, K., Golder, S., & Rodriguez-Lopez, R. (2014). Citation searching: A systematic review case study of multiple risk behaviour interventions. *BMC Medical Research Methodology, 14*, 73. doi:10.1186/1471-2288-14-73

INTERNET RESOURCES

Centre for Reviews and Dissemination: http://www.york.ac.uk/inst/crd

Cochrane Handbook for Systematic Reviews of Interventions: https://community.cochrane.org/book_pdf/764

Cochrane Library, Access Options for the Cochrane Library: www.cochranelibrary.com/help/access

Cochrane: www.cochrane.org

Evidence for Policy and Practice Information and Co-ordinating Centre (University of London), EPPI-Centre Methods for Conducting Systematic Reviews: https://www.betterevaluation.org/sites/default/files/Methods.pdf

Instant RSS Search: http://ctrlq.org/rss

The University of Adelaide, Joanna Briggs Institute: http://joannabriggs.org

U.S. National Library of Medicine: http://www.nlm.nih.gov

U.S. National Library of Medicine, PubMed Tutorial: www.nlm.nih.gov/bsd/pubmed_tutorial/ml001.html

CHAPTER 6

USING INFORMATION TECHNOLOGY TO IMPROVE POPULATION OUTCOMES

LAURA P. ROSSI | ANN L. CUPP CURLEY

INTRODUCTION

Information technology that is designed to guide healthcare decisions is now available to both clinicians and consumers. Technological innovations have revolutionized the ways that healthcare can be delivered. There are more choices to make about how to deliver care and information can be accessed faster than ever before. Technology has simultaneously made the lives of healthcare providers and healthcare consumers easier and more difficult. Scientific studies are being published at an exponential rate making it difficult for clinicians to synthesize diagnostic and treatment options across various specialties. Similarly, metrics related to provider performance and healthcare system access and quality are posted and regularly updated for viewing by the public. Various online search engines have expanded the choices that consumers have to find providers. While all of these data are intended to improve decision-making about health, the plethora of available data can be confusing, making it difficult for patients and families to make decisions. Innovative technologies are also being developed to increase consumers' abilities to access their health information and communicate directly with healthcare providers. Healthcare providers can now monitor physiologic and behavioral data in real time. From computers to smartphones, the recent explosion in technology constantly offers patients and their healthcare providers new opportunities to stay connected and to manage care (Elenko, Underwood, & Zohar, 2015).

The fourth competency for the Doctor of Nursing Practice (DNP) degree as outlined by the American Association of Colleges of Nursing (AACN, 2006) states, "DNP graduates are distinguished by their abilities to use information systems/technology to support and improve patient care and healthcare systems, and provide leadership within healthcare systems and/or academic settings" (p. 12). This chapter describes resources that can be found on the Internet, how to evaluate them for quality, and how they can be used in practice to enhance population-based nursing.

USE OF THE INTERNET TO OBTAIN HEALTH INFORMATION

The Internet has revolutionized the way that consumers worldwide access information and communicate with each other. According to Internet World Stats (2018), there are over 4.2 billion Internet users in the world with as much as 95% penetration in North America. A survey conducted by Rock Health (2018) found that almost 80% of people in the United States went online for health information in 2017, and between 2016 and 2018 close to a quarter of Americans used their cell phone and/or wearable devices to track their health habits. Facebook is a major vehicle for accessing information although there are now many channels available including Twitter, LinkedIn, YouTube, Instagram, and WhatsApp. There is also a proliferation of tablet and smartphone applications that provide scientific as well as self-help information to consumers and providers.

The Pew Internet Project tracks Internet use in many fields and reports that social determinants influence access to and use of online searches for health information. The digital divide is a term used to describe disparities in the use of the Internet and other forms of technology. It is often defined by age (younger people are more likely to use the Internet than older people), income (wealthier people are more likely to use the Internet than less wealthy people), geography (people living in urban or suburban areas are more likely to use the Internet than people in rural areas), and education (people who use the Internet tend to have attained higher degrees than people who do not). In general, individuals most likely to turn to online health information include adults aged 18 to 49 from higher income households and those with caregiving responsibilities. It is important to note that access is a key component of use. People living in rural areas have less access to broadband services, and people with low incomes are less likely to own cell phones, tablets, lap tops and other similar devices (Pew Research Center, 2018).

Race, ethnicity, and gender also appear to have an influence on the use of online resources with Whites and women among the highest frequency users. Findings from a 2013 Pew U.S. survey revealed that 29% of people who live in the United States and who prefer to speak or use Spanish are not Internet users, compared with 14% of all U.S. adults. In contrast, adults over the age of 65 or those living with a disability tend to use online resources less frequently (Pew Research Center, 2013). APRNs must understand the patterns of technology preferences and use among different groups in order to effectively plan for the use of technology in direct care or healthcare program planning.

Over the last several years, Internet searches have primarily focused on the need for information about a specific disease or medical problem followed by specific medical treatments or procedures. In addition, the Internet also serves as an important source of information about navigating the healthcare system including selection of providers, hospitals, and insurance use. Past surveys have indicated that there is an interest in using the Internet for topics such as food and drug safety, pregnancy and elder care issues such as dementia, chronic illness, long-term care, and end of life (Fox, 2011).

The increasing availability of cell phone technology worldwide offers tremendous potential for expanding access and use to increase patient engagement and participation in healthcare. In 2010, 17% of people who owned a cell phone in the United States used it to search for health information online. By 2012, that number had increased to 31%. Among smartphone owners, 52% reported using their phone to find health or medical information and 19% downloaded an app to track health or medical information. In 2018, 95% of Americans across all demographic sectors reported having a cellphone of some kind. Access to smartphone technology has doubled although ownership varies with age, education, and household income. Interestingly, 20% of American adults, particularly young adults, non-Whites and lower-income individuals rely solely on their "smartphones" for Internet access and have abandoned traditional broadband service at home. In addition, about 75% of U.S. adults own desktop or laptop computers, 50% own tablet computers, and 20% own small hand-held electronic reading devices (Pew Research Center: Internet and Technology, 2018).

A high proportion of Internet users (approximately 37%) have an interest in finding information related to medicine and health (Pew Research Center: Science and Technology, 2015). This tends to be more common among women than men. Many individuals report using the Internet to reach out to others with similar health conditions in order to learn about someone's health experience or to simply connect with others who have similar health concerns. People with health insurance tend to access online information in the form of email updates, application forms, and seeking support more frequently than those who do not have health insurance. Some Internet users post health-related questions online or share their own personal health experience, with the majority of those reaching out to a general audience of friends or other Internet users. Interestingly, consumers do not report using the Internet to seek out information on online rankings of health services as frequently as they do for other, more personal, reasons (Fox & Duggan, 2013).

An annual survey of breast cancer patients in Germany revealed that the percentage of such patients who searched disease-specific information on the Internet increased significantly from 27% in 2007 to 37% in 2013 (Kowalski, Kahana, Kuhr, Ansmann, & Pfaff, 2014). Researchers studied the use of mobile technology by a population of parents using pediatric care centers that serve primarily urban, low-income, African American patients. They found that a large majority (97.0%) reported owning a cell phone and that of those, 91.1% used their phone to text and 78.5% used it to access the Internet. Although these parents used technology primarily for social networking, the researchers determined that most parents were interested in receiving health information or utilizing social networking to learn more about health topics. They concluded that "[m]obile technology and social networks may be an underutilized method of providing health information to underserved minority populations" (Mitchell, Godoy, Shabazz, & Horn, 2014, Para 5).

Hitlin (2018) writes that the United States has reached a plateau in the number of people who access the Internet. This is due to the near saturation levels that have been reached. More than 90% of adults younger than 50 years are regularly online or use a smartphone, and there has been a marked shift in the number of people who rely solely on a smartphone to access the Internet. There are also new connected devices emerging for use in daily life such as smart TVs, wearable devices, household thermostats, and security systems.

With this general reliance on technology, there is a concern that many without access face additional barriers or difficulties during their healthcare experiences. Many people are still unable to afford or access technology; those in rural areas often cite limited high-speed Internet availability in their community as an issue. For others, especially the elderly, there are physical or emotional limitations affecting their willingness and/or ability to adopt new technology.

APRNs must be attentive to not only the disparities in access to technology but also the patient's abilities and motivation to use available technology. While there is a lot of valuable and high-quality information online, consumers can often be confused by the amount of data and unprepared to reconcile different facts in relation to their own conditions. There must be a realistic appraisal of the opportunities to use technology for self-care skill development in different populations. When there are limitations at the individual level, appropriate assistance for adoption or alternative sources of information must be available as systems increasingly shift to online materials and processes. Aggregating such utilization data (e.g., who uses the Internet, what types of information they are looking for, and what types of devices and methods they use to search for information) can provide insights into the needs for program development as discussed in Chapter 7, Concepts in Program Design and Development.

While access to timely information can be very beneficial, many websites are challenged to update their information and/or provide sufficient information for application in individual situations. An international survey commissioned by researchers at the London School of Economics determined that 81% of people with access to the Internet use it to search for advice about health, medicine, and medical conditions, but only about 25% of these users check where the information comes from. The countries that were surveyed for this study included Australia, Brazil, China, France, Germany, India, Italy, Mexico, Russia, Spain, the United Kingdom, and the United States (McDaid & Park, 2011). This underscores the imperative for APRNs to be knowledgeable and use discretion in selecting valid and reliable sources of information for use in guiding healthcare.

Accuracy of Internet Sites

People may find that they can access health information on the Internet more readily and conveniently than they can by reaching a healthcare provider. However, studies have shown that the Internet provides both accurate and inaccurate information. This requires that providers recommend appropriate sites and provide guidance to patients about how they can evaluate the various sources on online information sites. De Freitas,

Falls, Haque, and Bursztajn (2013) reviewed the literature related to online pharmaceutical marketing, undue influence and the psychology of decision-making among Internet users. Several factors appear to make the public more vulnerable to misinformation on such sites including the degree to which the individual may be socially isolated, dependent on the Internet, and excessively trusting in the veracity of online information. Frequently, people are unaware of a company's influence through advertising. Diviani, van den Putte, Giani, and van Weert (2015) examined health literacy and its effect on the ability of persons to evaluate the effectiveness and accuracy of online information. Not unexpectedly, they determined that effective and informed evaluation of online health information is negatively impacted by low health literacy. For these reasons, healthcare providers should not underestimate the need to assess a patient's vulnerability and ability to evaluate the appropriateness of a website.

Various social networking sites and communication methods, such as Facebook, LinkedIn, Pinterest, Tumblr, Twitter, Instagram, email, chat rooms, and texting, can also be used to exchange information with other people with similar health conditions. Farrell (2018) used Google to search for online discussion forums on common childhood ailments and evaluated five of them for accuracy of information. This author found that the majority of information on these sites was accurate and not a major problem for sharing of inaccurate information. While the social support aspects of social media can be both helpful and accurate, misinformation can be a concern because opinion and hearsay are often shared without scientific evidence or rebuttal.

There are many studies that illustrate the importance of being vigilant in knowing the patterns of Internet use by consumers. Modave, Shokar, Penaranda, and Nguyen (2014) completed an analysis of Internet sites that provide information on weight loss. Of the 103 websites that were analyzed, none scored the optimal 16 points on the researchers' scale. Only 5% of the websites scored at least an 8/12 on the section measuring physical activity, behavior, and nutrition content. Although government and university websites scored the highest on the researchers' evaluation scale, these sites tended to appear on pages 2 or 3 of the search. The researchers noted that the information that was most likely to be accessed by searchers is substandard because quality sites may be posted further down in the search. Narasimhulu, Karakash, Weedon, and Minkoff (2016) conducted a study to assess patterns of Internet use in pregnancy in a diverse inner-city population. They also examined the accuracy of pregnancy-related information obtained from the Internet. These researchers reported that the online information accessed by these women was not uniformly accurate.

Chan et al. (2012) searched the Internet using three different Internet search engines for websites that provide health-related information for gastrointestinal cancers. They assessed the websites using a scoring system that ranged from −84 (*poor*) to 90 (*very good*). The median score for the websites that they assessed was 53. The highest score was for pancreatic cancer (65) and esophageal cancer (61) sites. Rectal (50), gastric (49), and colon (48) sites scored the lowest. They also found that the best overall sites were charitable websites, which scored a median of 79. The authors noted that gastrointestinal cancers are the most common cancer for which Internet searches are performed.

Ten diabetes-focused social media sites were evaluated for quality of information and privacy protection of users (Weitzman, Cole, Kaci, & Mandl, 2011). The authors noted that only 50% of the sites presented evidence-based information, and inaccurate information about diabetes and ads for unfounded "cures" were found on three sites. In fact, of nine sites with advertising, transparency was missing on five. They also found that privacy protection was poor, "with almost no use of procedures for secure data storage and transmission; only three sites supported member controls over personal information" (p. 5).

Website development is in constant flux and somewhat inconsistent without any regulations for accuracy and quality. It is critical that APRNs understand how to evaluate websites for current and accurate information given the evidence that many Internet consumers do not confirm the validity of the Internet resources that they use. APRNs have an opportunity to better serve their population by helping consumers use the Internet wisely and directing them to sites that provide evidence-based information and privacy protection.

Evaluating Online Information

The Medical Library Association (MLA), the Health on the Net (HON) Foundation, and the U.S. National Library of Medicine (NLM) provide guidelines for evaluating online information. Links to these sites can be found in Table 6.1. The NLM has partnered with MedlinePlus to create a useful tutorial for all audiences entitled *Evaluating Internet Health Information: A Tutorial from the National Library of Medicine*, which is accessible through the NLM website at ods.od.nih.gov/Health_Information/How_To_Evaluate_Health_Information_on_the_Internet_Questions_and_Answers.aspx.

There are commonalities present in all of the guidelines. The following questions can be used to evaluate Internet sites for healthcare information.

TABLE 6.1 Links for Evaluating Online Information

RESOURCE	INTERNET ADDRESS	INFORMATION AVAILABLE
Medical Library Association	www.mlanet.org	Use the "For Health Consumers and Patients" link to find the MLA user's guide to finding and evaluating health information on the web, MLA's top health websites, and Deciphering Medspeak (What Did My Doctor Say?).
U.S. National Library of Medicine	www.nlm.nih.gov/hinfo.html	Use the health information site to find the guide to healthy web surfing, medical information on the Internet tutorial (from MEDLINE), Health Library Directory, dozens of links for safe health resources for consumers.
Health on the Net Foundation	www.hon.ch/HONcode/Patients/visitor_safeUse2.html	Includes guidelines for evaluating websites and the criteria for HONcode accreditation.

- Who runs the site?

  Check the address (uniform resource locator or URL) of the website. Government sites have *.gov* in the address, educational institutions have *.edu*, and professional sites have *.org* suffixes. Commercial sites have *.com* in the address. Commercial sites may exist for commercial reasons—to sell products—but many provide useful and balanced information. Go to the "About Us" page. The sponsor and the credentials of the people who run the site should be clearly identified. The site should also include a method for contacting the webmaster or the people responsible for maintaining the site.

- Why have they created the site?

  The site should identify its intended audience. Some sites have separate sections for consumers and for health professionals, whereas other sites are designed exclusively for either health professionals or consumers.

- Who is sponsoring the site? Does the information favor the sponsor?

  The website should disclose all financial relationships such as the source of funding for the site. Advertisements should be clearly labeled as such. Users should examine sites for balanced information that does not favor a sponsor.

- Where did the information come from? Is the information reviewed by experts?

  Websites should provide the credentials of contributors and the process for selecting information that is posted. Look for information on an editorial board; this can usually be found on the "About Us" page. Look for a statement that indicates that it is a peer-reviewed site. The information on the site should be presented clearly and should be factual, not opinion.

- Is it up to date?

  Websites, especially those that provide health-related information, should be current and updated on a regular basis. Dates should be clearly posted.

- What is the privacy policy?

  There should be a privacy policy posted on the site. Check the policy to see whether information is shared. Do not provide personal information unless the privacy policy clearly states what information is and is not shared (MLA, 2019; MedlinePlus, 2016).

The general public should be vigilant when using the World Wide Web. APRNs should provide their patients with a list of reliable health websites to visit, and patients should be encouraged to visit more than one site to check information. Patients can be taught to look for the seal of certification from an accrediting organization, such as the HON Foundation, and they need to be cautioned to avoid believing "claims or promises of miraculous cures, wonder drugs, and other extreme statements unless there is proof to these claims" (HON Foundation, 2010, para. 8).

The HON Foundation is a private organization that has created a code of conduct for medical and health websites (HONcode). It does not rate the quality of information but holds website developers to basic ethical standards in the presentation of information. Both APRNs and patients can look for HONcode certification when searching for reliable websites. Certification is free of charge. All HONcode-certified sites are reviewed annually. In addition to the annual review, the HON Foundation relies on users to report noncompliance with the HONcode and investigates complaints (HON Foundation, 2010). The HON Foundation code of conduct for medical and health websites can be found at www.hon.ch/HONcode/Webmasters/Conduct.html.

The Internet can be a very helpful tool for APRNs and their patients to use for monitoring and tracking progress as well as to explore alternative practices for the common goal of improving overall health. In recent years, there has been a proliferation of Internet applications (apps) intended to help patients with a variety of self-care tasks. While similar concerns about the accuracy of the evidence base and the lack of regulation exist, apps also require attention to usability, privacy, security, and functionality. Boudreaux et al. (2014) recommend several strategies to guide their evaluation and selection. Searching the scientific literature, app clearinghouses and app stores related to the use of a particular app can be useful in understanding a complete description of the app, any comparable products to address the specific self-care behavior, as well as user ratings and reviews. These search strategies are often limited by the lack of formal trials and standards and the difficulties in finding current information as new technology is almost continuously evolving. Using social media to query professionals and patient groups can provide guidance in the process of selecting an app for a particular population.

Perhaps the most effective techniques to guide selection of an app are in piloting its use and eliciting feedback from the patient population for whom the app is being selected. This will provide essential insights into the factors affecting the usefulness of the app for the targeted disease or health behavior and what might be required for successful implementation in the practice setting. More primary research is needed to determine the efficacy of health apps and their impact on health outcomes.

In the meantime, patients, consumers, and healthcare professionals need to be educated on good practices of data sharing and access when they go online or use an app. It is critical that APRNs encourage patients to discuss anything they learn on the Internet with their healthcare provider and confirm that their patients are capable of evaluating health-related websites. In particular, Staccini and Lau (2018) suggest there is a need for more emphasis on considering the privacy features in the app's design, specific approaches to consent and data sharing mechanisms for users, as well as any socio-demographic characteristics that may influence access to personal health information.

USING TECHNOLOGY TO IMPROVE POPULATION HEALTH

While new technologies are creating revolutionary changes in healthcare delivery and how healthcare is being delivered, they are not universally available or put into practice.

The current evidence suggests, however, that more technology will be introduced in the future to manage patient population health outcomes. This will be a key strategy to help improve access and communication with healthcare providers related to the assessment of health needs, symptom monitoring, and the evaluation of treatment responses. This section provides a brief summary of some of the technologies currently in use.

Telemonitoring and Telehealth Strategies

Telehealth is now considered a reliable and very promising method to increase access to populations particularly in rural and underserved areas. Healthcare providers working with various populations have reported excellent results when using technology in their practices to improve patient communication and population outcomes. Jones, Lekhak, and Kaewluang (2014) described a meta-review of the use of mobile telephony and short message service (SMS) to deliver self-management interventions for chronic health conditions. In their analysis of 11 systematic reviews, SMS texting improved adherence to appointment attendance and adherence with antiretroviral therapy and short-term tobacco smoking quit rates. Texting was considered to be an effective strategy regardless of age or socioeconomic status and allowed for individualization of the delivered message.

Wendel, Brossart, Elliot, McCord, and Diaz (2011) designed a program to increase access to mental health services in a rural Texas community and to address the obstacles including limited healthcare resources and a shortage of healthcare professionals. Rural settings have significant health disparities compared to urban communities, and one of the contributing factors is limited access to healthcare resources. Recognizing distance to medical clinics or hospitals was a key barrier to access for rural residents, the researchers evaluated a collaborative effort to improve transportation to services and combined this with a telehealth-based counseling program. Their experience led them to conclude that telehealth is a promising method for providing care to hard-to-reach patients. The authors note that it is imperative that there is a mechanism for secure transmissions and maintaining privacy when technology is used to transmit communications between providers and patients. They also reported that technical difficulties during the study caused some interruption in services. Protecting patient confidentiality and providing reliable services are hallmarks of good care. When planning services using advanced technologies, APRNs need to be aware of both the benefits and the barriers. It is essential that experts in the use of technology are included as team members to help design new interventions that incorporate the use of technology.

Avdal, Kizilci, and Demirel (2011) identified transportation as an important barrier to accessing care in rural communities and in urban areas with poor public transportation. They studied the use of telehealth in improving the outcomes of diabetic patients in Turkey. They explained that there is limited access to the Internet in Turkey. People with diabetes are monitored and treated in polyclinics that provide outpatient services for a wide range of health conditions. Polyclinics are often considered to be problematic due to overcrowding and patient difficulties reaching healthcare providers in a timely manner. In addition, people in Turkey must frequently travel long distances to reach polyclinics. The result is that people with diabetes are often poorly monitored. At baseline, hemoglobin A1C (HbA1C) levels were similar in both groups (non-telemed group and telemed group). Six months after the study began, HbA1C levels were significantly lower in the experimental group, whereas no changes were detected in the control group. The authors were encouraged by the results and concluded that telehealth is effective as a complementary tool to help patients manage their chronic health conditions.

Access is not always a function of the physical distance between aggregates and healthcare providers. In some cases, patients can become socially isolated because of their physical or financial limitations. The following are examples of how web-based technology has the potential to alleviate problems with access to services and to improve population outcomes. Oliver, Wittenberg-Lyles, Demiris, and Oliver (2010) carried out a project to engage residents in long-term care in "virtual" sightseeing. Their study was built on the work of earlier researchers who have demonstrated the positive effects of activity programs in long-term care facilities. The authors tested the feasibility of using live videoconferencing to establish communication between residents in a long-term care facility in Iowa and researchers in Athens, Greece. The overall goal of the study was to "open the world of travel for residents confined in long-term care settings and to engage residents in 'virtual' sightseeing of foreign settings" (p. 93). These authors documented that the residents who took part in this feasibility study became clearly engaged in the activity. They noted that, through technology, nursing homes can offer residents a way to explore the world outside of their usual environment, and they challenged researchers to build an evidence base to demonstrate the long-term value of this initiative on clinical outcomes for nursing home residents. Such studies offer tantalizing glimpses into the possibilities of using technology to enrich the lives of people in long-term care.

Many studies have also been conducted to determine how the use of technology can improve specific population outcomes and self-care behaviors alone and in combination with other interventions. Barnason et al. (2017) conducted a literature review of studies related to cardiovascular patient self-management. Based on this review, the authors recommend bundled strategies as the most beneficial method in optimizing self-care. Nurse practitioners completed a feasibility study using cell phones to improve medication adherence among a group of homeless individuals. The individuals in the study were given phones and the results proved promising as evidenced by improved medication adherence (Burda, Haack, Duarte, & Alemi, 2012).

Choi, Lee, Kang, Lee, and Yoon (2014) described the use of a web-based application to assist patients with metabolic syndrome in improving dietary behaviors. The 16-week, web-based nutritional program resulted in a decrease in overall body weight, waist circumference, body fat, and body mass index (BMI). Nothwehr (2013) investigated the feasibility of using remote coaching and a handheld electronic device to increase the consumption of fruits and vegetables and decrease television viewing in an adult population, with encouraging results. The author made an important point in writing that "[t]here may be a strong novelty factor to the technology that encourages use" (p. 23). Long-term follow-up and re-evaluation are important measures for confirming the results of any intervention in population health. This is a factor

APRNs should remember when evaluating the usefulness of new technologies. Haze and Lynaugh (2013) described a successful pilot study using smartphone technology to improve nurse–patient communication between nurses and teenagers with asthma who were enrolled in an asthma management program. The teenagers involved in the pilot reported that they felt more comfortable communicating through texting than by telephone calls and that they asked more questions when texting. Nurses were encouraged by the increase in communication with their patients. These examples provide a good illustration of the potential improvements that can occur as a result of effective technology use and underscores the need for nurses to consider the use of technology in designing new interventions for specific populations.

Mobile Technology

Mobile technology is being increasingly integrated into the care of patients to maximize the reach of healthcare services. Early work by Lorig, Ritter, Laurent, and Plant (2006) randomized patients with chronic diseases (heart, lung, or type 2 diabetes) to usual care control (501) or an intervention group (457) using an Internet program without face to face interaction. They used reminders to engage patients in learning about self-care management. When they compared the results of each group, they found comparable results. Free et al. (2013) completed a systematic review of the literature and concluded that text messaging is effective in facilitating behavior change to promote medication adherence and smoking cessation. Hilty, Chan, Hwang, Wong, and Bauer (2017) reviewed opportunities for integrating mobile technology into mental healthcare and identified the need for clinicians to develop skills in mobile health as well as a need for more research on such technologies with an emphasis on effectiveness.

Electronic Health Records and Health Information Exchange

E-health is a growing field. Technological innovation is transforming how healthcare is delivered and expanding the ways that APRNs can communicate with patients. There are a number of platforms that can connect APRNs to patients and/or other healthcare providers. Information can be exchanged via teleconferencing, webcasts, podcasting (delivery of audio, text, pictures, and/or video to a computer or mobile device), and Twitter (text-based messages sent through a social networking site), to name just a few. Communication devices range from tabletop home computers and laptops to tablets and smartphones. Recent evidence suggests that there are strong preferences for "how to" learning through video demonstrations rather than receiving information through printed text (Smith, Toor, & Van Kessel, 2018).

A nationwide random-digit-dial survey conducted in December 2011 revealed that most respondents believed that electronic health records (EHRs) and health information exchange (HIE) would improve healthcare quality especially when respondents' doctors had an EHR (Ancker, Silver, Miller, & Kaushal, 2013). EHRs are now in widespread use following the federal EHRs incentive programs designed to promote HIE. Many institutions have created patient portals that allow patients to communicate directly with providers, access health records, and make appointments. OpenNotes evolved as the result of an international movement that urges healthcare providers to make notes that are written during visits available to patients to read. OpenNotes is not a software program but rather a process that supports transparent communication between providers and patients (OpenNotes, 2019).

Tailoring the Approach for the Population

APRNs need to be mindful of both the usefulness and the limitations of technology. How much trust people have in information that they obtain online varies from individual to individual. Their level of trust can be influenced by their interest in the specific piece of information, their level of stress, their sense of urgency, and how engaged they are in their plan of care (Horrigan, 2017). It has been estimated that 49% of people can be characterized as relatively disengaged and not enthusiastic about obtaining additional information or education from online sources, while approximately 40% are very interested and engaged (Horrigan, 2017). Before making a decision about using online resources to supplement patient care, APRNs need to first assess how receptive patients are to this method of communication.

The examples cited in this chapter provide a glimpse into the opportunities open to APRNs for being creative in using technology to improve patient outcomes. Because this is a relatively new way to provide care, there is a dearth of literature on long-term follow-up to evaluate the impact of technology on patient outcomes, and few studies have been replicated. There are also barriers to the use of new technologies such as individual competency, system downtimes, privacy concerns, and disparities among groups related to availability and use patterns. Assessing populations for their patterns of technology use is an important part of the APRN's role. Equally important is the design of interventions that make use of new technologies while measuring the impact on relevant population outcomes. Research and program evaluations are needed to fully evaluate the advantages and disadvantages of using technology in populations to improve health while maintaining privacy and sustainability.

E-RESOURCES THAT SUPPORT POPULATION-BASED NURSING

There are many Internet resources identified throughout this text that can be used to support population-based nursing. Table 6.2 provides a number of such online sites. The list and the descriptions of the sites are not meant to be exhaustive, but can be used as a guide by APRNs to find sources of reliable health information.

The pre-eminent international source of health information is the World Health Organization (WHO). The U.S. Department of Health and Human Services (DHHS) is the U.S. government's principal agency for protecting the health of all Americans. It provides essential services (such as Medicare) and administers more grant dollars than all other federal agencies combined. Government sites (which have .gov in the

TABLE 6.2 Internet Resources That Support Population-Based Nursing

GOVERNMENT	LINK	DESCRIPTION
Agency for Healthcare Research and Quality	www.ahrq.gov	Information to guide consumers, employers, policymakers and healthcare provider in decision making including health information technology (IT) tools, recent research findings, available databases and funding opportunities for research.
Centers for Disease Control and Prevention	www.cdc.gov	Preeminent source of information for consumers, health professionals, policy makers, researchers, and educators including a large range of topics, including U.S. trend data and available clinical and educational tools (BMI calculator and educational slides) as well as professional reports (Emerging Infectious Diseases [EID], Morbidity & Mortality Weekly Report [MMWR], Preventing Chronic Disease [PCD], etc.)
Healthfinder.gov	https://healthfinder.gov	Easy-to-understand information about preventive health and how to access services. Health facilities and providers. A Guide to Everyday Healthy Living is available on various topics.
Let's Move!	https://letsmove.obamawhitehouse.archives.gov	Excellent resource accessible via Facebook, Twitter and Meetup related to First Lady Michelle Obama's campaign against obesity; provides nutritional information for consumers and healthcare providers specific to childhood obesity and increasing access to healthy foods and physical activities at school and in the community.
National Center for Complementary and Integrative Health	https://nccih.nih.gov/health/webresources	Source of information about research and application of complementary health products and practices.
National Center for Health Statistics	https://www.cdc.gov/nchs	Full range of statistical data produced by the federal government linking to more than 100 agencies that provide data and trend information on such topics as diseases, demographics, education, healthcare, and crime.
National Partnership for Action to End Health Disparities	https://minorityhealth.hhs.gov/npa	Guidance for various stakeholders on the reduction of health disparities with links to specific organizational efforts.
StopBullying.gov	http://www.stopbullying.gov	Information for all ages about the recognition, prevention and termination of bullying and available services.
The National Guideline Clearinghouse	www.guideline.gov	Public resource within AHRQ site for evidence-based practice guidelines. This site is no longer funded. Guideline acceptance ended in March, 2018.
The National Institutes of Health	www.nih.gov	Information about research funding and many science and health topics including slides and print material.
U.S. Department of Health and Human Services	www.hhs.gov	Broad range of information related to health care including programs, insurance, laws and regulations. Project funding announcements are also available.

(continued)

TABLE 6.2 Internet Resources That Support Population-Based Nursing (*continued*)

GOVERNMENT	LINK	DESCRIPTION
Education		
American Nurses Association	www.nursingworld.org	Official source of information for professional registered nurses in the United States with 54 constituent member nurses associations and affiliations with 35 specialty nursing and workforce advocacy affiliate organizations; outlines standards of practice, lobbies and regulatory agencies affecting nurses and the general public including an online consumer health resource developed and launched in 2011.
American Public Health Association	www.apha.org	Professional source of information for public health professionals whose goals are to increase access to healthcare, protect funding for core public health services, and eliminate health disparities.
HealthCareandYou.org	www.healthcareandyou.org	Explanation of the provisions and benefits in the Affordable Care Act by state in language and format accessible to consumers
Howard Gotlieb Archival Research Center, Boston University	hgar-srv3.bu.edu/collections/nursing	Widely respected source of nursing history addressing the early years of nursing and public health including a collection of personal and professional papers, including 250 of Florence Nightingale's letters and records of schools and organizations within this country and internationally.
National Academy of Medicine (formerly the Institute of Medicine)	https://nam.edu	Independent, nonprofit, nongovernmental source (within the National Academy of Sciences) with "unbiased and authoritative advice to decision makers and the public" responsive to mandates from Congress, federal agencies, and independent organizations; list of available reports published after 1998.
The American Nurses Credentialing Center, A Subsidiary of ANA	https://www.nursingworld.org/ancc	Source of standards for professional nursing certification, continuing nursing education accreditation, and oversight for the Magnet Recognition Program.
Nonprofit		
American Cancer Society	www.cancer.org	Independent, nonprofit source of science, practice guidelines and related health information for cancer prevention and treatment including resources and software applications for educators, consumers, and healthcare professionals at all levels.
American Heart Association	www.heart.org	Independent, nonprofit source of science, practice guidelines and related health information for prevention and treatment of cardiovascular disease and stroke including resources and software applications for educators, consumers, and healthcare professionals at all levels.
Asthma and Allergy Foundation of America	www.aafa.org	Independent, nonprofit source of science, practice guidelines and related health information for prevention and treatment of asthma and allergies including resources and software applications for educators, consumers, and healthcare professionals at all levels.

(continued)

TABLE 6.2 **Internet Resources That Support Population-Based Nursing (*continued*)**

GOVERNMENT	LINK	DESCRIPTION
The Pew Research Center, A Subsidiary of the Pew Charitable Trusts	www.pewresearch.org	Respected source of public information from polls, demographic research, media content analysis, and other empirical social science research reflecting the issues, attitudes, and trends shaping America and the world.
International		
World Health Organization (Arm of the United Nations)	www.who.int	Source of global health matters and technical support for different countries related to health trends including publications and resources in many languages on disease outbreaks, various health topics and evidence-based based clinical guidelines; multimedia site with information via podcasts and videos on various health topics for international travelers
Commercial		
Medscape	www.medscape.com	Online, peer-reviewed, free resource for health professionals including peer-reviewed original articles and continuing medical and nursing education; offers a customized version of the NLM's MEDLINE database, a drug interaction checker, and a drug reference, with free downloadable apps for health professionals. Copyright restrictions and privacy protection apply.
Analytic		
Epi Info	www.cdc.gov/epiinfo	A collection of free software tools available through the CDC website that can be used to create questionnaires, download data, and perform advanced statistical analyses and geographic information system (GIS) mapping that allows users to map trends in disease or outcomes of interest using zip codes or city boundaries and integrate data into a geographic map to summarize health services utilization data based on geographic location
The Visual Statistics System (ViSta)	www.uv.es/visualstats/Book	Free, downloadable statistical system that can be used for both descriptive and inferential analytic analyses. (copyright restrictions apply)

URL) are a rich source of information and offer a variety of resources for both consumers and healthcare providers. Nongovernmental websites are also a source of excellent information for healthcare providers and consumers. Sites with .edu in the address are owned by educational institutions. Many universities, particularly those that offer health-related degrees, have extensive resources available for people who are looking for information on health-related topics. Many professional organizations are operated as not-for-profits and work to further the interests of a profession and to protect the public. They are generally a rich source of information on the healthcare professions and usually have .org in the address. APRNs should search their specialty organizations for resources and information.

Nonprofit organizations use their earnings to pursue their goals by providing resources to support and disseminate new knowledge to professionals and the general public. Well-known examples are the American Heart Association (AHA), the American Cancer Society (ACS), and the Asthma and Allergy Foundation of America (AAFA). Many of these sites have an impressive amount of information and resources available, often free of charge. Most of these groups have .org in their URLs. Many commercial (.com) sites can also be useful but should be evaluated carefully to ensure balance and accuracy in the information provided.

The Not-So-Hidden Dangers of Social Media in Healthcare

Many professional organizations have written guidelines for the use of social media. It is critical that APRNs remember at all times that patient confidentiality is both a legal and an ethical responsibility. Complaints to state boards of nursing against nurses who use social media usually fall within the following areas (Spector & Kappel, 2012):

- Breach of privacy or confidentiality against patients
- Failure to report others' violations of privacy against patients
- Lateral violence against colleagues
- Communication against employers
- Boundary violation
- Employer/faculty use of social media against employees/students

There are a number of important considerations for APRNs who engage in an online presence. The Internet can be a valuable tool for patient care, communication, and social interaction and for boosting one's career, but nurses have also been fired, lost their licenses, and experienced bullying, all within the context of social media. The National Council of State Boards of Nursing (NCSBN) has produced social media guidelines for nurses. A video is available at www.ncsbn.org/347.htm, and *A Nurse's Guide to Professional Boundaries* (*NCSBN*) is located at www.ncsbn.org/ProfessionalBoundaries_Complete. pdf. Among the most important facts for people who use social media to remember is that once information is posted on the Internet, it is posted permanently and that privacy settings are not 100% effective.

SUMMARY

Technological innovation has led to a whole new lexicon for healthcare providers and has also provided new methods and opportunities for improving population outcomes. Email alerts, really simple syndication (RSS), podcasts, videoconferencing, and Twitter are efficient and cost-effective ways to "keep connected" and to deliver healthcare information to both consumers and healthcare professionals. E-health provides a means to bridge distances between patients and healthcare providers and is a creative option for providing patient care. In the fast-moving world of healthcare, technology provides a convenient way to keep up to date. Software apps that can be downloaded to mobile devices and updated on a regular basis make available immediate and important information (such as drug interactions/calculations) to APRNs and other healthcare providers.

To provide excellent and up-to-date clinical care, APRNs need to be technologically literate and willing to explore new ways to deliver healthcare. APRNs should evaluate their Internet and other technological resources carefully and use them to advance their practices to provide the latest evidence-based care possible. They also need to stay current in their knowledge of the latest technology and guide their patients to resources that are valid and useful. There are both challenges and opportunities to improve patient care through the use of new technology. Of primary concern are the legal and ethical responsibilities related to patient privacy. Regardless of these challenges, technology is here to stay, and it is the responsibility of APRNs to educate themselves and their patients on the many benefits of technology while adhering to patient privacy.

EXERCISES AND DISCUSSION QUESTIONS

Exercise 6.1 Online databases are a rich source of information for healthcare professionals. Use the following Centers for Disease Control and Prevention database to research the state that you live or work in: Go to https://www.cdc.gov/nchs/data-visualization/mortality-leading-causes/index.htm

- How do the leading causes of death in your state compare to U.S. figures?
- Identify five important risk factors that need to be targeted in your state.
- Identify vulnerable groups for whom targeted services need to be provided.

Exercise 6.2 Using the criteria and guidelines provided in this chapter, identify two credible websites for patients with a chronic illness who manage their own care at home. Consider sources that address self-management practices such as diet, activity, and medication management. What are the strengths and weaknesses of the sites that you found?

Exercise 6.3 Identify at least two technological innovations that are used to manage the care of the population that you serve. What factors influenced the choice of these particular innovations? How do you (or how do you plan to) evaluate their effectiveness? What outcomes do you hope to achieve through their use?

REFERENCES

American Association of Colleges of Nursing. (2006). *The essentials of doctoral education for advanced practice nursing.* Retrieved from http://www.aacn.nche.edu/DNP/pdf/Essentials.pdf

Ancker, J. S., Silver, M., Miller, M. C. & Kaushal, R. (2013). Consumer experience with and attitudes toward health information technology: A nationwide survey. *Journal of the American Medical Informatics Association, 20*(1), 152–156. doi:10.1136/amiajnl-2012-001062

Avdal, U., Kizilci, S., & Demirel, N. (2011). The effects of web-based diabetes education on diabetes care results: A randomized control study. *Computers, Informatics, Nursing: CIN, 29*(2), 101–106. doi:10.1097/NCN.0b013e3182155318

Barnason, S., White-Williams, C., Rossi, L. P., Centeno, M., Crabbe, D. L., Lee, K. S., . . . Wood, K. (2017). Evidence for therapeutic patient education interventions to promote cardiovascular patient self-management: A scientific statement for healthcare professionals from the American Heart Association. *Circulation: Cardiovascular Quality and Outcomes, 10*(6), 1–6. doi:10.1161/HCQ.0000000000000025

Boudreaux, E. D., Waring, M. E., Hayes, R. B., Sadasivam, R. S., Mullen, S., & Pagoto, S. (2014). Evaluating and selecting mobile health apps: Strategies for healthcare providers and healthcare organizations. *Society of Behavioral Medicine, 4*(4), 363–371. doi:10.1007/s13142-014-0293-9

Burda, C., Haack, M., Duarte, A. C., & Alemi, F. (2012). Medication adherence among homeless patients: A pilot study of cell phone effectiveness. *Journal of the American Academy of Nurse Practitioners, 24*(11), 675–681. doi:10.1111/j.1745-7599.2012.00756.x

Chan, D., Willicombe, A., Reid, T., Beaton, C., Arnold, D., Ward, J., . . . Lewis, W. (2012). Relative quality of Internet-derived gastrointestinal cancer information. *Journal of Cancer Education, 27*(4), 676–679. doi:10.1007/s13187-012-0408-2

Choi, Y., Lee M. J., Kang, H. C., Lee, M. S., & Yoon, S. (2014). Development and application of a web-based nutritional management program to improve dietary behaviors for the prevention of metabolic syndrome. *Computers, Informatics, Nursing: CIN, 32*(5), 232–241. doi:10.1097/CIN.0000000000000054

De Freitas, J., Falls, B., Haque, O. S., & Bursztajn, H. J. (2013). Vulnerabilities to misinformation in online pharmaceutical marketing. *Journal of the Royal Society of Medicine, 106*, 184–189. doi:10.1177/0141076813476679

Diviani, N., van den Putte, B., Giani, S., & van Weert, J. C. (2015). Low health literacy and evaluation of online health information: A systematic review of the literature. *Journal of Medical Internet Research, 17*(5), e112. doi:10.2196/jmir.4018

Elenko, E., Underwood, L., & Zohar, D. (2015). Defining digital medicine. *Nature Biotechnology, 33*(5), 456. doi:10.1038/nbt.3222

Farrell, A. (2018). Accuracy of online discussion forums on common childhood ailments. *Journal of the Medical Library Association, 106*(4), 455–463. doi:10.5195/jmla.2018.355

Fox, S. (2011). *Health topics.* Retrieved from Pew Research Center Science and Technology website http://www.pewinternet.org/2011/02/01/health-topics-2

Fox, S., & Duggan, M. (2013). *Peer-to-peer health care.* Retrieved from Pew Research Center Internet and Technology website http://www.pewinternet.org/2013/01/15/peer-to-peer-health-care

Free, C., Phillips, G., Galli, L., Watson, L., Felix, L., Edwards, P., . . . Haines, A. (2013). The effectiveness of mobile-health technology-based health behaviour change or disease management interventions for health care consumers: A systematic review. *PLoS Medicine, 10*(1), e1001362. doi:10.1371/journal.pmed.1001362

Haze, K., & Lynaugh, J. (2013). Building patient relationships: A smartphone application supporting communication between teenagers with asthma and the RN care coordinators. *Computers, Informatics, Nursing: CIN, 31*(6), 266–271. doi:10.1097/NXN.0b013e318295e5ba

Health on the Net Foundation. (2010). *The HON code of conduct for medical and health Web sites (HONcode).* Retrieved from http://www.hon.ch/HONcode/Webmasters/Conduct.html

Hilty, D. M., Chan, S., Hwang, T., Wong, A., & Bauer, A. M. (2017). Advances in mobile mental health: Opportunities and implications for the spectrum of e-mental health services. *mHealth, 3*(34). doi:10.21037/mhealth.2017.06.02

Hitlin, P. (2018). *Internet, social media use and device ownership in the U.S. have plateaued after years of growth.* Retrieved from Pew Research Center web site http://www.pewresearch.org/fact-tank/2018/09/28/internet-social-media-use-and-device-ownership-in-u-s-have-plateaued-after-years-of-growth

Horrigan, J. B. (2017). *How people approach facts and information.* Retrieved from Pew Research Center Internet & Technology web site http://www.pewinternet.org/2017/09/11/how-people-approach-facts-and-information

Internet World Stats. (2018). *Usage and population statistics.* Retrieved from https://www.internetworldstats.com

Jones, K. R., Lekhak, N., & Kaewluang, N. (2014). Using mobile phones and short message services to deliver self-management interventions for chronic conditions: A meta review. *Worldviews on Evidence-Based Nursing, 11*(2), 81–88. doi:10.1111/wvn.12030

Kowalski, C., Kahana, E., Kuhr, K., Ansmann, L., & Pfaff, H. (2014). Changes over time in the utilization of disease-related Internet information in newly diagnosed breast cancer patients 2007 to 2013. *Journal of Medical Internet Research, 16*(8), e195. doi:10.2196/jmir.3289

Lorig, K. R., Ritter, P. L., Laurent, D. D. & Plant K. (2006). Internet-based chronic disease self-management: A randomized trial. *Medical Care, 44*(11), 964–971. doi:10.1097/01.mlr.0000233678.80203.c1

McDaid, D., & Park, A. (2011). *Online health: Untangling the web.* Retrieved from https://www.researchgate.net/publication/232041614_Online_Health_Untangling_the_Web

Medical Library Association. (2019). For health consumers and patients: Find good health information. Retrieved from https://www.mlanet.org/page/find-good-health-information

MedlinePlus. (2016). *Evaluating Internet health information: A tutorial from the National Library of Medicine.* Retrieved from http://www.nlm.nih.gov/medlineplus/webeval/webeval.html

Mitchell, S. J., Godoy, L., Shabazz, K., & Horn, I. B. (2014). Internet and mobile technology use among urban African American parents: Survey study of a clinical population [Abstract]. *Journal of Medical Internet Research, 16*(1), e9. doi:10.2196/jmir.2673

Modave, F., Shokar, N., Penaranda, E., & Nguyen, N. (2014). Analysis of the accuracy of weight loss information search engine results on the Internet. *American Journal of Public Health, 104*(10), 1971–1978. doi:10.2105/AJPH.2014.302070

Narasimhulu, D. M., Karakash, S., Weedon, J., & Minkoff, H. (2016). Patterns of Internet use by pregnant women, and reliability of pregnancy-related searches. *Journal of Maternal Child Health, 20*, 2502–2509. doi:10.1007/s10995-016-2075-0

Nothwehr, F. (2013). People with unhealthy lifestyle behaviors benefit from remote coaching via mobile technology. *Evidence Based Nursing, 16*(1), 22–23. doi:10.1136/eb-2012-100953

Oliver, D. P., Wittenberg-Lyles, E., Demiris, G., & Oliver, D. (2010). Giving long-term care residents a passport to the world via the Internet. *Journal of Nursing Care Quality, 25*(3), 193–197. doi:10.1097/NCQ.0b013e3181d7964a

OpenNotes. (2019). *Everyone on the same page.* Retrieved from https://www.opennotes.org

Pew Research Center. (2013). *Who's not online? 5 factors tied to the digital divide.* Retrieved from http://www.pewresearch.org/fact-tank/2013/11/08/whos-not-online-5-factors-tied-to-the-digital-divide

Pew Research Center. (2018). *Digital divide persists even as lower-income Americans make gains in tech adoption.* Retrieved from http://www.pewresearch.org/fact-tank/2017/03/22/digital-divide-persists-even-as-lower-income-americans-make-gains-in-tech-adoption

Pew Research Center: Internet and Technology. (2018). *Mobile fact sheet.* Retrieved from http://www.pewinternet.org/fact-sheet/mobile

Pew Research Center: Science and Technology. (2015). *Public interest in science, health and other topics.* Retrieved from http://www.pewresearch.org/science/2015/12/11/public-interest-in-science-health-and-other-topics

Rock Health. (2018). *What 4K Americans think about digital health.* Retrieved from https://rockhealth.com/rock-weekly/what-4k-americans-think-about-digital-health

Smith, A., Toor, S., & Van Kessel, P. (2018). Many turn to YouTube for children's content, news, how-to lessons. Retrieved from Pew Research Center Internet and Technology website www.pewinternet.org/2018/11/07/many-turn-to-youtube-for-childrens-content-news-how-to-lessons

Spector, N., & Kappel, D. M. (2012). Guidelines for using electronic and social media: The regulatory perspective. *Online Journal of Issues in Nursing, 17*(3), 1. Retrieved from http://nursingworld.org/MainMenuCategories/ANAMarketplace/ANAPeriodicals/OJIN/TableofContents/Vol-17-2012/No3-Sept-2012/Guidelines-for-Electronic-and-Social-Media.html#NCSBN11e

Staccini, P., & Lau, A. Y. S. (2018). Findings from 2017 on consumer health informatics and education: Health data access and sharing. *Yearbook of Medical Informatics, 27*(1):163–169. doi:10.1055/s-0038-1641218

Weitzman, E. R., Cole, E., Kaci, L., & Mandl, K. D. (2011). Social but safe? Quality and safety of diabetes-related online networks. *Journal of American Medical Informatics Association, 18*(3), 292–297. doi:10.1136/jamia.2010.009712

Wendel, M. L., Brossart, D. F., Elliot, T. R., McCord, C., & Diaz, M. A. (2011). Use of technology to increase access to mental health services in a rural Texas community. *Family and Community Health, 34*(2), 134–140. doi:10.1097/FCH.0b013e31820e0d99

CHAPTER 7

CONCEPTS IN PROGRAM DESIGN AND DEVELOPMENT

LAURA ROSSI | ANN L. CUPP CURLEY

INTRODUCTION

Graduates of doctoral education for advanced nursing practice are expected to integrate nursing science with knowledge from other fields in order to provide the highest level of nursing care. They are also expected to develop and provide effective plans for "practice level and/or system-wide practice initiatives that will improve the quality of care delivery" (American Association of Colleges of Nursing [AACN], 2006, p. 11). In this chapter, the advanced practice registered nurse (APRN) will learn how to design new programs by addressing factors related to planning and organizational decision-making.

Effective program development requires the use of information that is accurate, pertinent, and timely. It is critical that programs be constructed in a way that takes into consideration factors that reflect the numerous internal and external forces that have the potential to impact the implementation and overall success of a program. Determining measures of success or desired outcomes when designing a program provides continuous check points for evaluation throughout program implementation. Program development, implementation, and evaluation will vary across geographic and practice settings because of the unique and varied characteristics of an APRN's practice.

SOURCES OF DATA

There are many stakeholders both within and outside of organizations whose support of a new program will be influenced by programmatic-related data. Clinical performance and patient outcomes data are often very meaningful to clinicians but that information must be assessed within the context of overall health outcomes and resource availability. Financial and health services utilization data are of critical importance to administrators who are challenged to support new program development while simultaneously managing the costs of care. Planners need to consider organizational goals to ensure a proper fit between an organization and a program. It is also important that they take into consideration the unique characteristics of the target population to ensure a proper fit between a program and a specific community. Data to guide program development are available from a number of sources.

Population-Level Data

Population demographics guide APRNs in the development of population-based programs. For example, communities have their own unique identifying characteristics. These characteristics include age, socioeconomic status, and ethnicity, among others. A program targeting the administration of the influenza vaccine during influenza season may look different when implemented in an urban area such as New York City versus a rural community such as farmland in Wisconsin. Information on population demographics as well as health service needs, utilization and performance trends are publicly available from many government websites. The U.S. Department of Health and Human Services (DHHS; www.hhs.gov/answers/research/find-social-service-research.html, healthdata.gov), the Agency for Healthcare Research and Quality (AHRQ; www.ahrq.gov/index.html) and the Centers for Disease Control and Prevention (CDC; www.cdc.gov/datastatistics) are three excellent sources of such information.

Existing data that can be used for benchmarking may be available to program planners and used to evaluate local health needs and program performance through registries that focus on the health status of a particular population, the care they receive, and their responses over a period of time. A recent survey (Blumenthal, 2017) identified a number of registries in the United States that are designed to capture broad scope data from a mix of automated and manual data capture methods. Among the most common registry elements are comorbidities, adverse events, organization demographics, patient-reported outcomes, laboratory and test imaging results, quality of life, pharmaceuticals, functional status, and patient experience. The American Medical Association (AMA) published *An Inventory of National Clinical Registries* (2015) on behalf of the National Quality Registry Network (NQRN) (tsihealthcare.com/wp-content/uploads/2014/05/National-Quality-Registry-Network-Listing.pdf). NQRN is a network of stakeholders who are interested in the development and use of registries for quality improvement purposes. Organizationally it operates within the Physician Consortium for Performance Improvement (PCPI®). For more information on NQRN, go to www.thepcpi.org.

Databases that address specific needs can also be developed by program planners. AHRQ provides guidance for the development of registries in their *AHRQ Registries for Evaluating Patient Outcomes: A User's Guide,* as well as access to existing databases (AHRQ Registry of Patient Registries) and standard data definitions that can facilitate analysis and comparisons across settings (www.ahrq.gov/news/blog/ahrqviews/disease-registries.html).

A complete assessment of patient/consumer needs and characteristics and comparisons of population outcomes against standard benchmarks provide necessary information for the planning of new programs.

Organization Level Data

APRNs are likely to develop new programs in the organization where they are employed. Often, there is organizational data that are available and accessible to guide the design of new programs or the restructuring of an existing program. For example, lengths of stay, readmissions, and other healthcare utilization data are a major focus for virtually all health systems. Developing programs to reduce lengths of stay and/or facilitate care transitions from hospital to home requires data related to the number of hospital discharges, disposition (e.g., home, rehabilitation, skilled nursing facility), patient demographics, primary discharge diagnoses, rehospitalization rate, and time from discharge to rehospitalization. A review of an organization's data might reveal a particular subset of patients with a specific need. For example, if a hospital's readmission rates for patients with heart failure trend above national benchmarks, an APRN could look at specific social determinants to determine which patients might benefit most from a transitional care program to minimize readmission rates. The introduction of the electronic health record provides new opportunities for evaluating patient populations and the impact of new programs within a specific organization or healthcare system. Close examination of the characteristics of a patient population (e.g., age, education, absence of insurance, access to a medical home) and the processes involved in discharge (e.g., ability to fill discharge medications, clear discharge instructions, medical equipment available for home use) can help guide the development of program components to reduce readmission rates. Having an understanding of the typical disease course for the patient population also helps in the identification of factors that contribute to readmission rates as well as the timing when a new program might be most beneficial. Organizational data also provide information that can be used to compare programs across specific agencies or health systems. Measuring program effectiveness is facilitated when standard benchmarks exist such as those that are available in national databases.

Consumer and Societal Trends and Demands

Consumer and societal trends and demands provide information or data that drive the rationale for designing a specific program. It is not cost-effective to support a program that does not meet an identified consumer need. A simple dictionary definition of a trend is the general direction in which something tends to move. In what direction is healthcare technology moving? In what direction are consumer attitudes and beliefs about disease prevention moving? Consumer and societal trends and demands are constantly changing, making it difficult to know which trends or demands to pay attention to and if they will continue and for how long. For example, in 2018 several IT trends were identified by HealthData Management including using IT to help achieve patient engagement and experience, protecting health information and data security, and rising importance of population health management (Bazzoli, 2018). Did these trends continue in 2020? Will they continue through 2021? Is a program designed in 2019 based on these trends still needed and viable in 2020? Will it be needed in 2021? It is critical for APRNs to examine on an ongoing basis the environment in which they practice to confirm the latest trends and demands or identify new ones.

Consumer attitudes and beliefs about how to access and manage healthcare are also changing. This creates a challenge in identifying which trends or demands to target in program development. As societal trends and demands shift, consumer needs and preferences also change, driving the demand for new programs. Consider the needs of an aging population in an era where hospital lengths of stay have declined and resources to provide care at home are limited. Changes in healthcare financing have resulted in higher copays for patients who may have multiple chronic conditions. It may not be cost-effective for health systems to develop or maintain programs that no longer meet an identified consumer or organizational need.

More than ever, consumers have access to information about the availability of healthcare services and programs. Quality and patient safety data related to institution and program performance are now publicly available on government, consumer, and institution websites. There is an expanding focus on transparency. The rapidly changing healthcare systems mandates that APRNs find ways to monitor and stay abreast of trends to confirm the viability of existing and/or new program opportunities in their practice environment. Involving consumers early in the program development process can be critical to developing a patient-centered process. Hibbard and Greene (2013) emphasize the evidence on the importance of patient engagement in healthcare reform and its potential for improving patients' outcomes and perceptions of their experience with services. While it is unclear how costs are impacted, they suggest that programs are most successful when they consider patient activation and flexible opportunities for tailored interventions. Such measures of patient activation can be useful in evaluating the intermediate outcomes of a program.

It is difficult to predict how long a trend will persist or endure, so staying abreast of consumer preferences and available options for care and self-management is essential. Programs are developed as a temporary bridge in anticipation of new technology becoming available. At other times, innovative programs can be nurtured and evolve as essential services that are available to a broader population. Careful consideration of the trends within and outside healthcare provide the basis for effective program development, sustainability, and growth.

INNOVATIVE CARE DELIVERY MODELS

Designing new programs requires creative thinking and innovation by nurse leaders to improve the outcomes of care within a cost- and resource-constrained environment. Most organizations now have an administrative structure that oversees efforts related to care redesign. Care delivery models or systems must operationalize the philosophy, values, and mission of an organization. Organizations place value on evidence-based practice, financial performance, program feasibility, and the achievement of improved outcomes of care. Programs must include rules and have structures that support accountability and operational processes. Specifically, they should identify who is accountable for expected outcomes and support strong relationships among key stakeholders and players.

A white paper commissioned by the Robert Wood Johnson Foundation outlined innovative care delivery models (2008). Twenty-four models were identified and categorized into acute care, bridging the continuum, or comprehensive care. Eight common elements or themes were noted throughout the models (Joynt & Kimball, 2008):

1. Elevated roles for nurses: nurses as care integrators

2. Migration to interdisciplinary care: team approach

3. Bridging the continuum of care

4. Pushing the boundaries: home as setting of care

5. Targeting high users of healthcare: elderly plus

6. Sharpened focus on the patient

7. Leveraging technology in care delivery

8. Driven by results: improving satisfaction, quality, and costs

The delivery of healthcare is an ever-changing process. Changes in the healthcare needs of a population should be addressed and routinely reassessed to ensure the program's original goals are being realized and the patients' needs are still being met. Iterative programmatic changes are often needed, but the end results must ultimately lead to improved patient health, decreased costs, and overall improved patient satisfaction. The process of care delivery in a specific program will vary with the population and service being provided. The white paper recommends nurse leaders consider the following elements in program development regardless of the type of care or method of its delivery:

- A specific population focus

- A team approach

- Consideration of the continuum of care, including the home environment

- Strategies to engage the patient/client

- Teaching or education

- A focus on results or outcomes

PROGRAM DEVELOPMENT: WHERE TO START

Justification

Program development requires considerable time and energy from many people. An important first step is assembling information gathered from various data sources. Establishing a data-driven justification is an important step in establishing need and securing necessary resources for moving ahead with program development. Justifying a program requires an articulation of scope and potential impact to engage stakeholders. Producing a well-defined set of expectations and value propositions will make key stakeholders feel confident about approving and funding a program. The identification of a trend (such as increasing readmission rates for a particular population) is one possible justification for a program, especially when the trend leads to increasing costs or morbidity/mortality. By conducting a literature search, an APRN might reveal evidence that transitional programs for patients with heart failure are successful in preventing readmissions. Transitional programs that already exist may be adapted to fit another patient population rather than designing a completely new program from scratch. Using evidence from the literature may reinforce the value or justification of such programs, especially if those programs have demonstrated success in achieving the desired outcomes such as reducing readmission rates and reducing overall healthcare costs. Friedan (2014) suggests the need for innovation as well as the use of a reasonable number of evidence-based interventions as a "bundle," which will likely produce a more significant impact than introducing isolated interventions.

Once a program is conceived and a literature review is completed, it is important to consider whether the program is feasible. A pilot or feasibility study can help frame the program structure and identify potential risks and barriers associated with implementation. Basic questions need to be addressed and answered in the preparation of a program justification, such as:

- Are other programs in place that serve a similar purpose?
- Are there other alternatives to the proposed program?
- Is the program economically and technically feasible in the proposed practice setting?
- Does the program make financial sense? A cost–benefit table can be used to list factors to compare program options and consider economic feasibility (Table 7.1).
- Is the program technically feasible?
- Is the program operationally feasible to implement?
- Is it possible to maintain and support the program once it is implemented?

Designing a program is different from implementing it; therefore, nurse leaders must determine whether the program can be effectively operated and supported. Critical issues such as operational and support issues must be considered. Table 7.2 offers a nonexhaustive list of examples.

TABLE 7.1 Potential Costs and Benefits of Proposed Program Worksheet

	POTENTIAL COSTS	POTENTIAL BENEFITS
Quantitative measures		
Qualitative themes		

TABLE 7.2 Operational and Support Issues for Designing New Programs

OPERATIONAL ISSUES	SUPPORT ISSUES
• What tools are needed to support the program, e.g., equipment and facilities? Do we currently have these resources? • What skills training does the staff need? • What procedures or processes need to be created and/or updated? • What will be needed to maintain and support the program once it is implemented?	• What support staff will be needed? • What program materials will the staff use? • What and how will staff training be provided? • How will changes be introduced and managed?

- Is the program politically feasible considering strategic goals and administrative directives? Nurse leaders must be cognizant of the political landscape surrounding the program.

- Will the program be allowed to succeed?

Nurse leaders must be cognizant of the organization's current strategic goals and administrative directives to determine whether or not the climate and the timing are appropriate for the program's development. The healthcare environment is in constant flux so it may be difficult to anticipate the number of external forces that may affect a program's acceptability. Being prepared with contingencies and adaptations to a program can be essential to gaining support to move ahead.

Programs with the potential to save money and improve patient outcomes are often very appealing. The Centers for Medicare & Medicaid Services (CMS) has tied reimbursement to certain key quality indicators. The Affordable Care Act (ACA) established the *Hospital Readmissions Reduction Program*, which requires the CMS to reduce payments to inpatient prospective payment system (IPPS) hospitals with excess readmissions. The ACA went into effect on October 1, 2012, and hospitals that were above the national average for 30-day readmission rates saw decreased reimbursement rates (CMS, 2019). Improving readmission rates makes good financial sense. Increasingly, healthcare financing strategies now consider the concept of value-based care. This approach to reimbursement calls for models in which healthcare providers are paid based on patient outcomes rather than the amount of service provided. "Value" is calculated by measuring the outcomes given the cost of producing these outcomes (*NEJM Catalyst*, 2017). The APRN should assess the community to determine whether other similar programs exist that would compete with the proposed program, or whether the proposed program could be built into an existing program. If a hospital has an existing community outreach department, the APRN could use the existing structure to house a new program.

In summary, justification of a program can be strengthened significantly by providing sound evidence such as a thorough review of the literature to establish the background of the problem and by examining current successful programs that may be applicable to the APRN's population of interest. Additionally, by following trends APRNs can compare outcome measures to national quality indicators (benchmarks) and follow these measures over time with a goal to improve patient outcomes and reduce costs. And finally, determining if the program is feasible will further strengthen the justification, as feasibility studies provide a systematic framework in which a program can be assessed and thoughtfully implemented or integrated into current practice. Outlining a system of accountability for the program through ongoing monitoring, evaluation and improvement is an essential component as it will inspire confidence in those who implement the program.

Identifying Key Stakeholders

The term *stakeholder* is commonly used in the business arena and refers to a person, group, or organization that has a direct or indirect stake in an organization because it can affect or be affected by the organization's actions, objectives, and policies. Stakeholders can be internal and external, but in either case, there is a synergistic two-way relationship between the organization and its program and the stakeholders. Nurse leaders strive to involve stakeholders who will support and facilitate successful program implementation. It is also important to know how and/or why some stakeholders may oppose the development of a program so that barriers can be anticipated and minimized. The following list of questions can guide identification of key stakeholders:

- Who will be affected by the program?
- Who can influence the program although not directly involved in its development, implementation, and evaluation?
- What group is interested in the program's success and outcomes?
- Who will be or could be impacted by the program?

There are many stakeholders in healthcare, but there are five important and powerful classifications of stakeholders that should not be ignored: patients/consumers, medical staff, agency management, professional staff, and boards of directors or trustees. Think broadly about the range of potential stakeholders, which may include government agencies, professional associations, present and prospective employees, local communities, the national community, the public at large, suppliers, competitors, the media, and future generations. Regular and timely communication with stakeholders about the program development and implementation process will be essential to ensure the engagement and commitment from those decision makers who allocate resources and provide support.

There may be considerable variability and/or overlap in stakeholders' expectations, including healthcare quality, support or adequacy of resources, as well as costs and profitability. Publicly reported indicators may impact consumers' perception of a hospital's quality of care. The board of trustees will be very invested in the organization's image, which can directly impact a consumer's decision about where to seek care—or a physician's decision about where to admit patients. Healthcare organizations have mission statements that reflect organizational values, and, in many cases, these statements reflect the value placed on the development of various programs.

The power or influence of stakeholders can vary as a result of the organizational makeup, their position in the organization, and their philosophy and values. These factors will drive the expectations of a new program so the justification should be consistent and fit with the existing culture. Addressing the concerns and expectations of stakeholders when designing a program can improve the likelihood of ongoing support and program success. The identification of program outcomes that stakeholders value can help win their support.

Assembling a Team

Program development requires a team of people who are directly familiar with each aspect of the process that will be part of the program. The composition of the team will depend on its scope and generally involves two types of staff: (a) individuals who will provide direct program services, and (b) staff who will support direct providers and program implementation. Those closest to the process provide essential information and support for making changes. The type and number of staff members needed to provide direct program services depends on the nature of the services that will be provided and the number of program locations. The same is true for the type and number of support staff needed for program implementation and evaluation.

There are many specific roles and tasks that individuals can assume during the program development phase in order to encourage shared commitment and to ensure broad ownership for success. An executive sponsor is very helpful to ensure resources such as protected staff time. The appointment of a process owner should also be considered. This team member could be an APRN with an administrative role in the program area who will ultimately be responsible for implementing and maintaining the program. These individuals can provide essential advice about internal and external forces that should be taken into account when designing a program.

A lead player is the program administrator or manager who will drive the project and manage the associated changes. Regardless of industry or setting, this essential role requires an individual who can provide oversight and direct the work of the team members' performance as well as monitor and provide ongoing feedback about the team's performance. This role usually involves the following common responsibilities:

- Identifies, researches, and solves program issues effectively
- Identifies the resources required for a program's success
- Recognizes and manages unanticipated issues and opportunities for improvement
- Documents and communicates operation of the program
- Ensures that the program complies with standards, regulations, and procedures
- Plans and sets timelines for program goals, milestones, and deliverables

Regardless of the number and type of team members, the program manager or administrator plays a critical role in building a successful team. A team that is effective and focused contributes to the success of the program. This requires attention to the charge to the team (sometimes referred to as the project charter), the expectations of individual team members, and the specific reasons/roles for the team's composition. A useful framework for building successful teams is described best by the acronym "together (T) everyone (E) achieves (A) more (M)." The origins of the model are difficult to trace, but its concepts are sound and used by many. Successful teambuilding requires attention to the following:

- Commitment
- Competence
- Control or sense of ownership
- Collaboration
- Communication
- Awareness of positive and negative consequences
- Coordination

Stakeholders, team leaders, and team players all play a critical role in the success and/ or failure of a program. Each member has a role and an expectation based on the anticipated outcome of a new program. Values sometimes play a role, and it is important to share these values and address them early on to ensure success. Often consideration of a new program requires creative thinking that could shift the culture and current thinking about how things are done. Engaging the team in consensus about this early on can be enabling and empowering as the program development process advances. Ultimately, commitment, communication, and collaboration are some of the most important characteristics a team requires for a successful program.

Structure

As the team moves forward, APRNs must be focused and cautious about employing complex approaches to program structure. Complex designs can lead to failure if discrete outcomes are not easily measured or if too many measures or variables are involved. The structure of a new program can be as simple or detailed as desired as long as there is clarity about the goals, components, and specific outcome measures that will determine success. For example, a simple approach might structure the program proposal around the following essential areas:

1. WHAT
   - What is the title of the program?
   - What is the focus of the program?
   - What are the goals of the program?
   - What are the objectives of the program?
   - What outcomes will be measured?
   - What is the budget for the program?
   - What is the timeline for program development, implementation, and evaluation?

2. WHERE
   - Where will the program take place?
   - Where is the program's base location?
   - Where will staff be housed?
   - Where will supplies or resources for the program be stored?

3. WHO
   - Who are the stakeholders?
   - Who is in charge of the program?
   - Who are the staff members involved in program development, implementation, and/or evaluation?
   - Who is the program attempting to reach?
   - Who will fund this program?

4. WHEN
   - When will the program be implemented?
   - When will the program end?

5. WHY
   - Why is the program needed (justification)?
   - Why might the program succeed or fail?

6. HOW
   - How will data be collected?
   - How often will data be collected?
   - How often will outcomes be examined?
   - How will the program be developed? Implemented? Evaluated?
   - How will the program sustain its funding or obtain future funding?
   - How will the program's success be determined?

This structure is the "skeleton" on which a program can be designed and can serve as a reference when planning resources, budgets, staffing, and operational procedures. A program's structure consists of the program's goals and objectives, which follow directly from strategic planning. The plan should include a description of the resources needed to achieve the goals and objectives, including necessary funding. A major component of these resources may include human resources described in terms of required skills and scope of practice. Technical resources for data, including their analysis and storage, will need to be considered when designing a program budget. Initial budget proposals for new programs usually estimate costs in broad categories. Final program budgets require careful attention to all aspects of program planning, implementation, and evaluation, and should estimate yearly costs as closely as possible. Funding is determined after a program budget is created. The source may be a state or federal grant, or it may be self-financed through health insurance held by consumers or a combination of funding sources. Whatever the source (or sources) for financing costs, a method of funding must be identified before the program can move forward.

Outcomes

Outcomes are often defined by regulatory, governmental, or certifying agencies such as The Joint Commission (TJC), the AHRQ, and the American Nurses Credentialing Center (ANCC). An outcome measure is often expressed as a rate or percentage and represents the end result of some process in a patient population over a set period of time. TJC often looks for the results of improvement projects designed to meet standards for accreditation. The ANCC manages the Magnet® designation program that provides a prestigious distinction to healthcare organizations for nursing excellence and high-quality patient care. To receive Magnet designation, the ANCC looks for systematic data collection related to outcomes of care for specific groups of patients and a demonstration that the majority of nursing units or practice arenas have outperformed the national benchmarks the majority of the time (ANCC, 2019). Performance on nurse sensitive indicators is often the focus. The AHRQ (2018) also provides guidance for the identification of quality indicators that can be used as outcome measures. For a complete list, go to www.qualityindicators.ahrq.gov/Default.aspx.

Often, the data used to justify the program's development and implementation can provide insights into the outcome data that are readily available. What does the program do? Why does the program exist? Outcomes are the measurable results of the program objectives. They provide a method of evaluating the success of a program. State and national statistics can be used as benchmarks when examining outcomes. Comparisons to quality indicators can also serve as benchmarks to evaluate success or progress in a program. Outcomes should be established for short-term, intermediate, and long-term objectives. The mnemonic SMART provides a template for writing such objectives (CDC, 2015).

- *Specific*: The outcome is well defined and unambiguous.
- *Measurable*: Concrete methods and criteria for assessing progress are used.
- *Achievable*: The goal can be a stretch but must be reasonable given the program's resources and sphere of influence. Reasonable goals and objectives must be motivational; they should provide incentives for the program staff and stakeholders.
- *Relevant*: The outcome must be relevant to the program's vision, mission, and goals. Outcomes must also be relevant to all people affiliated with or impacted by the program.
- *Time*: The time period for accomplishing goals and evaluating outcomes is reasonable.

Outcomes can be incremental and subtle. Framing personal observations or subjective experiences as concrete, specific, observable measures can be a daunting task. Hence, both quantitative and qualitative outcomes may be both helpful and necessary.

Impact is another tool used in recent years to measure program success. It uses qualitative and quantitative measures to establish its success by looking at broad-based outcomes. It is viewed in broader terms and is less specific than outcomes. Impact is defined as the difference in the changes in outcomes between those involved with the program and those not involved (Baker, 2000). It is the evaluation of the effects, both positive and negative, caused by a program. Impact evaluation is an effort to determine, in broad terms, whether a program has the desired effects on individuals, households, and institutions, and whether those effects are attributed to the interventions associated with the program. The following are examples of how the impact of a transitional program intended to reduce readmission rates for heart failure patients might be articulated in quantitative and qualitative terms:

- Within 1 year of the inception of the program, the hospital's heart failure readmission rate was reduced and outperformed the national benchmark.

- In a recent 10-month tracking period, more than 20 patients successfully completed the program.

- A patient's wife describes its value this way: "Thank you so much for your excellent program! I sincerely believe you and your team deserve an award for excellence in patient care. I don't know what we would have done without your support and guidance."

- The personal impact of the program and its professional staff is acknowledged by one participant: "[T]he staff helped me realize I was not eating as well as I should and got me moving in the right direction. Also, I noticed that when I eat so many fruits and vegetables, I don't have room for so much junk food. Before this program, I didn't realize how much salt was in the food I was eating."

On the other hand, program outcomes can illustrate whether or not the program is doing what it was intended to do. Outcomes should provide information that can be used for ongoing quality improvement. After defining program outcomes, consider using the SMART criteria stated previously to evaluate the program's stated outcomes. These questions may also be helpful:

- Is it clear what the program is assessing?

- Is the outcome measurable?

- Is the intended outcome measuring something useful and meaningful?

- How will the outcome be measured?

- Are the outcomes realistic for the time frame of the program?

Outcome data should be collected continuously at appropriately prescribed intervals (e.g., at specific milestones, quarterly). throughout the program implementation. All outcome data will not require the same frequency in order to monitor trends effectively.

For example, ensuring that program activities are being carried out may require more frequent monitoring in the initial stages where volume and patient experience ratings will have more relevance than once the program is felt to be up and running.

In summary, the outcome measures selected should show the progress (or ineffectiveness) of a program and allow for objective evaluation. Outcome measures must be clear, concise, measurable, and easily compared to quality indicators when possible. They should be realistic and time delimited. Evaluation of the impact of a program can also be helpful when dealing with qualitative and quantitative measures.

IMPLEMENTATION

Operating Policies and Procedures

Once the program proposal has taken shape, well-designed policies and procedures (P&P) will be important to guide implementation. These P&P should reflect the proposed structure, processes, and outcomes. Ensuring alignment with existing policies and compliance with regulatory mandates will help to ensure consistent performance and risk management while serving as a basis for evaluating process improvements. A program does not need a policy for every possible contingency. It should allow for flexibility in clinical decision-making and administrative operations. When developing P&P, the APRN should consider the following:

- Coordination of the writing and review of the P&P
- Providing administrative support and possible legal review
- Reviewing and discussing the P&P with the program staff
- Ensuring P&P are supported by evidence
- Interpreting and integrating the P&P into program practices
- Ensuring compliance with the P&P

Using the earlier example, if a program was designed for transitioning patients with heart failure from hospital to home, it would require a review of the literature to determine evidence-based strategies that have been used by other organizations to prevent or delay readmissions. Program planners would also need to review state and federal regulations related to important factors such as reimbursement for services and zoning requirements for program facilities. The synthesis of evidence provides a framework for the development of P&P for clinical services and program implementation.

A carefully constructed P&P manual is critical for program success. It can be modeled after evidence-based protocols and can provide the framework for consistent training of staff and community outreach workers. P&P also serve as a guideline for staff to follow to ensure delivery of quality care and consistent practices in the program.

Communications and Marketing

As mentioned previously, communication is essential to keep team members and stakeholders engaged. Similarly, there is no limit to the amount of communication that is needed during implementation. If a tree falls in the forest, but no one is around to hear it fall, does it make a sound? This question highlights a realistic problem that is faced when communicating about a program. You may have the best program in the world, but if you do not communicate the benefits and features of the program to the right audience, how are consumers going to find out about it? How are stakeholders and program team members going to buy into the program?

Marketing is an important component to consider in program design and development. It is important to be aware of not only your competitors but also what will appeal to your audience (e.g., potential participants). A strong marketing campaign can lead to long-term successes not only for your program but for future programs as well. Stakeholders will see the value in a well-constructed marketing plan, which ultimately is important for program sustainability. The American Marketing Association (2013) defines marketing as "the activity, set of institutions, and processes for creating, communicating, delivering, and exchanging offerings that have value for customers, clients, partners, and society at large" ("Marketing" section, para 1). Marketing requires activity and is not passive. It is a group effort involving a variety of individuals and groups, internal and external to the program or organization. Marketing is also process driven. Communication is essential to the process and can be delivered in many forms. The plan requires definition of the senders, receivers, and the media to be used. Consider the following basic questions when engaging in strategies to communicate about a program:

- Who will be responsible for communicating information about the program?
- What is the message being communicated?
- Who is the intended recipient of the communication?

For some programs, market research may be required to determine how interested patients/consumers and referring providers get information about the program. A well-mapped-out process for communication and marketing is critical for success. Advertising is only one part of marketing. The communication plan can include verbal and nonverbal communications. Verbal communication may include word of mouth, telephone voice messages, and presentations at meetings. Communication through nonverbal means includes ads in newspapers, information on an organization's website and Twitter account, newsletters, posters, text messages, and emails. Without clearly defined processes, responsible nurse leaders cannot plan effectively for launching the communication plan and will have difficulty determining what communication strategy is working and what is not.

Positioning is another concept nurse leaders must be aware of so that they can differentiate their programs from the competition. Positioning happens in one place, in the mind of the consumer, and occurs in a moment. Nurses must be prepared to present a "brand" of service in the healthcare market place to get the attention of the patients and/ or the referring providers who are the customers you are reaching out to. Interested customers will spend time and energy evaluating one program in relation to others before making a choice about which program to participate in. The following questions related to the concept of positioning can be helpful throughout the design and development phase but are particularly important during implementation (McNamara, n.d.):

- Who is the target market?
- Who are the competitors for the program?
- What should be considered when determining the logistics of the program, including costs?
- What should be considered when naming the program?

Programs are successful only if they attract the participation of the target population. There must be buy-in by its members, and without effective communication by a variety of modalities, this message may never reach the intended audience. As noted earlier, there are both verbal and nonverbal forms of communication. Verbal communication is probably the most effective for some populations, as the value of face-to-face interaction and relationship building is difficult to replace with nonverbal methods. With that said, communication requires an investment of both time and money, and these costs need to be included in the program budget.

Models for Program Design and Implementation

Various models can be used to guide the process of program development and implementation. Program planning models serve as organizing frameworks for developing a program from beginning to end, including planning, implementation, and evaluation. Nurse leaders may tailor these models to guide them in the design and development of their own programs. Some programs can take many years to implement depending on their focus and scope. Programs may be focused on individuals (patients or staff members), interpersonal processes (team communications), organizations (policy or practice development), communities (developing community resources), or environmental concerns (social determinants such as education and employment). APRNs should select a model based on the characteristics of the target population and/or the type of program they plan to develop. The *Healthy Populations* report (Siegel, Alderwick, Vuik, Ham, & Patel, 2016) recommends carefully considering the impact of social determinants on the population's health, and their ability to access and manage health (see Figure 4 on p. 24 at www.ge.com/sites/default/files/WISH_Healthy_Pop_26.07.pdf). All of the approaches described in the following are strongly focused on outcomes and program results.

The Logic Model

The *Logic Model*, developed by the W. K. Kellogg Foundation (2004), is commonly cited in the literature as a model for program planning. The model is used in program evaluation but is also useful and appropriate for program planning and management. It is a tool used to help shape a program. Additionally, logic models help leaders identify factors that may impact a program and enable them to forecast needed data and resources to achieve success. A logic model is a graphic display or "map" depicting the relationship among resources, activities, and intended results that identify underlying theory and assumptions.

The Logic Model is aligned with the scientific method. Just as a hypothesis is tested in research, program objectives are tested through program development, implementation, monitoring, and evaluation. The following steps outline the Logic Model program planning, clarifying program theory:

- Describe the problem(s) your program is attempting to solve or the issue(s) your program will address.

- Specify the needs and/or assets of your community that led your program to address the problem(s) or issue(s).

- Identify desired results by describing what you expect to achieve, short and long term.

- List factors you believe will influence change in the population or community.

- List successful strategies or "best practices" your research identified that helped address the targeted population and achieved results your program hopes to achieve.

- State assumptions underlying how and why the identified program will work.

The Logic Model provides a focus for leaders and helps to clarify program progress. Goals are easily identified, task responsibilities are assigned, and outcomes are clearly communicated. The Logic Model's graphic display helps key stakeholders and players visualize their roles and accountabilities so that collaboration and communication are enhanced.

Lane and Martin (2005) have described the successful application of the Logic Model by three APRNs who designed and evaluated a breast health program for rural, underserved women. According to the authors, "The Logic Model was most useful in outlining the program, guiding the first year, and identifying needed direction for the future of the program. It was at the heart of the program development and served as the visual schemata" (p. 110).

Developing a Framework or Model of Change

The Model of Change builds on the Logic Model and incorporates best practices to promote change and improvement in the community (Community Toolbox, 2018). This innovative model provides a road map for creating a new program by outlining the relationships among inputs, such as resources, outputs or the proposed interventions, impact (e.g., immediate results), and outcomes, including community or behavioral change. The Community Toolbox, created as a public service sponsored by the University of Kansas, is an online resource for individuals interested in promoting community health and development. Developing a Framework or Model of Change is a 12-step process that organizes thinking and orients program development through intended outcomes. The steps include the following:

- Analyzing information about the problem or goal

- Establishing a vision or mission

- Defining organizational structure and operating mechanisms

- Developing a framework or model of change

- Developing and using action plans
- Arranging for community mobilizers
- Developing leadership
- Implementing effective interventions
- Ensuring technical assistance
- Documenting progress and using feedback
- Making outcomes matter
- Sustaining the work

Activities outlined in the Developing a Framework or Model of Change process reinforce a focus on collective thinking to create a common understanding and ensure commitment. The steps set the stage for strategic action incorporating comprehensive evidence-based interventions that provide a clear rationale for programs to facilitate funding opportunities and inform the need for data collection and outcome measurement. Using and developing best practices ensures that interventions will have the desired impact on outcomes and, more important, advance the science of healthcare. Several examples of how the model has been used to plan, develop, implement, and evaluate successful community programs are available on the Community Toolbox University of Kansas website (www.ctb.ku.edu).

The PRECEDE–PROCEED Model

The *PRECEDE–PROCEED Model* of health program planning and evaluation is another design model evolved at Johns Hopkins University based on the work by Green and Kreuter (1992). It is founded on epidemiological principles; social, behavioral, and educational sciences; and health administration. The two fundamental propositions underlying this model are (a) health and health risks are caused by multiple factors, and (b) because of this, efforts to impact change must be multidimensional. Consequently, the model's goals are twofold: (a) to explain health-related behaviors and environments, and (b) to design and evaluate interventions that influence both behaviors and the environment.

The model follows a continuous cycle linking the information gathered in the PRECEDE steps with the actions in the PROCEED process. Experience in the PROCEED process in turn provides additional information to re-initiate the PRECEDE process for iterative changes. The PRECEDE (*Predisposing, Reinforcing,* and *Enabling Constructs in Educational Diagnosis* and *Evaluation*) process outlines the following program planning steps:

1. Determine population needs.
2. Identify health determinants of these needs.
3. Analyze behaviors and environmental determinants of health needs.
4. Outline factors that predispose, reinforce, or enable behaviors.
5. Ascertain interventions best suited to change behaviors.

The PROCEED (*P*olicy, *R*egulatory, and *O*rganizational *C*onstructs in *E*ducational and *E*nvironmental *D*evelopment) process defines four steps to program implementation and evaluation:

1. Implement interventions.

2. Evaluate interventions.

3. Evaluate the impact of interventions on the health behaviors and factors supporting the behaviors

4. Evaluate outcomes.

Ahmed, Fort, Elzey, and Bailey (2004) used the PRECEDE–PROCEED Model to study the barriers that underserved women had to overcome in order to be screened for breast cancer. Once these barriers were identified, recommendations were made to improve healthcare system procedures. Box 7.1 summarizes how the model was used by these researchers. Another example of how the PRECEDE–PROCEED Model can be used was illustrated by Allegrante, Kovar, MacKenzie, Peterson, and Gutin (1993), who implemented and evaluated a walking program for patients with osteoarthritis of the knee. They found success with their program and suggest that the intervention strategies designed around this model are readily adaptable for a wide range of settings.

An Evaluation Framework for Community Health

Produced by the Center for Advancement of Community Based Public Health and based on work by the CDC, Framework for Program Evaluation in Public Health (2000) is another model that can be used for program development, implementation, and evaluation. This systematic approach involves procedures that are useful, feasible, ethical, applicable, and accurate. Evaluation is the driving force for planning effective programs, improving existing programs, and demonstrating results to justify investment in resources. The framework comprises six interdependent steps that build on one another and facilitate understanding of the program context, including its history, setting, and organization. The steps are as follows:

- Engage stakeholders (those involved in the program, those served or affected by the program)

- Describe the program (needs, expected effects, activities, resources, stages of program development, operational chart)

- Focus the evaluation design (program purpose, users, uses, questions, methods, agreements)

- Gather credible evidence (program indicators, sources, quality, quantity, logistics of data collection)

- Justify conclusions (program standards, analysis and synthesis, interpretation, judgments, recommendations)

- Ensure use and share lessons learned (program design, preparation, feedback, follow-up, dissemination, additional uses).

A more detailed checklist is summarized at prevention.sph.sc.edu/Documents/CENTERED%20Eval_Framework.pdf

BOX 7.1

APPLICATION OF THE PRECEDE–PROCEED MODEL

Case Study: Use of the PRECEDE Model to Explore How Underserved Women Overcame Barriers to Mammography Screening. What Must Precede the Outcome?

PRECEDE

Step 1: Determine population needs.
The authors note that mammography can reduce breast cancer mortality and that rates of regular screening are very low in the general population. Efforts to improve rates have had varying results.

Step 2: Identify health determinants of these needs.
The authors conducted focus group discussions with women from underserved populations who themselves obtain regular screenings. The goal of the focus groups was to identify facilitators and barriers to mammography screenings.

Step 3: Analyze behaviors and environmental determinants of health needs.
Two themes emerged from the discussions. The first is related to the environment and the second to behavior: (a) the role of the healthcare system in preventive health behaviors and practices and (b) personal factors (the woman's responsibility).

Step 4: Outline factors that predispose, reinforce, or enable behaviors.
The authors note that lack of insurance used to be viewed as one of the major barriers to obtaining mammography—but even with the removal of this barrier, rates remain low. The focus of this study was on the behavioral factors influencing mammography screening. The authors report that the women in the focus groups described characteristics that influence them to obtain regular screenings: (a) awareness, knowledge, and trust—they understood cancer risks (some had personal experiences with family members who had cancer; some had healthcare providers who were receptive and encouraging); (b) personal responsibility—they demonstrated attitudes that support proactive behaviors, and this behavior developed within their families or through interaction with others; and (c) pride in self and satisfaction—these women found satisfaction with being role models for others.

Step 5: Ascertain interventions best suited to change behaviors.
To increase screening rates in underserved populations, the authors recommend providing information on risks and the importance of mammography in early detection (education) and inviting adherent women to act as role models. They further emphasized the importance of involving the media in providing information, as many of the women in the focus groups reported getting their information about mammography from television.

Source: Adapted from Ahmed, N., Fort, J., Elzey, J., & Bailey, S. (2004). Empowering factors in repeat mammography: Insights from the stories of underserved women. *Journal of Ambulatory Care Management, 27*(4), 348–355.

OVERCOMING BARRIERS AND CHALLENGES

The first step in overcoming barriers is assessing and identifying obstacles to program development, implementation, and evaluation. Insight into obstacles can pave the way toward developing action plans to overcome barriers and challenges. Is the challenge in the design of the program? Is the challenge the competition? Is the challenge related to resources, including time? Is the challenge due to the data being collected or the process of data collection? Gaglio, Shoup, and Glasgow (2013) explain that areas that correspond to the structure, process, and outcome components of a program should guide program administrators during the quality improvement process. For example, one area that should be scrutinized is adoption. Adoption is the absolute number, proportion, and representativeness of settings and intervention agents who are willing to initiate a program. Another important area that they have identified is maintenance, which is a reflection of implementation and represents the extent to which a program or policy becomes institutionalized or is assimilated into routine organizational practices and policies.

The plan–do–check–act (PDCA) model used in quality improvement can be used to identify obstacles and plan for subsequent actions. In 1980, NBC TV aired a program called "If Japan Can. . .Why Can't We?" It highlighted Japan's rise as an economic power from not just virtual, but actual, ashes. The program featured W. E. Deming, a statistician who taught quality control to Japanese manufacturers. That program and Deming are often credited with bringing quality-improvement initiatives to the attention of corporate America (Walton, 1991). Deming believed that American thinking was too "linear" and that it should be more circular. The PDCA model is a Deming creation based on work by Andrew Shewhart.

- *Plan*: Plan the change.

- *Do*: Do it.

- *Check*: Check the results, then tailor your action based on the results.

- *Act*: Act to stabilize the change or begin to improve on the change with new information.

An example of the successful use of the PDCA model to improve the quality of care in an acute care hospital is provided by Saxena, Ramer, and Shulman (2004). A collaborative team was formed in an acute care hospital and charged with improving blood-administering practices using the FOCUS-PDCA method. FOCUS is the acronym for *F*inding a process to improve, *O*rganizing a team familiar with the process, *C*larifying the current situation, *U*nderstanding causes of variation, and *S*tarting the PDCA cycle. The hospital identified a need to improve blood-administering processes (F) and formed a collaborative team that included nursing representatives, quality improvement, and laboratory and pathology personnel (O). They reviewed all of the P&P related to blood transfusions (C), had independent auditors assess current practices (U), then trained nurses to observe and assess the dispensing and administering of blood products to determine adherence to P&P (S). They found that continuous, direct observational audits using the PDCA method improved compliance with P&P, thus reducing risks related to transfusion error.

The PDCA model is an iterative process. The point is to strive toward continuous improvement or quality through ongoing assessment and improvement of structure, process, and outcomes. Quality-improvement models such as this can provide a framework to assist APRNs in addressing some of the barriers that may be encountered in program development

SUMMARY

In this chapter, APRNs and nurse leaders are given the tools to design and develop comprehensive programs that address multiple components of program development ranging from the identification of key stakeholders to marketing and communication strategies. Program designs that address consumer and societal trends are more likely to be successful and produce improved quality of care. Ultimately, the goal is to generate improved patient outcomes. Successful programs must incorporate knowledge from many fields in order to address issues related to the structure, process, and outcomes involved in program planning, development, implementation, and evaluation. Various program models provide a standard and tested method for helping nurse leaders throughout the process of program implementation.

EXERCISES AND DISCUSSION QUESTIONS

Exercise 7.1 Using data that can be found on the DHHS or the CDC websites, identify trends in population demographics and health in an area that you serve.

- What are the implications for healthcare providers?
- What type of healthcare services and programs are needed right now?
- What type of services do you believe will be needed in 10 years?
- From a demographic point of view, in 10 years, what will be the important characteristics of the population that you serve if you continue to practice in this geographic region?

Exercise 7.2 You are interested in developing a program to reduce the rate of readmissions for heart failure who have been hospitalized in an urban academic medical center. There have been many prior initiatives to address this issue. Explain the process you will undertake to develop an effective program including consideration of established best practices and the outcomes of past initiatives.

- What are the important characteristics of the population you are serving in this geographic region?
- Consider the data you will need and how you will obtain it.
- How would you go about the analysis of the data?
- What steps would you take to identify the priority needs your program will be addressing?
- Using the "SMART" method, write short-term, intermediate, and long-term objectives for the program.
- How might you use the PRECEDE–PROCEED Model to plan, implement, and evaluate the program?
- How will you market the program?

REFERENCES

Ahmed, N. U., Fort, J., Elzey, J., & Bailey, S. (2004). Empowering factors in repeat mammography: Insights from the storied of underserved women. *Journal of Ambulatory Care Management, 27*(4), 348–355. doi:10.1097/00004479-200410000-00007

Allegrante, J. P., Kovar, P. A., MacKenzie, C. R., Peterson, M. G., & Gutin, B. (1993). A walking education program for patients with osteoarthritis of the knee: Theory and intervention strategies. *Health Education Quarterly, 20*(1), 64–81. doi:10.1177/109019819302000107

Agency for Healthcare Research and Quality. (2018). *AHRQ quality indicators.* Retrieved from www.qualityindicators.ahrq.gov/Default.aspx

American Association of Colleges of Nursing. (2006). *The essentials of doctoral education for advanced practice nursing.* Retrieved from https://www.aacnnursing.org/Portals/42/Publications/DNPEssentials.pdf

American Marketing Association. (2013). *Definitions of marketing.* Retrieved from https://www.ama.org/AboutAMA/Pages/Definition-of-Marketing.aspx

American Medical Association. (2015). *An inventory of national clinical registries.* Retrieved from the National Quality Registry Network website http://tsihealthcare.com/wp-content/uploads/2014/05/National-Quality-Registry-Network-Listing.pdf

American Nurses Credentialing Center. (2019). *Frequently asked questions about ANCC's 2019 Magnet recognition program manual.* Retrieved from https://www.nursingworld.org/organizational-programs/magnet/magnet-program-faq

Baker, J. L. (2000). *Evaluating the impact of development projects on poverty: A handbook for practitioners.* Washington, DC: The World Bank.

Bazzoli, F. (2018). *12 trends that will dominate healthcare IT in 2019.* Retrieved from the HealthData Management website https://www.healthdatamanagement.com/list/12-trends-that-will-dominate-healthcare-it-in-2019

Blumenthal, S. (2017). The use of clinical registries in the United States: A landscape survey. *EGEMS The Journal for Electronic Health Data and Methods, 5*(1), 26. doi:10.5334/egems.248

Center for Advancement of Community Based Public Health. (2000). *An evaluation framework for community health.* The Center for Advancement of Community Based Public Health, University of North Carolina. Retrieved from http://prevention.sph.sc.edu/Documents/CENTERED%20Eval_Framework.pdf

Centers for Disease Control and Prevention. (2015). *Develop SMART objectives.* Retrieved from https://www.cdc.gov/phcommunities/resourcekit/evaluate/smart_objectives.html

Centers for Medicare & Medicaid Services. (2019). *Hospital readmissions reduction program (HRRP).* Retrieved from http://www.cms.gov/Medicare/Medicare-Fee-for-Service-Payment/AcuteInpatientPPS/Readmissions-Reduction-Program.html

Community Toolbox. (2018). *Tools to change our world.* Retrieved from http://ctb.ku.edu/en

Friedan, T. R. (2014). Six components necessary for effective public health program implementation. *American Journal of Public Health, 104*, 17–22. doi:10.2105/ajph.2013.301608

Gaglio, B., Shoup, J. A., & Glasgow, R. E. (2013). The RE-AIM framework: A systematic review of use over time. *American Journal of Public Health, 103*, e38–e46. doi:10.2105/ajph.2013.301299

Green, L. W., & Kreuter, M. W. (1992). CDC's planned approach to community health as an application of PRECEDE and an inspiration for PROCEED. *Journal of Health Education, 23*(3), 140–144. doi:10.1080/10556699.1992.10616277

Hibbard, J. H., & Greene, J. (2013). What the evidence shows about patient activation: Better health outcomes and care experiences; Fewer data on costs. *Health Affairs, 32*(2), 207–214. doi:10.1377/hlthaff.2012.1061

Joynt, J., & Kimball, B. (2008). *Innovative care delivery models: Identifying new models that effectively leverage nurses* [white paper]. Princeton, NJ: Robert Wood Johnson Foundation.

Lane, A., & Martin, M. (2005). Logic model use for breast health in rural communities. *Oncology Nursing Forum, 32*(1), 105–110. doi:10.1188/05.onf.105-110

McNamara, C. (n.d.). *Designing and marketing your programs.* Retrieved from the Free Management Library website http://managementhelp.org/np_progs/mkt_mod/market.htm

NEJM Catalyst. (2017). *What is value-based healthcare?* Retrieved from https://catalyst.nejm.org/what-is-value-based-healthcare

Saxena, S., Ramer, L., & Shulman, I. (2004). A comprehensive assessment program to improve blood-administering practices using the FOCUS-PDCA model. *Transfusion, 44,* 1350–1356. doi:10.1111/j.1537-2995.2004.03117.x

Siegel, S., Alderwick, H., Vuik, S., Ham, C., & Patel, H. (2016). Healthy Populations: Designing strategies to improve population health. Report of the WISH Healthy Populations Forum 2016. Retrieved from https://www.ge.com/sites/default/files/WISH_Healthy_Pop_26.07.pdf

Walton, M. (1991). *Deming management at work.* New York, NY: Perigee Books.

W. K. Kellogg Foundation. (2004). *Logic model development guide.* Retrieved from https://www.bttop.org/sites/default/files/public/W.K.%20Kellogg%20LogicModel.pdf

INTERNET RESOURCES

Agency for Healthcare Research and Quality: https://www.ahrq.gov/index.html

AHRQ, Quality Indicators: www.qualityindicators.ahrq.gov/Default.aspx

AHRQ Registries for Evaluating Patient Outcomes: A User's Guide: https://www.ahrq.gov/news/blog/ahrqviews/disease-registries.html

An Inventory of National Clinical Registries (AMA and NQRN): http://tsihealthcare.com/wp-content/uploads/2014/05/National-Quality-Registry-Network-Listing.pdf

Centers for Disease Control and Prevention (CDC): https://www.cdc.gov/DataStatistics

Community Toolbox: https://ctb.ku.edu/en

PCPI, NQRN: https://www.thepcpi.org

The Center for the Advancement of Community Based Public Health, *An Evaluation Framework for Community Health Programs:* http://prevention.sph.sc.edu/Documents/CENTERED%20Eval_Framework.pdf

The U.S. Department of Health and Human Services: https://healthdata.gov

WISH Healthy Populations Forum 2016, *Healthy People Report:* https://www.ge.com/sites/default/files/WISH_Healthy_Pop_26.07.pdf

CHAPTER 8

EVALUATION OF PRACTICE AT THE POPULATION LEVEL

BARBARA A. NIEDZ

INTRODUCTION

Early in their careers, nurses often have an enthusiasm and energy for caring for one patient at a time. Over the years that focus broadens as the more experienced nurse embraces a role that is more expansive and addresses issues at a population level. As administrators, leaders, educators, and managers, the advanced practice registered nurse's (APRN's) scope of practice widens even further. Quality nurse professionals expand their view to the entire organization and across departments. Nurses have, over the years, moved in many diverse directions. We not only care for patients at the bedside, but in their homes, businesses, schools, prisons, rehabilitation settings, as well as in outpatient and mental health facilities. Nurses also serve in settings that may be considered more "nontraditional"; for example, working for managed care organizations (MCOs) by providing utilization management, and designing and implementing case and disease management (DM) programs. Another critical responsibility of APRNs is the oversight of clinical outcomes at the population level.

The advancement of many educational opportunities for nurses has moved our profession into new and exciting places. The advent of the advanced practice licensure designation has opened doors for nurses that did not exist 20 years ago. Nursing is proactive and responsive to the needs of the healthcare environment and to the needs of patients. APRN status and licensure expand the nursing role to include status as primary care providers, and APRNs are recognized in many preferred provider networks across the country, receiving appropriate reimbursement. Our potential to influence the health of patient populations has expanded accordingly.

This chapter describes ways to evaluate population outcomes, systems changes, as well as effectiveness, efficiency, and trends in care delivery across the continuum.

Strategies to monitor healthcare quality are addressed, as well as factors that lead to success. Most importantly, these concepts are explored within the role and competencies of the APRN. Specifically, this chapter addresses at least three of the American Association of College of Nursing (AACN) Doctor of Nursing Practice (DNP) Essentials (AACN, 2006). These are: (a) clinical scholarship and analytical methods for evidence-based practice (Essential III), (b) clinical prevention and population health for improving the nation's health (Essential VII), and (c) advanced nursing practice (Essential VIII).

MONITORING HEALTHCARE QUALITY

Nurses have been concerned about the quality of patient care for many years. Although our definitions of quality have varied, at the heart of this discussion is our collective desire to continuously improve patients' health and management of various disease states, regardless of where a given patient fits on the continuum.

Definitions of Quality and Theoretical Models

Just as nurses have cared for one patient at a time, initial models for quality dealt with individual patient reviews. Donabedian (1980) defines quality in broad terms: "Quality is a property that medical care can have in varying degrees" (p. 3). His definition holds that "attributes of good care . . . are so many and so varied that it is impossible to derive from them either a unifying concept or a single empirical measure of quality" (p. 74). This notwithstanding, Donabedian's (1980) model of structure, process, and outcome addressed how quality can be maximized in organizations, and continues to be used today to structure research on quality methods throughout the globe (Ayanian & Markel, 2016; Berwick & Fox, 2016; Rowe, McCarty, & Huett; 2018).

In recent years, Donabedian's influence continues in the way organizations are required to demonstrate their quality endeavors. For example, most accrediting bodies, such as The Joint Commission (TJC), the National Committee for Quality Assurance (NCQA), and the Utilization Review Accreditation Commission (URAC), all require evidence of a quality structure. Trilogy documents (a program description for quality, the annual work plan, and an annual program evaluation) are developed and reported through a committee structure that provides insight into the quality program from frontline staff through governance. In addition, process indicators of quality, such as whether or not the patient with an elevated ST segment and positive troponin is provided with aspirin on admission to the emergency department (ED), are a mandate within the core measure set for acute myocardial infarction (AMI). Finally, the emphasis of outcomes in recent years also emerges from the Donabedian model. The model provides for a robust relationship between structures and processes, which, taken together, enhance the potential for maximizing outcomes, such as reducing the incidence of significant cardiac damage in AMI.

Nash, Reifsnyder, Fabius, and Pracilio (2011) explain that the concept of population health includes an integrated system of care across the continuum. The population health model "seeks to eliminate healthcare disparities, increase safety, and promote effective, equitable, ethical and accessible care" (p. 4). They explain that quality is defined in terms of clinical data and outcomes, both economic and patient centered. In their view, "quality is founded on evidence-based medicine" (p. 5) and describes the relationship between quality of care and the cost of care; if the quality of care improves, the cost of care is reduced (Nash et al., 2011). Nash et al. (2011) describe the importance of prevention, screening, and patient self-care management. They describe the importance of identifying risk factors to the development of chronic illness and the influence of the community, the availability of and access to various programmatic elements that can help manage and reduce the cost of care. The incidence of diabetes mellitus could potentially be reduced by getting control of the rampant obesity problem across the United States. As an example of a prevention indicator of quality for health plans, monitoring the patient's body mass index (BMI) is an important Healthcare Effectiveness Data and Information Set (HEDIS, 2018) measure and is also included in the Centers for Medicare & Medicaid Services Five-Star Quality Rating System (CMS STARs) measures. Preventing the incidence of diabetes mellitus can potentially result in reducing its short- and long-term complications, which could subsequently save thousands, perhaps hundreds of thousands, of healthcare dollars. As an example, consider the impact of preventing the incidence of type 2 diabetes mellitus on end-stage renal disease (ESRD), and the cost of dialysis alone. In 2016, Medicare expenditures for outpatient dialysis were $11.4 billion (Medicare Payment Advisory Committee, 2018).

The Institute for Healthcare Improvement (IHI) puts the ideas of Nash et al. (2011) into action in the Triple Aim initiative. The goals of the Triple Aim are (a) better health, (b) better experience of care, and (c) lower cost. The Triple Aim framework serves as the model for many organizations and communities (Bisognano & Kenny, 2012). The Triple Aim site can be accessed at www.ihi.org/Topics/TripleAim/Pages/default.aspx. Similarly, national healthcare reform has brought this issue front and center. Baehr et al. (2016) describe key components or units that provide for breadth of coverage, the extent to which they accurately address healthcare needs, provide for the funding of care, and the coordination of care. Though no one present unit possesses all of the features needed, the role of accountable health organizations (ACOs) in total population health is explored. (See Chapter 9, The Role of Accreditation in Validating Population-Based Practice/Programs for more information on ACOs.)

Juran (DeFeo, 2014; DeFeo, 2017) offers a definition of quality that is both parsimonious and applicable across disciplines. He defines quality in terms of the customer and explains that a product or service has quality if it is "fit for use" in the eyes of the customer. Goonan (1995) and Dienemann (1992) have applied Juran's definition to healthcare scenarios. Patients, as consumers of healthcare products and services, fit the definition of customers, regardless of the payment source. Juran (DeFeo, 2014; DeFeo, 2017) explains that for a product or service to meet the needs of the customer, it must have the right features and must be free from deficiencies.

In Juran's view (DeFeo, 2017), new features (such as new cardiac surgical equipment or the capacity to provide outpatient dialysis) may require capital and operating expenses. Deficiencies or defects in our healthcare products or services always contribute to the cost of poor quality, and although there might not be an outlay of dollars, there are still financial consequences. In years past, hospitals were reimbursed for service provided regardless of the outcome. However, as we turned into the new millennium, cost avoidance awareness became more and more noticeable in the literature. For example, the cost of one hospital-acquired pressure ulcer has been estimated at $127,185 for a stage IV hospital-acquired pressure ulcer, and $124,327 for a stage IV community-acquired pressure ulcer (Brem et al., 2010). Today hospitals are no longer reimbursed for the cost associated with the development of a III- or IV-degree pressure ulcer in a patient if that ulcer was hospital-acquired and not present on admission. The CMS, which functions under the aegis of the U.S. Department of Health and Human Services (DHHS), promulgated rules to this effect in 2008 (see www.cms.gov/HospitalAcqCond). The development of a hospital-acquired III- or IV-degree pressure ulcer is also included in the National Quality Forum's (NQFs) list of "never events" ("The Power of Safety," 2010). In recent years, the CMS has dictated by law and regulation that hospitals will not be reimbursed for care related to 14 of these never-event conditions that occur during an inpatient admission (CMS, 2018a). In the 10 years since this reimbursement change, researchers have started to observe changes in rates, demonstrating that by tying reimbursement to quality, improvements become noticeable (Peasah, McKay, Harman, Al-amin, & Cook, 2013). Other preventable outcomes that contribute to the cost of poor quality have consequences that go beyond dollars and cents. Deficiencies that result in complications and even deaths arise from poor systems and human failures. These have gotten significant and appropriate attention through the patient safety movement (Institute of Medicine [IOM], 1999, 2001). Through TJC and the National Patient Safety Goals, attention to hospitals and other healthcare organizations has resulted in significant strides toward reducing deficiencies. The importance of improving quality by avoiding the "never events" and reducing deficiencies has reinforced the necessity of accurate and thorough documentation and medical decision-making by all healthcare providers.

Although Juran's definition of quality does have merit and application in healthcare (Kaplan, Bisgaard, Truesdell, & Zetterholm, 2009; Muerer, McGartland-Rubio, Counte, & Burroughs, 2002), capturing ways and means to measure both outcome and process indicators of quality have emerged from an evidence-based approach. For example, research literature has shown that in order to decrease the incidence of congestive heart failure (CHF) hospital readmission rates, inpatient discharge instructions should capture key components, including (a) discharge medications, (b) the importance of weight tracking and documenting daily, (c) diet control, (d) what to do if symptoms worsen, (e) activity level restrictions, and (f) follow-up care instructions (Centers for Disease Contol and Prevention [CDC], 2018a; Yancy et al., 2017). Lack of any of these components is clearly seen as a "deficiency" and should be captured across aggregate data sets in hospitals (see http://www.jointcommission.org/). Thus, measurement mechanisms emerge from Juran's definition of quality (2010), which also fit with Donabedian's (1980) framework of structure, process, and outcome and Nash et al.'s (2011) view of population health.

Organizational Models for Excellence

Nurses provide the backbone of healthcare organizations, whether inpatient, outpatient, rehabilitation, home care, community health, or in an MCO. Services can be provided in person or sometimes via the telephone. In certain circumstances, nurses provide support by developing and monitoring telehealth programs. As such, understanding the organizational framework that can maximize positive outcomes and minimize deficiencies through the role of the nurse has value. The APRN, in particular, adds value, particularly through oversight and development of these newly emerging models of care.

Both Juran (DeFeo, 2017) and Donabedian (1980) put the concept of quality into the framework of an organization. Care of a patient across the wellness–illness continuum requires consistent and cogent processes and systems. Accordingly, Donabedian's view is that healthcare organizations require appropriate structure and key processes. Taken together, the structure and processes assist the organization in producing desired outcomes for their patients (Donabedian, 1980). Juran characterizes organizations as high functioning and marked by positive outcomes if features are maximized and deficiencies are minimized. In order to accomplish this, organizations plan for, control, and continuously improve quality. Both clinical and service quality characteristics are defined in terms of customers' needs and expectations. Others have made similar observations in applying Juran's organizational model in healthcare organizations (Best & Neuhauser, 2006; Goonan & Scarrow, 2010; Maddox, 1992). In 1987, the federal government instituted the Malcolm Baldrige Award, which recognizes those organizations that demonstrate principles characteristic of high performance and achieve significant business results through quality-improvement techniques. This award is based on seven key guiding principles and embodies the theoretical model of quality that Juran honed throughout his career (DeFeo, 2017; National Institute of Standards and Technology [NIST], 2018). In the late 1990s, this award was opened to healthcare organizations. Between 2002 and 2017, there were 21 winners of the Baldrige Award in the healthcare division (NIST, 2018).

In order for organizations to maximize positive outcomes and minimize deficiencies, planning must take on a strategic focus. Leadership and governance have responsibility and oversight for quality, and are essentially responsible for organizational planning. Quality planning, according to Juran (DeFeo, 2014; DeFeo, 2017), provides depth, breadth, and scope of how the product or service is designed, developed, and implemented. Key quality characteristics in the form of measurable goals and objectives for the organization and for patient outcomes are designed in the system or process before that product or service begins. Once that product or service is in operation, customers' needs and expectations (whether in the form of clinical quality, customer satisfaction, core business processes, or utilization of healthcare resources) can be understood, defined, and measured. External benchmark comparison data can be helpful in goal setting and in evaluating the extent to which a product or service meets customers' expectations. Juran's model (DeFeo, 2014; DeFeo, 2017) holds that all products and services are delivered to the customer employing various processes and systems. High-performing organizations design processes and systems to meet customer needs consistently, reducing variation in outcomes and minimizing defects. Juran calls this piece of the puzzle "quality control."

For example, hospitals have put tremendous effort into improving patient flow in recent years: meeting patient (as customer) expectations for reducing delays in the emergency department (ED) and physician (as customer) expectations for radiology results reporting in a timely manner. The advent of the electronic health record (EHR) in hospitals and other healthcare organizations is another example of an efficient way to capture documentation and evidence of the patient's history across the continuum of care as well as contribution to overall patient safety and reduction of medical error. These complex operational processes in hospitals exemplify organizational processes and systems that can address key customer groups' needs: patients and providers.

W. Edwards Deming (Moen & Norman, 2010) developed similar theories of quality and consistently modeled the theme of reducing variation and building quality into a product or system so that there is less need to depend on inspection (after the fact). Deming's model was also influenced by the work of other quality giants like Shewhart and Feigenbaum ("Guru Guide," 2010). Ishikawa ("Guru Guide," 2010) paved the way for Japan's economic turnaround after World War II, largely based on the work of both Juran and Deming, who were sent by the U.S. government to support Japan after the war. These models rely heavily on the theory that all of quality is measurable and that reducing variation in processes holds a vital role in reducing the incidence of defects and, ultimately, ensuring better outcomes.

Berwick, Godfrey, and Roessner (1990) were pre-eminent in applying these theoretical models to healthcare. Six leading healthcare organizations were armed with a national demonstration grant from the Robert Wood Johnson Foundation; within this seminal work, the authors cataloged the experiences of these organizations in applying this theoretical approach to quality. Their experiences clearly indicate that the models and tools had merit and value in reducing defects, improving processes, and maximizing outcomes (Berwick et al., 1990). This landmark work demonstrated that what had been shown repeatedly in manufacturing and in service industries throughout the country (and, in fact, worldwide) could be repeated in healthcare, and laid the groundwork for potential application throughout the healthcare industry. Deming's model has been applied in nursing, and the literature is replete with references depicting its application (Gavriloff, 2012; IHI, 2018a).

The IHI has put Deming's model into action. The IHI's rapid cycle improvement model is based on iterative cycles of "plan, do, study, act" (PDSA). This model encourages small tests of change; implementation of bundles is built on this concept. The bundle concept is the development of a small number of evidence-based key components, which, implemented organizationally using iterative PDSA cycles, result in a desired outcome. There are five key components in the central line bundle: (a) hand hygiene, (b) maximal barrier precautions, (c) chlorhexidine skin antisepsis, (d) optimal catheter site selection, and (e) daily review of line necessity. The "how to guide" includes detail as to how an organization can successfully implement the bundle, using iterative PDSA cycles. For example, the CLABSI (central line-associated bloodstream infection) bundle encourages the use of a checklist. So one of the PDSA cycles included to guide the implementation of the bundle relates to the use of this checklist. Other implementation strategies include developing measurement mechanisms and ensuring adequate supplies to guarantee sterile technique on insertion and availability of chlorhexidine and other important adjuncts to reducing the CLABSI rate in hospitals (CDC Healthcare Infection Control Practices Advisory Committee, 2018b).

Deming (Moen & Norman, 2010), Juran (DeFeo, 2017), Crosby ("Guru Guide," 2010), and others explain that reducing variation is a continuous task, even when a given product or service is exceeding the needs of customers and especially when a given product or service is not competitive in the marketplace. The Six Sigma movement (DeFeo & Barnard, 2004; Pyzdek & Keller, 2014) emerged from a quality-improvement initiative at General Electric in the 1980s and set out to reduce defects or deficiencies to fewer than 3.4 defects per 1,000,000 opportunities. In essence, this model for quality improvement and planning is built on the work of Juran, Deming, Crosby, Ishikawa, Feigenbaum, and others ("Guru Guide," 2010). Although it is clear that Donabedian's work is theoretically sound, it also resonates with this thinking. In designing an influenza vaccination process for employees using the Six Sigma approach, Kaplan et al. (2009) applied the model to a population health issue. Many others have applied the Six Sigma theoretical model to various healthcare processes. For example, Kuwaiti and Subbarayalu (2017) applied the model in Saudi Arabia to reduce the falls rate. Loftus, Tilley, Hoffman, Bradburn, and Harvey (2015) used the model to improve the central line bloodstream infection rate. This model has significant application for process improvement across the spectrum of healthcare processes (Corn, 2009). To illustrate the application of process improvement theory and the use of Six Sigma models, consider the studies presented in Box 8.1.

BOX 8.1

EXAMPLES OF PROCESS IMPROVEMENT THEORY AND THE USE OF THE SIX SIGMA MODEL

1. Anderson-Dean (2012) described the application of lean (which is a variation of Six Sigma model, focusing on eliminating waste and "nonvalue added" steps in a given process) principles in nursing informatics.

2. Drenckpohl, Bowers, and Cooper (2007) used the method to reduce errors related to breast milk identification processes in the neonatal intensive care unit (NICU).

3. Breslin, Hamilton, and Paynter (2014) applied the Lean Six Sigma model to care coordination processes.

4. Corn (2009) described the history of the model and its application in healthcare.

5. Fairbanks (2007) applied Six Sigma and Lean methodologies to improve operating room delays in throughput.

6. Stankovic and DeLauro (2010) used the model to improve timeliness and reduce errors in the laboratory in processing specimens.

7. Yun and Chun (2008) applied the design aspect of Six Sigma to telemedicine service processes.

8. Kuwaiti and Subbarayalu (2017) applied the model in Saudi Arabia to reduce the falls rate.

9. Loftus et al. (2015) used the model to improve central line bloodstream infection rate.

Developing a Six Sigma approach works best when it is done broadly, across the entire organization. When a Six Sigma approach is well defined for a given organization, the impetus and funding source for the program comes directly from governance and cascades from the senior leadership team throughout, to the frontline employees, who use the systems and processes within them on a day-to-day basis. Deciding which projects are convened and which are not is also a governance process, and would likely emerge out of the quality infrastructure. Governance provides for an educational process to learn and apply the use of the many tools in the Six Sigma tool chest, many of which have a heavy statistical process control overlay. Six Sigma leadership uses an educational process in the form of various "belts" for certification. For example, a master black belt possesses the skills to oversee multiple Six Sigma projects simultaneously. The black belt is typically the project facilitator; green belts are often process business owners and may serve as the team lead in a Six Sigma team. The yellow belt is the team member who will also be schooled in the use of many of the tools (Pyzdek & Keller, 2014).

The patient safety movement in healthcare has given rise to a wider application of the Six Sigma model. In addition, the language of defects and deficiencies, though developed out of manufacturing and other types of product development, has resulted in consistent thinking that complications heretofore considered risks of procedure or hospitalization are now considered preventable (Courtney, Ruppman, & Cooper, 2006). The patient safety movement in the United States emerged largely due to TJC and their attention to sentinel events (Joint Commission Resources, 2003). In addition, the consensus report "To Err Is Human," published by the IOM in December 1999, provides a focus on the potential for preventable error. One of the most telling comments early in the report explains that there are between 44,000 and 98,000 preventable medical errors annually in the United States that lead to patient deaths (IOM, 1999). The variability in the range is significant. Measurement mechanisms that would provide accurate descriptions of these sentinel events did not exist at that time. In the language of the process improvement gurus, these are defects and deficiencies. Applying these theoretical models to healthcare has tremendous potential in accurately describing quality of care by improving outcomes through attention to process.

Kaplan and Norton (1996, 2001) take measurement in organizations a step further and link progress against the strategic planning cycle to organizational goals and objectives. Their "balanced scorecard" model lends itself to healthcare well, and has been applied internationally (Chu, Wang, & Dai, 2009; Moulin et al., 2007; Potthoff & Ryan, 2004; Yap, Siu, Baker, Brown, & Lowi-Young, 2005). In fact, the Malcolm Baldrige Award has several specific criteria (see www.nist.gov/baldrige/publications/hc_criteria.cfm), and one of the most important is the recognition of "results." The results criteria require evidence of measurement and improvement of quality across organizations and systems. A well-defined scorecard at the enterprise level, which is balanced across several categories relating to the customer's experience, is a useful and important tool for senior leadership and governance. As we move into a discussion about planning, controlling for, and improving quality across the entire patient population, understanding theoretical models for process improvement and their application become not only useful and accepted, but necessary and, most important, lead to improved outcomes of care.

Process Improvement Models and Tools

The literature provides applied evidence of various process improvement models that have many commonalities. Deliberate and thoughtful use of applied evidence and the use of process improvement models can result in reduction of defects and deficiencies to levels that meet and exceed customers' expectations, whether those expectations surround clinical quality, customer satisfaction, core business process, or utilization of healthcare resource expectations. The "plan, do, check, act" (PDCA) process improvement model (Moen & Norman, 2010); the Juran Six-Step Quality Improvement Process model (DeFeo, 2017); or Six Sigma's define, measure, analyze, improve, and control (DMAIC) model all have common features and they are all problem-solving models that drive measurable improvement when used properly. They can facilitate a thought process and require a team initiative. They will work whether the problem is related to clinical quality, customer satisfaction, core business processes, or utilization of healthcare resources. They work inside and outside of healthcare, whether the problem is simple or complex and whether one is concerned about the care of patients or developing tangible products for retail sale. Box 8.2 describes characteristics that are commonly found in process improvement models.

All process improvement models have these common characteristics. In addition, a variety of tools support the quality professional along the process improvement path. Tools such as process flow charting, barriers and aids charts, cost–benefit analyses, data-collection tools and statistical methods, SIPOC (suppliers–inputs–process–outputs–customers)

BOX 8.2

CHARACTERISTICS AND COMMONALITIES OF PROCESS IMPROVEMENT MODELS

1. The problem is defined in measurable terms.

2. The problem is stated in terms of the customer's needs and expectations.

3. External comparative benchmark data are sometimes drawn on to help set the goal for the project.

4. Members of the team have well-defined responsibilities.

5. Most teams should have 6–10 members. Larger teams may not be able to control the problem process and might need to break into smaller groups to be effective. Smaller teams may have inadequate representation to fully address all facets of the problem.

6. The team includes an executive sponsor to usher the project as a priority in the organization.

7. Other team roles include business process owner as team leader, internal or external consultant as facilitator, and clearly described roles for remaining team members.

8. There is an analysis phase. This phase employs both qualitative and quantitative methods to arrive at barriers, obstacles, and root causes of the problem.

(continued)

9. The analysis phase should be well supported with qualitative data (like a cause–effect diagram) and quantitative "theory testing" data (like a diagnostic study of the root causes of the process problem).

10. Remedies that address both the qualitative and quantitative barriers are designed.

11. A plan for piloting or testing the remedies is well defined, engages the full team, considers the cost of implementation and decision-making therein, and defines whether or not they are sufficient to achieve the desired improvement.

12. A measurement mechanism is designed to evaluate the effectiveness of the change strategy and the degree to which an additional remedial plan is needed.

13. A mechanism for evaluating ongoing data collection, day to day and month to month, is put in place, to ensure that the gains are held constant.

14. In order to provide an effective use of a process improvement model, the focus must be clear and well defined. Teams must sometimes winnow down a larger project to its smaller component parts. At the end of a successful process improvement project, consider going back to revisit other improvement opportunities, which may have been set aside from the focal interest.

analyses, project planning tools, lean thinking, and many others provide useful insight and drill closer to improvement goals (Balanced Scorecard Institute, 2018; DeFeo & Barnard, 2004; Pyzdek & Keller, 2014; Womack & Jones, 2003).

Population-Based Models

On a continuum from health and wellness (H&W) products to complex care management, a variety of population-based models have emerged over recent years (Box 8.3). Patients move across a continuum from good health to the end of life and enter a variety of settings in doing so. Programs are designed to offer both telephone care and field-based approaches to prevention, DM, care coordination, case management (CM), and care integration. Patients are identified through predictive models and other stratification methods. The extent of outreach is determined by various levels of acuity, and the frequency of patient contact may depend on clinical assessment and care planning. Motivational interviewing and health education are primary strategies to engage patients into modifying their behaviors, but a hallmark of all of these programs is ultimately a change in health behaviors, which leads to desired outcomes. Preventive strategies such as smoking-cessation programs, as well as care coordination strategies such as identifying a medical home and ensuring medical transportation to an outpatient facility, combined with condition-specific strategies in the presence of various chronic disease states, to reduce the incidence of ED usage for primary care and reduce inpatient admissions are all examples of ways to improve access to care in the hopes of ensuring overall quality of care (Kitzman, Hudson, Sylvia, Feltner, & Lovins, 2017; McClure et al., 2018; Scherz et al., 2017). Research has shown that disease and CM programs are effective in reducing the trajectory of chronic disease by providing less utilization of healthcare resources and providing enhanced patient satisfaction by improving the patient's ability to perform activities of daily living and improving her or his ability to manage chronic diseases (self-efficacy) (Jones et al., 2017; Kalter-Leibovici et al., 2017; Russo et al., 2017).

BOX 8.3

POPULATION HEALTH MODELS

1. *Health and Wellness (H&W):* These programs are primarily telephonic, and may have a biometric screening component; program awareness and patient education materials are often part of a direct-mail campaign. These programs aim at identifying patients with significant health risk and encourage patient participation in screening. Completion of a health risk assessment is often a key component of lifestyle management programs. Smoking cessation, weight reduction, and attendance at preventive care visits are examples of desired outcomes for this patient population. Although significant health risks may emerge here, this patient population is essentially healthy without the presence of diagnosed disease states; the focus of H&W programs is aimed at identifying risks, with prevention of chronic illness as the ultimate target.

2. *Disease Management (DM):* These programs are likely to be telephonic, field based, or a combination of both. Patients qualify for DM programs on the basis of identified disease states, singly or in combination. Most DM programs target at least five or six disease conditions: persistent asthma, COPD (chronic obstructive pulmonary disease), CAD (coronary artery disease), diabetes mellitus, CHF (congestive heart failure), and depression. Other programs are broader and capture superutilizers—high-risk patients with varied chronic disease states. DM programs often have a care coordination component, which can provide such things as assistance in placing patients in a medical home, medical transportation (to help reduce the overuse of emergency medical services and ED care), or help in finding funding sources for medication management (to avoid disease exacerbations due to medications not being filled), and so on. Examples of outcomes for this patient population include, but are not limited to, (a) ensuring that a diabetic patient gets HbA1C testing done at least annually, (b) ensuring that a patient with persistent asthma has a prescription for controller medications, and (c) confirming that a CHF patient knows the importance of measuring his or her daily weight and what to do if symptoms worsen. For example, when a patient who has CHF and an ejection fraction of less than 40% is being discharged from the inpatient setting with proper discharge plans and instructions, we ensure that the patient is appropriately prescribed an angiotensin-converting enzyme (ACE) inhibitor and knows the importance of weighing himself or herself daily. In summary, care coordination ensures that the patient has the ability to fill the prescription (has transportation to obtain and financial resources to buy), has a scale at home or the means to purchase one, and has transportation to the doctor's office for follow-up or preventive care.

3. *Case Management (CM):* These programs capture patients who have complex needs and multiple health conditions. These patients are often high risk and high cost, and come to the surface in stratification and predictive models because of overutilization of EDs and multiple admissions due to poor outpatient management or lack of a medical home. These patients account for a very small percentage of the total population, but account for more than 60% of the total healthcare dollar. Models that integrate care across various specialties for a given patient set (e.g., patients with severe mental illness who also have multiple medical disease conditions) are emerging.

One of the most interesting recent trends in population-based care management is care integration. Care integration is a concept that is well known to nurses but may not be as familiar to other health professionals. Here is an example: A patient is admitted to an inpatient acute care hospital with a significant drug overdose subsequent to an attempted suicide. This long-standing behavioral health (BH) patient has been managed "on and off" by a variety of BH professionals, and has been receiving various psychotropic medications. In addition, the patient has a medical history that includes long-standing diabetes and coronary artery disease; other healthcare professionals have managed these aspects of the patient's healthcare. In fact, the medical professionals have not been in touch with the BH professionals, at the patient's request. In the ED, the BH professionals' role is pre-empted as the patient's overwhelming medical needs are the priority. When the patient is admitted to the intensive care unit (ICU), a host of consultants are brought to the case, and after being "cleared medically," the patient is transferred to the inpatient BH unit. Care is sometimes fragmented and the BH needs are addressed separately and apart from the medical needs of the patient. The primary care provider may not be involved until after discharge and may not have a clear sense of the many issues that play a role in the complete care of this patient. Although there is no question about the prioritization of care, there is also no integration of care. The patient's experience is divided into two distinctly different phases, in some ways compromising effective use of healthcare resources. This is where the importance of the medical home comes into play. Length of stay is clearly segmented into two sequential phases rather than managed in parallel. Although this inpatient example is a familiar one, lack of care integration is a common problem also on the outpatient side of the care continuum. Processes of care that appropriately integrate care have been somewhat problematic in the U.S. healthcare system in the past. In recent years, it has become apparent that care integration needs to improve, which would improve the quality of care, resolve access issues, and reduce over-utilization of healthcare resources (Cornwell, Brockmann, Lasky, Mach, & McCarthy, 2018; Guerrero et al., 2017; Thomas et al., 2017).

Two recent initiatives bring these ideas into sharp perspective. The first is the concept of the patient-centered medical home (PCMH). Within this model, care integration services are well defined and the process of bringing care to the patients where, when, and how they need it becomes not only possible but practical. The NCQA promulgates standards that describe this initiative (see www.ncqa.org/tabid/1302/Default.aspx). Accountable care organizations (ACOs) provide another model that incorporates these ideas into organized systems of care with healthcare providers, PCMHs, and hospitals partnering together. This is a program furthered by the CMS (see www.cms.gov/Medicare/Medicare-Fee-for-Service-Payment/ACO/index.html.)

Nurse-Sensitive Process and Outcome Indicators at the Population Level

Many authors have promulgated ways to organize measures, as taken together they represent a picture of quality. Kaplan and Norton (1996, 2001) suggest four generic categories that could work for any organization, including organizations that focus on healthcare. These perspectives include (a) internal business processes, (b) customer focus, (c) learning and growth, and (d) financing. The NCQA places the HEDIS measures into categories as well. The HEDIS categories include (a) effectiveness of care, (b) access/availability of care, (c) satisfaction with the experience of care, (d) use of services, and (e) cost of care (NCQA, 2018d). The complete list of categories can be found at http://www.ncqa.org/hedis-quality-measurement/hedis-programs.

Although the list of possible indicators used to measure population health and population health nursing may seem endless, four categories of measures, metrics, and indicators emerge. These broad categories are clinical quality, customer satisfaction, core business processes, and utilization of healthcare resources. Loosely based on Kaplan and Norton (1996, 2001) and the NCQA HEDIS frameworks, an organizing framework for evaluating population health nursing emerges. As these categories are of use in organizing our thinking regarding quality in the inpatient setting, they also have merit in outpatient settings, and as we consider care of the entire population with a given disease condition, these categories continue to add value to this discussion as an organizing framework. For the purpose of this discussion, the words "measures," "metrics," and "indicators" are used interchangeably. As we have put forward a definition of quality that is "measurable," our measures are quantifiable, a set of metrics that indicate the presence or absence of quality, and degrees on that continuum.

Whenever possible, standardized data definitions are essential. This sets up a level playing field for comparisons. Since the late 1990s, data sets, external comparisons, and guidance for standardized numerator and denominator have emerged across the patient continuum of care. As our industry has become more accountable to the public for outcomes, this kind of standardization has been essential, facilitating external comparisons on the basis of data sets. In addition, these numerators and denominators are described in detail, right down to the technical specifications. These technical specifications describe what types of codes are included in the numerator and which are included and excluded in the denominator. These codes have become widely accepted, the application of which results in fair and appropriate comparisons and rankings. Various groups (both governmental and private) have defined measures, specified the technical mechanics of counting and determining rates, and applied these measures across the industry. These include, but are not limited to: (a) CMS (www.cms.gov/center/quality.asp), (b) TJC (www.jointcommission.org), (c) the Agency for Healthcare Research and Quality (AHRQ) (https://www.ahrq.gov), (d) NCQA (www.ncqa.org), (e) the National Quality Forum (NQF) (www.qualityforum.org), and (f) the National Database of Nursing Quality Indicators (NDNQI) (www.pressganey.com/ourSolutions/performance-and-advanced-analytics/clinical-business-performance/nursing-quality-ndnqi).

Measures have also emerged over time. As our foray into this area of accountability for outcomes has been heightened by legislators, policy makers, and the public at large, the connection between the cost of poor quality in healthcare and healthcare reform has become more explicit. Although it might require capital and operational outlay of funding to develop a specific product or service with the right features within the healthcare industry, the cost of poor quality adds a substantial burden to the cost of healthcare. For example, when a patient in a hospital setting experiences a delay in obtaining a diagnostic procedure that is essential to the appropriate management of his or her disease state, this core business process can delay decision-making, causing a longer length of stay for the patient in the hospital. This delay may also lead to disease progression and result in complications that otherwise might have been prevented. Another question that should be addressed is whether these types of delays are due to the type of insurance, underinsurance, or lack of insurance. As discussed in Chapter 2, Identifying Outcomes in Population-Based Nursing, an important component of APRN practice is the need to recognize and address issues related to healthcare disparities.

When patient safety is compromised in hospitals, the result can be substantial. The example of delayed diagnostic testing may not only hinder the determination of a patient's diagnosis but may lead to patients receiving inaccurate medications or treatments or errors, such as a patient identification mix-up, that can result in loss of life. Over time, we are better able to identify the impact of the cost of poor quality by capturing and quantifying these indicators of quality in the aggregate. Sorting out "what counts and what doesn't" helps to provide clarity and a clearer view of quality across the board.

Clinical Quality

Nurse-sensitive indicators of population health that relate to clinical quality can be seen in a number of the metrics recognized by external organizations with available external benchmarks. In the HEDIS (NCQA, 2018a) data set created and maintained by the NCQA, there are several benchmarks that relate to chronic disease conditions. Nurses who are in the field or on the phone in telephone call centers reach out to patients with the intention of helping them wade through the various resources made available to them through private and public means to manage their overall health, given the presence of various disease states. The most common disease states managed by DM programs include: (a) diabetes mellitus, (b) persistent asthma, (c) COPD, (d) CAD, and (e) CHF. Other chronic disease conditions also may be of interest. In CM programs, the complexity of care is heightened by the number and acuity of the chronic conditions coexisting in a patient's profile. Social problems, housing, transportation, and pharmacy costs often emerge in CM programs. Similarly, the emphasis from a clinical quality perspective in H&W programs is on preventive care, early recognition of emerging disease, and use of appropriately placed screening tools.

With the agreement of the NCQA, the CMS has adopted the use of HEDIS in its STAR rating program for various types of MCOs. For example, each Medicare Advantage Health Plan licensed by the CMS is rated on a five-point star system. Clinical quality measures include process indicators collected through administrative means that contribute to a given health plan's STAR rating. For example, whether or not the patient with a diagnosis of diabetes mellitus has a hemoglobin A1C (HbA1C) test done at least annually tells us something about the care that a patient with diabetes receives. CMS weights each one of the STAR measures as to its importance. This process indicator of clinical quality that is determined by the presence or absence of an administrative claim or encounter for an outpatient laboratory test (in this case HbA1C) is weighted with 1 point toward the health plan's overall STAR rating. However, the actual value of the HbA1C is a component of "comprehensive diabetes care," a HEDIS measure, which is included in HEDIS, and another STAR measure for Medicare Advantage health plans in Part C. We know from scientific research that patients who maintain lower HbA1C levels (less than 8.0%) have fewer complications, a better quality of life, and longer life expectancy than do patients who are poorly controlled (CMS, 2018b). This makes HbA1C levels a significant clinical outcome indicator. Health plans collect actual HbA1C levels through a rigorous process and through a variety of means, including EHR data, providers' outpatient medical records, or actual laboratory data feeds. Most importantly, these data are weighted at three times the value of a process indicator in the overall STAR rating. In order to score at the highest, 5-star rating, Medicare Advantage health plans strive to have a significant percentage of their patients score less than 8% on the HbA1C test.

Box 8.4 lists several examples of clinical quality measures that are sensitive to the APRN role at the population health level in DM, CM, and lifestyle management or H&W programs, whether their intervention is on the telephone, in person in any setting, or via a telehealth program. APRNs who have responsibilities regardless of the setting can strengthen a program design by ensuring that outcome measures are used in evaluating program effectiveness and incorporating a blend of process and outcome measures in quality program development.

BOX 8.4

SAMPLE NURSE-SENSITIVE CLINICAL QUALITY MEASURES IN DM, CM, AND H&W PROGRAMS

1. HEDIS Comprehensive Diabetes Mellitus Care: Did the patient have at least one HbA1C level drawn in a 12-month period?

2. CMS STARs HEDIS: Comprehensive Diabetes Care: Did the patient, aged 65 or older, show good control, through HbA1C levels of 8% or less?

3. HEDIS Asthma Care: Did the patient diagnosed with chronic persistent asthma have prescriptions for the appropriate medications to manage chronic persistent asthma?

4. AHRQ Prevention Quality Indicator of Congestive Heart Failure: What is the annual inpatient admission rate per 100,000 (at the population level) for CHF?

5. AHRQ Prevention Quality Indicator of Chronic Obstructive Pulmonary Disease: What is the annual inpatient admission rate per 100,000 (at the population level) for COPD?

6. HEDIS: Did the patient diagnosed with CAD and an LDL (low-density lipoprotein) level of >100 mg/dL have a prescription for a statin or HMG-CoA (3-hydroxy-3-methylglutaryl-coenzyme A) reductase inhibitor?

7. HEDIS: Did the infant have appropriate well-child visits during their first year of life?

Source: Adapted from Healthcare Effectiveness Data and Information Set. (2018). Narrative, technical specifications, and survey measurement (Vols. 1–3). Washington, DC: National Committee for Quality Assurance. Retrieved from http://ncqa.org/tabid/59/Default.aspx

Utilization of Healthcare Resources

One of the many important goals for nurses who work in DM, CM, and H&W programs is to direct patients to use healthcare resources in the most cost-effective way. In the context of population health, the most expensive healthcare resources include the use of the ED and inpatient stays. By ensuring that the patient's discharge plan coming out of the inpatient setting is fully executed, one can reduce the risk of rehospitalization. By ensuring that patients have transportation and other care coordination needs met, it is to be hoped that we can reduce or eliminate emergency medical service (EMS) utilization for a ride to the local ED for primary care issues. The two metrics that are the most useful and sensitive to the nursing role in DM and CM programs are inpatient admissions per 1,000 members and ED visits per 1,000 members. In some ways, this work is an extension of the work that nurses have participated in for years in utilization management (UM) programs based in hospitals, for health plans, and for other providers of healthcare benefits. However, DM, CM, and H&W nurses take UM to the next step and ensure that patients have the means, insight, and knowledge to carry out their healthcare needs with some degree of independence and autonomy. By reviewing care needs and targeting the right level of care, and matching it to the appropriate venue, we reduce the inappropriate use of these very costly services.

An evaluation of the utilization of healthcare resources is often included in a given DM or CM contract as a "return on investment" (ROI) analysis as evidence of financial performance. The bulk of the healthcare dollar primarily resides in the use of two resources: ED visits and inpatient stays. Both may be misused in the absence of an effective medical home or with poor access to primary care. At the population level, measuring the impact of population health models on the utilization of these two key healthcare resources is a very important component of any population health evaluation method. Three possibilities present themselves in an ROI evaluation; rigorous methodology is a component of well-designed DM and CM models. First, an estimation of cost avoidance involves using historical data to predict the number and percentage of ED utilizers and inpatient admissions in a given patient population that are likely to occur after a year of DM intervention. For example, after 1 year of investment in a telephonic nursing DM program, it is reasonable to predict that patients will be linked into a medical home and lessen their risk of admissions for preventable primary care conditions such as uncontrolled diabetes, asthma, or even CHF. These strategies also have the potential to prevent the use of EDs for primary care. Another method to evaluate ROI is to predict a trend and trajectory based on the baseline history of a given set or population of patients. A typical data set for comparison is a 12-month period of time, used as the starting point or baseline for comparisons moving forward. A third option to calculate the ROI of a DM population health nursing program posits that as a result of DM intervention, certain specific events will not occur. These are examples of rate changes that could (potentially) be the subject of an ROI calculation: a reduction in the readmission rate, reduction of the rate of patients per 1,000 with multiple admissions in a given year, or reduction of patients with admissions for ambulatory-sensitive conditions (ASCs). ASCs are also described by AHRQ as preventive quality indicators. (Visit www.ahrq.gov for more information on these important indicators.)

In recent years, two additional areas were identified for cost-savings indicators: reducing the incidence of readmissions to the inpatient setting within 30 days of discharge and reducing the cost of pharmaceuticals by developing an appropriate formulary and applying rigorous criteria for medical necessity of pharmaceuticals. APRNs can take a key role in reducing inappropriate use of healthcare resources by ensuring that care coordination tasks are addressed across the continuum, particularly at the point of transition from one setting to another, and by building and tapping into community resources as well as medication management (Moye, Chu, Pounds, & Thurston, 2018; Shah, Forsythe, & Murray, 2018). All-cause readmissions within 30 days are emerging as a significant measure of healthcare resource usage, and is another example of a CMS STARs outcome measure that is weighted more heavily in a given health plan's overall STAR rating. Finally, although readmission after discharge from an acute care facility has long been an area of focus, in recent years, unplanned acute care readmissions within 30 days of discharge from a rehabilitation setting and from long-term care hospitals (LTCHs) have also received attention (CMS, 2018c). Additionally, significant efforts have been made to reduce the utilization of expensive medications in pharmacy benefit programs and specialty pharmacy programs alike. Innovative programs, driven by pharmacists, which target long-term control of chronic conditions and the role of the clinical pharmacist, are emerging. Medication therapy management (MTM) programs for patients with chronic illness and complex medication profiles are becoming more of a mandate and less of a luxury (CMS, 2018b).

Measures that relate to medication usage such as medication reconciliation, particularly in the chronically ill and the elderly, are included in CMS STARs, as Plan D measures (part of the pharmacy benefit) and selected measures in Plan C, the medical benefit. There are also pharmacy measures that relate to special needs patient population plans for those patients who are dually eligible for both Medicare and Medicaid (CMS, 2018d).

It could be argued that many of these measures fall into both the clinical quality and the utilization of healthcare resource categories. They not only improve the clinical quality of care received and serve to prevent short- and long-term complications, but also reduce inpatient hospitalizations for patients with chronic illness and an acute need, as well as reduce the cost of care. It is also interesting that many of these clinical and utilization of healthcare resource measures also emerge for Medicare patients who are members of ACOs. ACOs are formed to address the needs of direct, fee-for-service Part A and Part B Medicare patients. These ACOs mandate at least 5,000 Medicare patients for a 3-year term. In order to achieve the incentives, these ACOs must demonstrate the same type of improvement in similar measures as Medicare Advantage health plans (CMS, 2018e).

Customer Satisfaction

For many years, patients have been identified as important consumers of healthcare products and services and, accordingly, have been defined as "customers" and important stakeholders in DM and CM organizations (NCQA, 2018b; URAC, 2018). Accordingly, key metrics that are sensitive to the nursing role can tell us something about the degree to which our patients, as customers, have had a positive experience with our nurses, whether those nurses practice in hospitals, in DM organizations, or at MCOs. How frustrating is it when a customer makes a telephone call to any company and ends up in a hold queue for long periods of time? Two call center metrics are often cited as important: (a) average speed of answer (ASA) and (b) call abandonment rate (ABN) (Cross, 2000; Del Franco, 2003; Formichelli, 2007; Gustafson, 1999; Hudson, Gonzalez-Gomez, & Rychalski, 2017; Saberi, Hussain, & Chang, 2017). This literature is replete with guidance on how long it should take to answer inbound telephone calls in order to meet or exceed customers' expectations. The industry standard for ASA is fewer than 30 seconds and that for ABN is less than 5%. That is, less than 5% of calls should be lost when a customer abandons the call due to a prolonged waiting time (Cross, 2000; Del Franco, 2003; Formichelli, 2007; Gustafson, 1999; Hudson et al., 2017; Saberi et al., 2017). Akin to waiting for a response to a call light in an inpatient setting, prolonged wait times on the phone are a primary source of customer dissatisfaction. In recent years, the advent of multiple phone trees, predictive dialing, and interactive voice response (IVR) use in call centers has added technology and options aimed at improving the customer's experience. Call wait times and abandonment rates continue to be important drivers of customer satisfaction (Hudson et al., 2017; Khudyakov, Feigin, & Mandelbaum, 2010; Mandelbaum & Zeltyn, 2013; Saberi et al., 2017; Whiting & Donthu, 2009). Ensuring that staffing levels (for both licensed and nonlicensed staff members) are appropriate, that technology provides adequate tools for observing the call queue, and using data down to the level of the staff member are important oversight supervisory functions for ensuring telephonic DM or CM care in a way that meets or exceeds customer satisfaction.

Monitoring, managing, and measuring complaints are additional ways to tap into the customer's experience. Customer complaints, whether from patient as customer or provider as customer, can be an insightful means to understanding patterns and trends of care delivery, and can be the key to improvement. Customer complaints can be very serious and can lead to a written complaint or, if a patient is not satisfied with the resolution offered, the launching of a formal grievance process. Customer complaints that are resolved by the nurse on the call are important to document and are worth tracking. Sometimes, complaints come into a DM call center that might be serious, but the target of the complaint is not the DM organization. In this case, these complaints are also valuable indicators of quality and should be referred to an appropriate authority or organization. Again, tracking and trending the nature of the complaint and the agency or organization to which the complaint was referred (rather than resolution) may be all that is required.

Various techniques are available for tracking patient, provider, and client satisfaction for DM programs. Annual surveys are the most frequent vehicle used, and the Population Health Alliance provides patient and provider surveys to organizational members (www.populationhealthalliance.org). These surveys have established reliability and validity. The surveys include items that measure the overall satisfaction of the patient with the services provided by the DM organization, but also tap into the "likelihood to recommend."

Satisfaction with the skills and techniques employed in the service of DM programs by the individual nurse can also be assessed. Accordingly, these items are "nurse sensitive." Examples include items that evaluate the nurse's willingness to "listen" as well as provide information that can influence the patient's behavior in the interest of better management of specific chronic disease states.

Measuring customer satisfaction through a survey process has long been established as an important function, whether that measurement occurs in a hospital or in a population health setting, like a DM program. Many hospitals use a variety of prominent vendors for patient satisfaction monitoring such as Press Ganey™ Associates (www.pressganey.com/index.aspx), Healthstream® Research (www.healthstream.com/index.aspx), and many other research groups that specialize in healthcare survey processes. In recent years, the CMS has mandated the use of an agreed-upon set of questions administered in a consistent way regardless of the vendor. In the inpatient venue, the CMS survey titled the Hospital Consumer Assessment of Healthcare Providers and Systems (HCAHPS) is widely used (HCAHPS, 2018). Although individual vendors, such as Press Ganey, offer comparisons based on various methods, the HCAHPS survey offers broad comparisons across the country on an agreed set of questions, worded the same and applied using the same mandated research methods.

Surveys targeted at primary care providers, specialists, and other providers of healthcare services that evaluate the extent to which the DM organization provides services to them in the interests of their patients, are another important tool to gauge overall effectiveness. Annual surveys of providers as customers can also be insightful to a DM organization. The IHI also provides some insight into the usefulness of provider satisfaction assessment (IHI, 2018b). Other proprietary organizations provide additional insight (see also www.rand.org/content/dam/rand/pubs/research_reports/RR400/RR439/RAND_RR439.pdf).

Phone automated surveys and IVR surveys are also available, and a variety of telephone services provide this capability. This type of data collection and these methods have been used extensively because they provide timely feedback that is relevant on an ongoing basis. They do present advantages over annual surveys, in that a data stream is available with data summaries on six to eight items at weekly, monthly, even daily frequency, with assignment right to the level of the nurse. Survey research is fraught with both opportunity and challenge. Careful attention must be paid to sample size, response rate, generalizability of the findings, frequency of assessment, reading level of written surveys, and so on. In short, survey research requires the same rigor as a well-designed research study if the results are expected to reflect services rendered accurately and point to quality-improvement initiatives.

In recent years, the CMS has launched a customer satisfaction survey that taps into a given patient's level of satisfaction with the benefits and administration of the health plan. This tool, titled the Consumer Assessment of Healthcare Providers and Systems (CAHPS), has been developed in conjunction with the NCQA (2018c). Technical specifications on the use of this survey tool can be found at HEDIS (2018). Some of these measures do evaluate patients' health behaviors (e.g., if the patient has obtained a flu shot) and their overall experience with the healthcare industry in general. Although the CAHPS tool does not specifically measure DM or CM, some of the items on the instrument may be nurse sensitive and may be of value because of available comparative data and because some health plans bundle DM into their services. For example, some of the questions on the adult CAHPS tool refer to specific aspects of care rendered by the doctor or other healthcare provider (nurses are not included as a separate type of healthcare provider). Other questions refer to the extent to which advice has been offered by healthcare providers on such things as smoking cessation and hypertension and cholesterol management, all of which may relate to the nursing role in disease prevention/management or H&W programs that encourage self-care management.

Patient self-reported outcomes are captured in survey form by the CMS in the form of the Health Outcomes Survey (HOS), which is administered to a defined cohort of CMS members every 2 years. These self-reported outcomes include measures on the extent to which patients perceive their overall physical and emotional health status over the 2-year period of time. HOS measures also contribute to CMS STAR measures for managed Medicare health plans and for special needs plans for the dually eligible (CMS, 2018f).

Core Business Processes

Nurses are supported in many ways by the systems and processes through which they provide care. Although this is true in any direct care setting, it also has merit in telephone care and field-based DM and CM programs. While in hospitals, there might be some value to considering how acuity influences staffing levels; in the DM industry, acuity levels and ratios of staff to patients in DM programs are useful data. At the same time, because nurses are supported by job descriptions that are accurate and competency based, they are evaluated on their performance on a regular and ongoing basis. This is sound human resource practice, regardless of the setting or care type. Similarly, productivity levels are very important in all settings in which nurses practice. Can a given nurse manage a patient care assignment that is appropriate to the setting and meet all of the patient care requirements in a given time frame? This important question in the DM and CM industry might be answered by examining not only how many patients can be cared for per nurse per day, but how many active minutes of the day the nurse is talking with patients on the telephone. Although in hospitals, outpatient settings, and rehabilitation facilities there is a "hands on" nature to the care, in telephonic DM programs both "calls per nurse per day" and "talk time in minutes" are direct measures of nursing productivity. Clinical quality and utilization of healthcare resource outcomes may be the best overall indicators of the quality of care, but these indirect measures also have merit. In other words, for a nurse to be effective in managing the care of an entire population of patients across the continuum of care, volume and focus matter. In order to measure overall effectiveness of a group of nurses in DM programs, these measures of core business processes, when taken with clinical quality, customer satisfaction, and utilization of healthcare resources, can add to the panel of metrics that bring depth and understanding to managing the care of hundreds of thousands of patients across an entire population.

Other measures that are reflective of core business processes have value in evaluating the role of the nurse. In population health, DM, and CM processes, APRNs are interested in finding those patients for whom they can have an impact on their healthcare behaviors and make a difference in the way in which they manage their day-to-day care. A patient with diabetes and advanced comorbidities, who has not been in an ED or admitted (even for short- or long-term complications) to an inpatient facility, may not have obvious gaps in treatment (i.e., this patient is well managed without any help from the DM nurse). Suppose that a given diabetic patient is well managed (on his or her own), has an annual checkup with the primary care provider, and whose last Hb1C was less than 7%. This patient may have very little actionable need for a conversation with a nurse in a DM program other than an introduction, consent, a condition-specific assessment, written materials, and encouragement to stay the course. Contrast this to a newly diagnosed 55-year-old patient with an HbA1C of over 11%, with poor nutritional habits, who has just started on insulin and was just discharged from the hospital for "uncontrolled diabetes." Patients such as these have more actionable needs and are at risk for readmission if no DM assessments and interventions are put into place. Finding these patients, teeing them up for the nurse, and ensuring that we have accurate call information are all strategies that are collectively called "patient identification" and "acuity stratification" processes. Oftentimes, DM and CM companies and MCOs use sophisticated information technology processes to identify patients for the nurse to call. A resulting engagement rate that measures the percentage of patients who are identified with one or more of the disease conditions under study and the percentage of patients who complete an enrollment and condition-specific assessment process with a nurse is a useful indicator of the degree to which the DM and/or CM programs are reaching the intended population. This is a type of volume indicator that, when taken together with productivity metrics, can provide some evaluation of the impact of the role of the nurse on population health in DM and CM programs.

In summary, about 20 to 25 metrics in the four categories of (a) clinical quality, (b) customer satisfaction, (c) utilization of healthcare resources, and (d) core business processes taken together would provide an organization with a keen and parsimonious panel of metrics. This panel of metrics described in detail earlier provides the reader with possibilities for evaluating the totality of any given population health nursing program, whether DM, CM, or all three program types. Kaplan and Norton (1996, 2001) describe this idea of a panel of metrics to guide the strategy of the organization as "the balanced scorecard." The examples provided earlier and from these four categories fit the evaluation need in DM, CM, and H&W programs, but neither the categories nor the example metrics are the only possibilities. In general, metrics and measures should be easily found using existing measurement mechanisms and standardized data definitions, which can be compared against national standards and are representative of the nurse's role in improving the health of the population. A parsimonious set is useful; it is often the case that in healthcare we measure too many things. In tracking countless indicators without intention or purpose, we lose the ability to make the measures meaningful and may miss the overall strategic goals of the organization.

Data Sources

Administrative data sets have been criticized in the past for not providing useful information and for not serving as accurate measures of quality ("Case-Mix Measurement," 1987). However, a broader understanding of the usefulness of administrative data has emerged in more recent times, particularly when evaluating quality at the level of the population (Jha, Wright, & Perlin, 2007; Schatz et al., 2005). Claims data have also been called "administrative data." Encounter data are another type of administrative data that are captured for patients in "at risk" health plans, that is, plans that are capitated or partially capitated. Administrative data are rich in various coding types, including, but not limited to, the *International Classification of Diseases*, 10th Edition (ICD-10) (CDC, 2018c), codes, Current Procedural Terminology or CPT codes, or the CMS's Healthcare Common Procedure Coding System (HCPCS) codes. Used as the basis for electronic billing, these codes are rich in information about the patient and have been refined through the years to provide even more information (American Academy of Professional Coders, 2018). In DM, the ICD-10 codes, demographics, and patient experiences as captured through the administrative process provide an outline of care that affords the opportunity not only to identify patients with the most actionable need but also to find patients with those gaps in treatment. In the past, the evaluation of quality required detailed and sometimes tedious chart reviews, with random samples of charts pulled from various patient types. The effective use of administrative data is providing a rich source of information on the effectiveness of DM programs in shaping patients' health behaviors and habits over time (NCQA, 2018a).

In most DM programs, some type of documentation is required to track the patient's progress with an educational approach and the degree to which a behavior is shaped. So, although it is most important for the nurse to document an educational session on, for example, the importance of asthma controller medications, it may be just as important to hold a three-way call with the patient's primary care provider to identify the need to move from frequent use of a short-acting beta agonist to an inhaled corticosteroid and to document this action. The measure of the true outcomes (such as the claim for the prescription or no documented ED visits for the remaining year) may come through that administrative data set later on, but the role of the nurse is and should be accurately captured in written or electronic documentation. The review of the nurse's documentation from a clinical perspective is no less important in call center and field-based DM programs than it is in the hospital, in an outpatient setting, or in a direct-care home setting. This documentation needs to be audited on a regular and ongoing basis; this supervisory function can also provide rich evidence of the productivity and role of the nurse. It is an important precursor to those outcomes that may be measured through claims or other sources.

Patient self-reported data may also be useful, but this source of information may be risky as it introduces bias (recall bias, information bias, etc.; see Chapter 4, Epidemiological Methods and Measurements in Population-Based Nursing Practice: Part II). Patients' recollection of a given result may be colored by their own resistance to a change in health behavior, by their lack of knowledge, or by very strong denial defense mechanisms that develop along what may be a very difficult diagnosis to accept. Consequently, there are times when self-report data may not be useful. For the NCQA to award the status of Accredited With Performance Reporting, certain measures must be met that include actual laboratory results, and patient self-report is not permitted. Data-collection methods using the HEDIS "hybrid" method require actual provider-held chart reviews (for a random sample) or data on laboratory results that come directly through a link to the laboratory that performed the test. Two examples that exemplify the use of laboratory data include the collection of HbA1C annual results in the patient with diabetes and the annual LDL levels in the CAD patient. The HEDIS technical specifications provide a depth of rigor on these data-collection methods that is intense and appropriate. On the other hand, HEDIS recognizes that claims data on flu shots are very unreliable. Appropriately, patients are offered flu shots on a seasonal basis at health fairs, county-run clinics, during an inpatient stay, or at a local pharmacy (Pollert, Dobberstein, & Wiisanen, 2008). It may be the case that in these venues, there may be no claim submitted for the flu shot, considerably reducing the accuracy of the claims data on the incidence of obtaining flu shots in various patient populations. For most adults, the accuracy of the data on whether or not a patient has received a seasonal flu shot may be maximized by asking them. Self-report may be the best source of data available but is still not ideal. Data sources abound for key metrics in a panel of indicators that are both nurse sensitive and descriptive of population-based nursing. The CMS recognizes the value of self-reported data and has incorporated a variety of measures in the Health Outcomes Survey (Health Services Advisory Group, 2018).

Quantitative Strategies for the Evaluation of Outcomes

One significant advantage of the study of health at the population level is the ample access to large populations of electronic data, allowing for a large sample size for analysis. Certainly, nursing's role in population health is enhanced by our ability to measure and track key characteristics of the patient population that are indicative of clinical quality and utilization of healthcare resources. Administrative data sets and access to an electronic medical record (EMR) in a given venue, or an EHR that has the potential to "follow" the patient across various inpatient and outpatient settings, have enhanced our collective ability as a profession to evaluate nursing's role in providing care and service by allowing us to use large data sets to analyze patterns of care and disease in the populations we serve.

Data Availability

The advent of the universal electronic billing process became a reality many years ago in the United States with the advancement of Medicare legislation. The CMS, known at the time as the Healthcare Financing Authority (HCFA), launched an electronic billing process for hospitals in the early 1990s. The electronic format emerged from a device called the "universal bill." This universal bill, issued in 1992 (UB92), was the first vehicle to provide a rich source of demographic, diagnostic, and procedural data. In more recent years, ways and means to measure quality through this data set and other claims from individual providers, from outpatient venues of all types, as well as from rehabilitation settings and other posthospital venues, have been continually refined. Administrative data do provide some practical application. Although the usefulness of these data has been qualified and challenged over time, there is a fair amount of consensus that the information included in claims and encounters can be useful in determining the overall health of a given population of patients with certain chronic conditions (e.g., CHF, CAD, asthma, COPD, and diabetes). These data also illustrate nursing's role regardless of venue in influencing outcomes for these patients ("Case-Mix Measurement," 1987; Jha et al., 2007; McCarthy, Bihrle Johnson, & Audet, 2013; Schatz et al., 2005).

Because of the very nature of lifestyle management (H&W), DM, and CM programs, data collection on large data sets becomes possible. Although there are methodological considerations for appropriate hypothesis testing of these data, developing processes for determining the impact of the nursing role on outcomes becomes possible without extensive and tedious chart review and manual data collection.

Electronic systems for facilitating both EMR and EHR also raise the bar on the potential for outcomes research related to nursing's role in population health. In H&W, DM, and CM programs, the nursing role in providing guidance for patients' self-management of their disease conditions is documented in such a way that these "self-reported" data on milestones for patient care management are adequately captured for electronic reporting, theory testing, and hypothesis evaluation. For example, nurses who are involved in lifestyle management and H&W programs that include such things as smoking-cessation programs are able to interact with patients telephonically to ascertain their progress with smoking cessation, and these interactions are captured in electronic reporting for later analysis. Our ability to evaluate whether or not the patient has filled a smoking-cessation prescription or is using a smoking-cessation treatment may be facilitated if pharmacy claims are available, but in general, we have no idea whether the patient filled the prescription and is taking it without a self-report. The patient's report on 7-day prevalence ("Have you smoked a tobacco product in the past 7 days?") is the type of data available only through self-report or direct observation. These data can also be easily captured in EMR databases, and although it is still patient self-reported data, it is extremely useful and can be used in measurement submission, for example, in selected HEDIS measures (NCQA, 2018a).

In 2009, and through the Affordable Care Act (ACA), incentive monies became available to organizations to implement electronic means and to advance the use of the EMR and EHR systems as part of the HITECH (Health Information Technology for Economic and Clinical Health) Act. The program was called "Meaningful Use," and organizations were required to use these information systems and, once implemented, submit data to the CMS on quality process and outcomes measures (CMS, 2018g).

Hybrid data collection is a method proffered in the HEDIS data-collection model. For some of the metrics, securing the data may require samples of outpatient charts with designated data collectors to provide specific data that are not available through electronic means. Here is an example. Some programs may have the ability to secure electronic results of laboratory data. So the HEDIS measure called "comprehensive diabetes care" includes several components. One measure includes the extent to which patients who have been diagnosed with diabetes were able to secure an HbA1C test within a 12-month period. This HEDIS metric can easily be compiled through quantitative methods if claims data are available. However, unless laboratory data are also available, the actual value of the HbA1C is not forthcoming. An alternative to this is found in the hybrid method of data collection. HEDIS provides for a method of random sample selection and sample size. Data collectors are deployed, and collect the needed information by hand. For this measure and for several others in the HEDIS data set, patient self-reported data are not acceptable. In order to sort out the impact of a nursing DM strategy on patients' ongoing diabetes management, it is essential to be able to determine not only whether the patients have an annual HbA1C test performed but also the results of that test. More important, once you have those data, one has the ability to analyze which patients have good control (HbA1C less than 7% or 8% depending on defined metrics for your population) and which patients have poor control (HbA1C > 9%), and this can lead to identification of the strengths or weaknesses in a DM program. Without actual laboratory results in an electronic feed or hybrid data collection, claims data are limited in providing this insight. With good reason, and because of the significant dollars at risk, as incentives are provided for those organizations demonstrating improved outcomes in population health, audit validation procedures are rigorous.

The CMS has, over time, refined billing practices and requirements for appropriate documentation in the electronic invoicing processes for inpatient facilities and independent providers of care. Accordingly, these changes have helped to capture useful information not only in claims and encounters but also in provider practices, and to make connections for patients across the continuum of care. Incentives have been developed in recent years to reward positive practices and to better align payment with outcomes. For example, years ago UM practices for Medicare required payment only when the appropriate patient placement and level of care in an acute care setting occurs, whereas individual provider reimbursement for an inpatient stay occurs regardless of denied payment to the facility. TJC and the CMS have now aligned their processes around the core measures project, holding hospitals accountable for process of care measures (e.g., getting the AMI patient with ST elevation to the catheter laboratory within 90 minutes of arrival to the hospital). In the past, no incentives were given to physicians who achieved the less-than-90-minute goal. Similarly, keeping a patient in the hospital longer for a hospital-acquired complication (e.g., removal of a retained instrument) had no consequences. In 2009, the CMS began to limit reimbursement to hospitals that demonstrate these "never events" (CMS, 2018a). As a result, 14 conditions were identified in this category. Similarly, in 2006 a drive by the CMS to "pay for performance" was launched, encouraging individual providers to capture data in their billing practices that demonstrate patient outcomes and preventive measures in their outpatient practices, with a resultant financial reward (CMS, 2018d). For example, providers who can demonstrate (through their CMS billing) that a certain percentage of their diabetic patients have had an HbA1C test done annually, and a significant proportion of that patient population has results below 7% or 8% depending on the nature of their patient population, receive additional reimbursement.

The ease of access to administrative data sets and claims data has appropriately led to legislation that is intended to protect the integrity of these electronic data. The Health Insurance Portability and Accountability Act (HIPAA) was passed in 1996, and has resulted in a number of requirements across the country and in any venue or service related to the patient's right to confidentiality and privacy protections. Highlights of these regulatory requirements include the following concepts: (a) annual training for all staff members (whether involved in patient care or not) regarding protected health information; (b) signed business associate agreements ensuring that these protections transverse various vendors and clients; (c) adequate auditing, policies, and procedures are in place to ensure that the extent and spirit of the regulations are met (Brown, 2009; DHHS, 2018).

National Trends and Healthcare Reform

Data availability, whether from electronic, self-report, or hybrid data, has changed the nature of the healthcare landscape, and the accessibility and reliability of these data have been influenced by powerful market pressures. Certainly, the CMS has had a significant impact on healthcare in the United States since Medicare legislation in the 1960s first guaranteed healthcare as a right to all Social Security recipients over the age of 65 (Social Security, n.d.). In recent years, evolving legislation linked the issue of availability of healthcare to the quality of healthcare and recognized the inherent relationship between cost and quality. As quality improves, the cost of care is reduced. As measurement mechanisms and the availability of data have developed over the past 20 years, so has the collective wisdom. At the end of 2009, it was almost impossible to pick up a newspaper or read about the latest political debate without time and attention brought to "healthcare reform." Although pundits deconstruct the key elements of the current need for healthcare reform, all agree that the cost of providing healthcare in the United States has escalated. One can only hope that accessibility has improved for increasing segments of our society, but there are still significant disparities throughout regions of the country with a shortage of both primary care and subspecialty providers. There continues to be broad disagreement over the way in which healthcare reform was enacted despite legislation passed in 2010. Regardless of the ongoing debate about this legislation, data availability as a result of claims, in patient self-reporting, in hybrid data collection, and as a result of provider P4P (pay for performance) initiatives makes the measurement of quality considerably more elegant, more reliable, and clearer than it has ever been in the United States in estimating the impact of nursing's role in improving population health.

Since its enactment in 2010, the debate regarding healthcare reform has continued to mark the political landscape. By the end of 2014, a number of states had chosen to refrain from opting into the program. The consequences of these states' decisions remain controversial 10 years after the ACA was signed into law. After the presidential election in 2016, the ACA continued to be the source of debate and efforts to legislate the reversal of the ACA were largely unsuccessful. As of this writing, the ACA remains in force and provides healthcare insurance coverage for a disenfranchised segment of the U.S. population

(CMS, 2018h) Regardless of the political debate, data on clinical outcomes are equally available for Medicare and Medicaid programs across the United States.

Standardized Data Definitions and Comparative Databases

A theme that is consistent in this chapter on evaluation methods is that measurement methods have evolved for the better over the course of the past 20 to 30 years. Clearly, the information technology age and the availability of administrative data sets are related to the present state of data availability. In addition, clinicians have provided adequate guidance through professional organizations on both process and outcome indicators of quality and have evolved data definitions that have methodological rigor and standardization. This agreement and standardization give rise to the potential for comparisons that are methodologically sound.

Standardized data definitions are made available by the NCQA (HEDIS volumes are available for purchase at www.NCQA.org) and include detailed technical specifications. The NCQA is a leader in the field and provides not only technical specifications and guidance on hybrid data collection and sample size but certifications for HEDIS auditing capabilities. In addition to this functionality, the NCQA provides annual data comparisons with actual percentile rankings on the HEDIS measures for Medicare, Medicaid, and commercial lines of business. These are published on its website annually. Purchase of the Quality Compass makes regionalized comparisons possible and provides the percentile ranking comparisons a little sooner than they become public. Metrics with standardized data definitions are available from private and public groups, including, but not limited to, the NQF (www.qualityforum.org/Home.aspx), the CMS (www.cms.gov/center/quality.asp), TJC (www.jointcommission.org/), and specialty groups such as the American College of Cardiology, the Society of Thoracic Surgeons, and many others.

Qualitative Strategies for the Evaluation of Program Outcomes

Significant strides in nursing have been made (that did not exist 40 years ago) to improve measurement methods and use quantitative means to evaluate population health. This notwithstanding, qualitative methods are also a source of rich and useful information in this evaluation process.

Accreditation and Certification

Accreditation and certification programs offer a systematic review of a given organization's ability to provide evidence of compliance with standards. Standards define the required elements to accreditation success, and these organizations provide both rigor and agreed-upon methodologies in pursuit of organizational distinction. Although many would argue that the process itself is more quantitative than qualitative, most would agree that the result is a credential that is desirable, often sought after, and sometimes a mandate. Most accreditation and certification programs provide various levels of review and accept both depth and breadth in terms of evidence permitted. (See Chapter 9, The Role of Accreditation in Validating Population-Based Practice/Programs for more information on accreditation and certification.)

Community Advisory Boards

As DM, CM, and UM programs have within their essential construct the total health of the population at large as a key benefit, oftentimes representative members of that patient population are sought after to provide insight into the effectiveness and usefulness of these programs as benefits. These committees or boards meet on a regular basis (as frequently as quarterly to as seldom as annually or "ad hoc," depending on the need) and provide qualitative insight as to the impact of the program on patients' lives, as well as insight into enhancements. Telephonic services, written materials, field-based options, communication devices, and program changes are often reviewed with these boards to anticipate patient response. Certainly, members of the benefit program (patients and families) and local community groups representing the various segments of the community affected by the benefit might be included in the membership roster.

Provider Advisory Committees

Providers across specialties and venues, from nurses to physicians to hospitals, health systems, public health agencies, and managed care plans, are key components to the overall success in improving the health of the patient population in its entirety. Telephonic nursing provides options for care that did not exist in the past. However, face-to-face communications from nurse to primary care provider become more complex in this environment. In addition, quantitative methods have the potential to supply providers with data on their care practices that may or may not demonstrate the achievement of improvements in patient outcomes. Providing feedback to primary care providers in a systematic and patient-centered way is a strategy that can be of tremendous benefit. Consequently, devising a vehicle to enhance communications with healthcare providers in a formal setting, such as through committees, can be of significant value.

Provider advisory committees come in all shapes and sizes and meet with varying frequency. Shalala (2010) advises that APRNs who are in private practice represent an important enhancement to our ability to extend primary care capacity across the country (Naylor & Kurtzman, 2010). Representative providers, including APRNs, can "weigh in" on data presentation; they can provide advice on ways and means to make sound use of these data in a global way, as well as help to anticipate reaction. These forums serve as educational opportunities for the DM program and can enhance practice management as well as demonstrate how the EHR across the continuum of care can enhance communication processes among all members of the healthcare team as well as maximize patient outcomes. Provider advisory committees provide depth to a DM program, which is not easily found through quantitative methods.

SUMMARY

APRNs play an increasingly important role in evaluating the quality and effectiveness of healthcare delivery systems. As APRN roles have expanded into this area, it is paramount that APRNs understand the ways and means used to evaluate population health outcomes, as well as the systems of care that provide population health services. Various definitions of quality have been presented, and several theoretical frameworks are available for evaluating quality. Nurse-sensitive indicators of quality can be described using the following categories: (a) clinical quality, (b) utilization of healthcare resources, (c) core business processes, and (d) customer satisfaction. APRNs hold various roles, both clinical and administrative, in a variety of settings. Regardless of role or setting, measurement and improvement of quality with its broad definitions remain paramount. In the past, measurement systems were limited, and manual data collection was the primary method of gaining insight and information as to the outcomes of clinical care, management of chronic illness, and the patient's experience. As nurses strive to make an impact on the overall health of the population, reduce the cost of care, and improve the patient's experience of their healthcare, APRNs' roles expand.

EXERCISES AND DISCUSSION QUESTIONS

Exercise 8.1 You are a staff nurse working in a busy internist's medical practice. You've been a nurse for more than 30 years, and about 3 years ago, you decided to pursue an advanced degree in a RN to DNP program. You have about 2 years to go; you have just finished a course in Epidemiology and you are intrigued by the total population health model. You believe it could serve as a good framework for your DNP project. The physician who you work for is excited about your educational advancement and is willing to support your idea of constructing your DNP project in this practice. You've noticed that you have quite a few patients with type 2 diabetes mellitus in the practice; many of these patients have Medicare, some have Medicaid, and most have been diagnosed for more than the 5 years that you have been with the practice.

The practice is not automated; though there is a beginning electronic medical record, this practice has a 30-year track record, and most of the files are handwritten. This notwithstanding, you have a good relationship with the practice manager, who does the billing for the practice.

To further the possibility of framing your DNP project and to better grasp how to evaluate this practice at the population level, answer the following questions:

1. What measurements would be important to framing a DNP practice problem, and how would you go about doing this in your practice?

2. How could you determine, more specifically, the nature of the problem?

3. What is the gap in your practice and what qualitative and quantitative measures can shed insight?

Exercise 8.2 You are a staff nurse working in a large community hospital on a medical-surgical unit that has primarily elderly cardiac patients. You have worked part time at this hospital for more than 20 years, and now that your children have finished college, you have decided to pursue an advanced degree. You enrolled in an RN to DNP program as you have always wanted to remain clinically connected. You have no interest in pursuing an administrative role, but cardiac patients have always interested you. You note that many of your cardiac patients are familiar; there seems to be a bit of a revolving door, and many patients seem to be readmitted.

Your nurse manager knows that you are pursuing an advanced degree and has suggested that reducing readmissions within 30 days for congestive heart failure (CHF) would make a good DNP project. Furthermore, she's mentioned that the quality improvement (QI) department is very interested in this and will be supportive of your efforts as this is an organizational priority.

To further the possibility of framing your DNP project and to better grasp how to evaluate this practice at the population level, answer the following questions.

1. What measurements would be important to framing a DNP practice problem, and how would you go about doing this for the patients in the hospital, and on your unit?

2. How could you determine, more specifically, the nature of the problem?

3. What is the gap in practice at your organization (and on your unit), and what qualitative and quantitative measures can shed insight?

REFERENCES

American Academy of Professional Coders. (2018). *What is medical coding?* Retrieved from https://www.aapc.com/medical-coding/medical-coding.aspx

American Association of Colleges of Nursing. (2006). *The essentials of doctoral education for advanced nursing practice.* Retrieved from http://www.aacn.nche.edu/DNP/pdf/Essentials.pdf

Anderson-Dean, C. (2012). The benefits of Lean Six Sigma for nursing informatics. *American Nursing Informatics Association, 27*(4), 1, 6–7.

Ayanian, J. Z., & Markel, H. (2016). Donabedian's lasting framework for health care quality. *The New England Journal of Medicine, 375*, 205–207. doi:10.1056/NEJMp1605101

Baehr, A., Holland, T., Biala, K., Margolis, G. S., Wiebe, D. J., & Carr, B. G. (2016) Describing total population health: A review and critique of existing units. *Population Health Management, 19*(5), 306–314. doi:10.1089/pop.2015.0105

Balanced Scorecard Institute. (2018). *Handbook for basic process improvement.* Retrieved from https://balancedscorecard.org/Resources/Articles-White-Papers/Process-Improvement-Tools

Berwick, D., & Fox, D. M. (2016) Evaluating the quality of medical care: Donabedian's classic article 50 years later. *The Millbank Quarterly, 94*(2), 237–241. doi:10.1111/1468-0009.12189

Berwick, D. M., Godfrey, A. B., & Roessner, J. (1990). *Curing health care: New strategies for quality improvement.* San Francisco, CA: Jossey-Bass.

Best, M., & Neuhauser, D. (2006). Joseph Juran: Overcoming resistance to organizational change. *Quality and Safety in Health Care, 15*(5), 380–382. doi:10.1136/qshc.2006.020016

Bisognano, M., & Kenney, C. (2012). *Pursuing the Triple Aim.* San Francisco, CA: Jossey-Bass, Wiley.

Brem, H., Maggi, J., Nierman, D., Roinitzky, L., Bell, D., Rennert, R., . . . Vladeck, B. (2010). High cost of stage IV pressure ulcers. *American Journal of Surgery 200,* 473–477. doi:10.1016/j.amjsurg.2009.12.021

Breslin, S. E., Hamilton, K. M., & Paynter, J. (2014). Development of Lean Six Sigma in care coordination: An improved discharge process. *Professional Case Management, 77*(2), 77–83. doi:10.1097/NCM.0000000000000016

Brown, J. (2009). *The healthcare quality handbook* (24th ed.). Pasadena, CA: JB Quality Solutions.

Case-mix measurement and assessing quality of hospital care [Annual supplement]. (1987). *Health Care Financing Review, 1987*(Suppl), 39–48.

Centers for Disease Control and Prevention. (2018a). Division for heart disease and stroke prevention: Heart failure fact sheet. Retrieved from https://www.cdc.gov/dhdsp/data_statistics/fact_sheets/fs_heart_failure.htm

Centers for Disease Control and Prevention, Healthcare Infection Control Practices Advisory Committee. (2018b). *Guidelines for the prevention of intravascular catheter-related infections.* Retrieved from http://www.cdc.gov/hicpac/pdf/bsi/bsi-guidelines-2011.pdf

Centers for Disease Control and Prevention. (2018c) International Classification of Diseases, tenth revision, clinical modification (ICD-10-CM). Retrieved from https://www.cdc.gov/nchs/icd/icd10cm.htm

Centers for Medicare & Medicaid Services. (2018a). *Hospital acquired conditions (present on admission indicator)*. Retrieved from http://www.cms.gov/HospitalAcqCond

Centers for Medicare & Medicaid Services. (2018b). *Quality measures and performance standards*. Retrieved from http://www.cms.gov/Medicare/Medicare-Fee-for-Service-Payment/sharedsavingsprogram/Quality_Measures_Standards.html

Centers for Medicare & Medicaid Services. (2018c). LTCH Care Data Set Version 4.00. Retrieved from https://www.cms.gov/Medicare/Quality-Initiatives-Patient-Assessment-Instruments/LTCH-Quality-Reporting/Downloads/Final-LTCH-CARE-Data-Set-Version-400-Change-Table-Effective-July-1-2018.pdf

Centers for Medicare & Medicaid Services. (2018d). *Part C and D performance data*. Retrieved from http://www.cms.gov/Medicare/Prescription-Drug-Coverage/PrescriptionDrugCovGenIn/PerformanceData.html

Centers for Medicare & Medicaid Services. (2018e). *Part C reporting requirements*. Retrieved from http://www.cms.gov/Medicare/Health-Plans/HealthPlansGenInfo/ReportingRequirements.html

Centers for Medicare & Medicaid Services. (2018f). *Physician quality reporting system*. Retrieved from https://www.cms.gov/Medicare/Health-Plans/HealthPlansGenInfo/ReportingRequirements.html

Centers for Medicare & Medicaid Services. (2018g). EHR incentive programs; 2018 program requirements. Retrieved from https://www.cms.gov/Regulations-and-Guidance/Legislation/EHRIncentivePrograms/2018ProgramRequirements.html

Centers for Medicare & Medicaid Services. (2018h). Affordable Care Act regulations and guidance. Retrieved from https://www.cms.gov/cciio/resources/regulations-and-guidance/index.html

Chu, H. L., Wang, C. C., & Dai, Y. T. (2009). A study of a nursing department performance measurement system: Using the balanced scorecard and the analytic hierarchy process. *Nursing Economics, 27*, 401–407.

Corn, J. B. (2009). Six Sigma in health care. *Radiologic Technology, 81*(1), 92–95.

Cornwell, B. L., Brockmann, L. M., Lasky, E. C., Mach, J., & McCarthy, J. F. (2018) Primary care–Mental health integration in the Veterans Affairs Health System Program. *Psychiatric Services, 69*, 696–702. doi:10.1176/appi.ps.201700213

Courtney, B. A., Ruppman, J. B., & Cooper, H. M. (2006). Save our skin: Initiative cuts pressure ulcer incidence in half. *Nursing Management, 37*(4), 36, 38, 40. doi:10.1097/00006247-200604000-00010

Cross, K. F. (2000). Call resolution: The wrong focus for service quality? *Quality Progress, 33*(2), 64–67.

DeFeo, J. A. (2014). *Juran's quality essentials for leaders*. New York, NY: McGraw-Hill.

DeFeo, J. A. (2017). *Juran's quality handbook: The complete guide to performance excellence* (7th ed.). New York, NY: McGraw-Hill.

DeFeo, J. A., & Barnard, W. W. (2004). *Juran Institute's Six Sigma's breakthrough and beyond: Quality performance breakthrough methods*. New York, NY: McGraw-Hill.

Del Franco, M. (2003). Cutting back on call abandonment. *Catalog Age, 20*(7), 59–60.

Dienemann, J. (Ed.). (1992). *Continuous quality improvement in nursing*. Washington, DC: American Nurses Publishing.

Donabedian, A. (1980). *The definition of quality and approaches to assessment*. Ann Arbor, MI: Health Administration Press.

Drenckpohl, D., Bowers, L., & Cooper, H. (2007). Use of the Six Sigma methodology to reduce incidence of breast milk administration errors in the NICU. *Neonatal Network, 26*, 161–166. doi:10.1891/0730-0832.26.3.161

Fairbanks, C. B. (2007). Using Six Sigma and Lean methodologies to improve OR throughput. *AORN Journal, 86*(1), 73–82. doi:10.1016/j.aorn.2007.06.011

Formichelli, L. (2007). By the numbers. *Multichannel Merchant, 24*(4), 44–45. doi:10.1109/MSPEC.2007.369262

Gavriloff, C. (2012). A performance improvement plan to increase nurse adherence to use of medication safety software. *Journal of Pediatric Nursing, 27*, 375–382. doi:10.1016/j.pedn.2011.06.004

Goonan, K. J. (1995). *The Juran prescription*. San Francisco, CA: Jossey-Bass.

Goonan, K. J., & Scarrow, P. (2010). Interview with a quality leader: Kate Goonan and performance excellence. *Journal for Healthcare Quality, 32*(3), 32–35. doi:10.1111/j.1945-1474.2010.00091.x

Guerrero, A. P. S., Takesue, C. L., Medeiros, J. H. N., Duran, A. A., Humphry, J. W., Lunsford, R. M., . . . Hishinuma, E. S. (2017) Primary care integration of psychiatric and behavioral health services: A primer for providers and case report of local implementation. *Hawaii Journal of Medicine and Public Health, 76*(6), 147-151.

Guru guide: Six thought leaders who changed the quality world forever. (2010). *Quality Progress, 43*(11), 14–21.

Gustafson, B. M. (1999). A well-staffed PFS call center can improve patient satisfaction. *Healthcare Financial Management, 53*(7), 64–66.

Health Services Advisory Group. (2018). *Medicare Health Outcomes Survey.* Retrieved from https://www. hosonline.org

Healthcare Effectiveness Data and Information Set. (2018). *Narrative, technical specifications, and survey measurement* (Vols. 1–3). Washington, DC: National Committee for Quality Assurance. Retrieved from http://ncqa.org/tabid/59/Default.aspx

Hospital Consumer Assessment of Healthcare Providers and Systems. (2018). *CAHPS hospital survey.* Retrieved from https://www.ahrq.gov/cahps/surveys-guidance/hospital/index.html

Hudson, S., Gonzalez-Gomez, H. V., & Rychalski, A. (2017). Call centers: Is there an upside to the dissatisfied customer experience? *The Journal of Business Strategy, 38*(1), 39–46. doi:10.1108/JBS-01-2016-0008

Institute for Healthcare Improvement. (2018a). Retrieved from http://www.ihi.org/Pages/default.aspx

Institute for Healthcare Improvement. (2018b). *Provider and Staff Satisfaction Survey.* Retrieved from http:// www.ihi.org/resources/Pages/Tools/ProviderandStaffSatisfactionSurvey.aspx

Institute of Medicine. (1999). *To err is human; building a safer health system. A consensus report.* Retrieved from http://www.nationalacademies.org/hmd/~/media/Files/Report%20Files/1999/To-Err-is-Human/ To%20Err%20is%20Human%201999%20%20report%20brief.pdf

Institute of Medicine. (2001). *Crossing the quality chasm: A new health system for the 21st century.* Washington, DC: National Academy Press.

Jha, A. K., Wright, S. M., & Perlin, J. B. (2007). Performance measures, vaccinations, and pneumonia rates among high-risk patients in Veterans Administration health care. *American Journal of Public Health, 97,* 2167–2172. doi:10.2105/AJPH.2006.099440

Joint Commission Resources. (2003). *Root cause analysis in health care; tools and techniques* (2nd ed.). Oakbrook, IL: Author.

Jones, L. K., Greskovic, G., Grassi, D. M., Graham, J., Halyan, S., Gionfriddo, M. R., . . . Evans, M. A. (2017). Medication Therapy disease management: Geisinger's approach to population health management, *Journal of Health-System Pharmacy 74,* 1422–1435. doi:10.2146/ajhp161061

Kalter-Leibovici, O., Freimark, D., Freedman, L. S., Kaufman, G., Siz, A., Murad, H., . . . Silver, H. (2017). Disease management in the treatment of patients with chronic heart failure who have universal access to health care: A randomized controlled trial. *BMC Medicine, 15*(90), 1–13. doi:10.1186/ s12916-017-0855-z

Kaplan, S., Bisgaard, S., Truesdell, D., & Zetterholm, S. (2009). Design for Six Sigma in healthcare: Developing an employee influenza vaccination process. *Journal for Healthcare Quality, 31*(3), 36–43. doi:10.1111/j.1945-1474.2009.00029.x

Kaplan, R. S., & Norton, D. P. (1996). *The balanced scorecard.* Boston, MA: Harvard Business School Press.

Kaplan, R. S., & Norton, D. P. (2001). *The strategy-focused organization.* Boston, MA: Harvard Business School Press.

Kitzman, P., Hudson, K., Sylvia, V., Feltner, F., & Lovins, J. (2017) Care coordination for community transitions for individuals post-stroke returning to low-resource rural communities. *Journal of Community Health, 42,* 565–572. doi:10.1007/s10900-016-0289-0

Khudyakov, P., Feigin, P. D., & Mandelbaum, A. (2010). Designing a call center with an IVR (interactive voice response). *Queueing Systems, 66,* 215–237. doi:10.1007/s11134-010-9193-y

Kuwaiti, A. A., & Subbarayalu, A. V. (2017) Reducing patients' falls rate in an academic medical center (AMC) using Six Sigma "DMAIC" approach. *International Journal of Health Care Quality Assurance, 30*(4), 373–384. doi:10.1108/IJHCQA-03-2016-0030

Loftus, K., Tilley, T., Hoffman, J., Bradburn, E., & Harvey, E. (2015) Use of Six Sigma strategies to pull the line on central-line associated bloodstream infections in a neurotrauma intensive care unit. *Journal of Trauma Nursing, 22*(2), 78–86. doi:10.1097/JTN.0000000000000111

Maddox, P. J. (1992). Successful implementation of a CQI process. In J. Dienneman (Ed.), *Continuous quality improvement in nursing* (pp. 115–124). Washington, DC: American Nurses Publishing.

Mandelbaum, A., & Zeltyn, S. (2013). Data-stories about (im)patient customers in tele-queues. *Queueing Systems, 75*, 115–146. doi:10.1007/s11134-013-9354-x

McCarthy, D., Bihrle Johnson, M., & Audet, A. M. (2013). Recasting readmissions by placing the hospital role in community context. *Journal of the American Medical Association, 309*, 351–352. doi:10.1001/jama.2013.1

McClure, J. B., Bush, T., Anderson, M. L., Blasi, P., Thompson, E., Nelson, J., & Catz, S. L. (2018). Oral health promotion and smoking cessation program delivered via tobacco quitlines: The Oral Health 4 Life Trial. *American Journal of Public Health, 108*(5), 689–695. doi:10.2105/AJPH.2017.304279

Medicare Payment Advisory Committee. (2018). *Report to the Congress: Medicare payment policy*. Retrieved from http://www.medpac.gov/-documents-/reports

Moen, R. D., & Norman, C. L. (2010). Circling back: Clearing up myths about the Deming cycle and seeing how it keeps evolving. *Quality Progress, 43*(11), 22–28.

Moulin, M., Soady, J., Skinner, J., Price, C., Cullen, J., & Gilligan, C. (2007). Using the public sector scorecard in public health. *International Journal of Health Care Quality Assurance, 20*, 281–289. doi:10.1108/09526860710754352

Moye, P. M., Chu, P. S., Pounds, T., & Thurston, M. M. (2018) Impact of a pharmacy team-led intervention program on the readmission rate of elderly patients with heart failure. *American Journal of Health-Systems Pharmacy 75*, 183–190. doi:10.2146/ajhp170256

Muerer, S. J., McGartland-Rubio, D., Counte, M. A., & Burroughs, T. (2002). Development of a healthcare quality improvement measurement tool: Results of a content validity study. *Hospital Topics, 80*(2), 7–13. doi:10.1080/00185860209597989

Nash, D. B., Reifsnyder, J., Fabius R. J., & Pracilio, V. P. (2011). *Population health: Creating a culture of wellness*. Sudbury, MA: Jones and Bartlett Learning.

National Committee for Quality Assurance. (2018a). HEDIS and performance measurement. Retrieved from http://www.ncqa.org/hedis-quality-measurement/hedis-programs

National Committee for Quality Assurance. (2018b). *Standards and guidelines for the accreditation and certification of disease management*. Washington, DC: Author.

National Committee for Quality Assurance. (2018c). *Tell us your opinion!* Retrieved from http://ncqa.org

National Committee for Quality Assurance. (2018d). *Technical specifications for health plans* (Vol. 2). Washington, DC: Author.

National Institute of Standards and Technology. (2018). *Baldridge performance excellence program*. Retrieved from http://www.nist.gov/baldrige/publications/hc_criteria.cfm

National Quality Forum. (2010). *Quality connections: The power of safety: State reporting provides lessons in reducing harm, improving care*. Retrieved from http://www.qualityforum.org/Publications/2010/06/Quality_Connections__The_Power_of_Safety__State_Reporting_Provides_Lessons_in_Reducing_Harm,_Improving_Care.aspx

Naylor, M. D., & Kurtzman, E. T. (2010). The role of nurse practitioners in reinventing primary care. *Health Affairs, 29*, 893–899. doi:10.1377/hlthaff.2010.0440

Peasah, S. K., McKay, N. L., Harman, J. S., Al-amin, M., & Cook, R. L. (2013) Medicare non-payment of hospital-acquired infections: Infection rates three years post implementation. *Medicare & Medicaid Research Review, 3*(3), 1–13. doi:10.5600/mmrr.003.03.a08

Pollert, P., Dobberstein, D., & Wiisanen, R. (2008). Jumping into the healthcare retail market: Our experience. *Frontiers of Health Services Management, 24*(3), 13–22. doi:10.1097/01974520-200801000-00003

Potthoff, S., & Ryan, M. J. (2004). Leadership, management, and change in improving quality in healthcare. *Frontiers of Health Services Management, 20*(3), 37–41. doi:10.1097/01974520-200401000-00007

Pyzdek, T., & Keller, P. (2014). *The Six Sigma handbook* (4th ed.). New York, NY: McGraw-Hill.

Rowe, A. D., McCarty, K., & Huett, A. (2018) Implementation of a nurse driven pathway to reduce incidence of hospital acquired pressure injuries in the pediatric intensive care setting. *Journal of Pediatric Nursing, 41*, 104–109. doi:10.1016/j.pedn.2018.03.001

Russo, A. N., Sathiyamoorthy, G., Lau, C., Saygin, D., Zioazhen, H., Ziao-Feng, W., . . . Hatipogiu, U.(2017). Impact of a post discharge integrated disease management program on COPD hospital readmissions, *Respiratory Care, 62*, 1396–1402. doi:10.4187/respcare.05547

Saberi, M., Hussain, O. K., & Chang, E. (2017) Past, present and future of contact centers; a literature review. *Business Process Management Journal, 23*, 574–597. doi:10.1108/BPMJ-02-2015-0018

Schatz, M., Nakahiro, R., Crawford, W., Mendoza, G., Mosen, D., & Stibolt, T. B. (2005). Asthma quality-of-care markers using administrative data. *Chest, 128*, 1968–1974. doi:10.1378/chest.128.4.1968

Scherz, N., Bachmann-Mettler, I., Chmiel, C., Senn, O., Boss, N., Bardheci, K., & Rosemann, T. (2017) Case management to increase quality of life after cancer treatment: A randomized controlled trial. *BMC Medicine, 17*(223), 1–8. doi:10.1186/s12885-017-3213-9

Shah, B., Forsythe, L., & Murray, C. (2018). Effectiveness of interprofessional care teams on reducing hospital readmissions in patients with heart failure: A systematic review. *Medical Surgical Nursing, 27*(3), 177–185.

Shalala, D. (2010). *Group recommends expanding nurses' role in primary care.* Retrieved from http://thefutureofnursing.org/recommendations

Social Security. (n.d.). *Legislative history.* Retrieved from http://www.ssa.gov/history/tally65.html

Stankovic, A. K., & DeLauro, E. (2010). Quality improvements in the preanalytical phase: Focus on the urine specimen flow. *MLO: Medical Laboratory Observer, 42*(3), 22, 24–27.

Thomas, M., Hutchison, M., Castro, G., Nau, M., Shumway, M., Stotland, N., & Spielvogel, A. (2017) Meeting women where they are: Integration of care as the foundation of treatment for at-risk pregnant and postpartum women. *Maternal Child Health, 21*, 452–457. doi:10.1007/s10995-016-2240-5

U.S. Department of Health and Human Services. (2018). *Health information privacy.* Retrieved from https://www.hhs.gov/hipaa/for-professionals/security/laws-regulations/index.html

URAC. (2018). *Case management accreditation.* Washington, DC: Author. Retrieved from https://www.urac.org/programs/case-management-accreditation

Whiting, A., & Donthu, N. (2009). Closing the gap between perceived and actual waiting times in a call center: Results from a field study. *Journal of Services Marketing, 23*, 279–288. doi:10.1108/08876040910973396

Womack, J. P., & Jones, D. T. (2003). *Lean thinking.* New York, NY: Free Press.

Yancy, C. W., Jessup, M., Bozkurt, B., Butler, J., Casey, D. E., Drazner, M. H., & Johnson, M. R. (2017). 2017 Update ACCF/AHA guideline for the management of heart failure: Executive summary: A report of the American College of Cardiology Foundation/American Heart Association Task Force on practice guidelines. Retrieved from https://www.acc.org/latest-in-cardiology/ten-points-to-remember/2017/04/27/15/50/2017-acc-aha-hfsa-focused-update-of-hf-guideline

Yap, C., Siu, E., Baker, G. R., Brown, A. D., & Lowi-Young, M. P. (2005). A comparison of systemwide and hospital-specific performance measurement tools. *Journal of Healthcare Management, 50*, 251–263. doi:10.1097/00115514-200507000-00007

Yun, E. K., & Chun, K. M. (2008). Critical to quality in telemedicine service management: Application of DFSS (design for Six Sigma) and SERVQUAL. *Nursing Economics, 26*, 384–388.

INTERNET RESOURCES

Agency for Healthcare Research and Quality (AHRQ): www.ahrq.gov

ASQ: www.asq.org/learn-about-quality/iso-9000/overview/overview.html

Baldiage Performance Excellence Program: www.nist.gov/baldrige/publications/hc_criteria.cfm

CMS "Accountable Care Organizations" (ACOs): https://www.cms.gov/Medicare/Medicare-Fee-for-Service-Payment/ACO/index.html

CMS "Hospital-Acquired Conditions (Present on Admission Indicator)": www.cms.gov/HospitalAcqCond

CMS "Quality Care Center": www.cms.gov/center/quality.asp

CMS, The Center for Consumer Information & Insurance Oversight": https://www.cms.gov/cciio/resources/regulations-and-guidance/index.html

Healthcare Facilities Accreditation Program (HFAP): https://www.hfap.org

HealthStream: www.healthstream.com/index.aspx

National Committee for Quality Assurance (NCQA): www.ncqa.org

National Database of Nursing Quality Indicators (NDNQI; http://www.pressganey.com/ourSolutions/performance-and-advanced-analytics/clinical-business-performance/nursing-quality-ndnqi

National Quality Forum (NQF): www.qualityforum.org

NCQA "HEDIS and Performance Measurement": http://www.ncqa.org/hedis-quality-measurement/hedis-programs

Population Health Alliance: www.populationhealthalliance.org

Press Ganey™: www.pressganey.com/index.aspx

Rand Health "Factors Affecting Physician Professional Satisfaction and Their Implications for Patient Care, Health Systems, and Health Policy": www.rand.org/content/dam/rand/pubs/research_reports/RR400/RR439/RAND_RR439.pdf

The Commission on Accreditation of Rehabilitation Facilities (CARF): www.carf.org/Accreditation

The Joint Commission (TJC): http://www.jointcommission.org

Triple Aim: www.ihi.org/Topics/TripleAim/Pages/default.aspx

URAC: www.urac.org

CHAPTER 9

THE ROLE OF ACCREDITATION IN VALIDATING POPULATION-BASED PRACTICE/PROGRAMS

EILEEN M. HORTON

INTRODUCTION

This chapter addresses the role of specialty accreditation and certification in population-based healthcare. The scope of advanced practice nursing continues to evolve and expand throughout a variety of clinical practice sites such as acute care hospitals, long-term care facilities, subacute/rehab facilities, long-term acute care (LTAC), ambulatory health, public health, and behavioral health settings. Irrespective of the setting, the expectation for the advanced practice registered nurse (APRN) is a working knowledge of the required program accreditations for licensing and reimbursement. Also important is an understanding of the role of certification in validating patient care and quality outcomes.

The Institute of Medicine's (IOM) seminal work, *The Future of Nursing* (2010), defines the roles that APRNs should have in the design of future healthcare models. The IOM report identifies the need for healthcare organizations to support nurses as leaders in the development and adoption of innovative models of patient-centered care. The report further specifies all of the responsibilities of agencies, including the federal government, to support these efforts. APRNs receive significant academic preparation focusing on advanced clinical practice. Such nurses also require knowledge on operationalizing and implementing clinical programs.

The American Association of Colleges of Nursing (AACN) identifies the eight essential areas of educational content for a doctorate in nursing practice (DNP). Developing programs and working toward program accreditation requires competence in each of the essentials. Essential II, *Organizational and Systems Leadership for Quality Improvement,* focuses on leadership, and the APRN's ability to "develop and evaluate care delivery approaches that meet the current and future needs of patient populations based on scientific findings in nursing and other clinical sciences, as well as organizational, political, and economic sciences" (AACN 2006, p. 10). This core competency of DNP education best addresses the abilities that are required to lead organizations seeking accreditation.

A set of standards is the primary hallmark of a credentialing program. Whether evaluation of a given program is housed in a facility (like an acute care hospital accredited through The Joint Commission [TJC]), a public health agency, or a disease management (DM) program, both accreditation and certification are considered to be measures of quality. For example, TJC's certification program for congestive heart failure (CHF) is offered in conjunction with the American Heart Association and offers this certification based on standards and outcomes (TJC, 2018). As nurses practice and provide nursing care within and throughout these facilities and programs, accreditation is an indirect measure of the quality of nursing practice. The processes used within an accrediting program are also variable, but are often characterized by common features: (a) written documentation is submitted for review; (b) site visits comprise an overview of the program, its capabilities and outcomes, and staff interviews; and (c) chart or file reviews of some kind are included in the accreditation process validating that as nurses we provide evidence-based care.

Accreditation and certification are mechanisms for evaluating the processes and outcomes of clinical programs. Accreditation is positively associated with the establishment of organizational structures and processes, the existence of quality and safety cultures, improved patient care and outcomes, as well as other benefits. During the process of accreditation there is hardly a time when an organization must not produce metrics that are sensitive to the nursing role, demonstrate patient characteristics, and quantify patient outcomes. The accrediting process becomes qualitative as the evaluation of the quality of the program may or may not show actual improvement in defined patient care indicators. Many accrediting bodies are not prescriptive in the application of their standards; this is in no way a detracting characteristic. In fact, the latitude in the application of the standards (the "how") is often desirable as there are many ways to achieve the same outcome. Examples of accrediting bodies and the type of programs that they accredit or certify are provided in Exhibit 9.1. This list is not intended to be exhaustive but simply illustrative. Each includes standards that evaluate the outcome of nursing care in some way.

The effectiveness of patient care is evaluated by measuring patient outcomes; similarly, clinical programs are validated by measuring programmatic outcomes. Some accreditation and certification programs are essential requirements for clinical practice while others are voluntary additional credentials. The following information is a sampling of the various types of credentials that need to be considered when developing a new population-based clinical program or working within an established one.

EXHIBIT 9.1

EXAMPLES OF ACCREDITING BODIES AND THE TYPES OF PROGRAMS THEY ACCREDIT

The Joint Commission (TJC) accredits acute care hospitals and provides certification to a number of specialty hospitals and programs, many of which have a patient focus that goes well beyond the patient's inpatient experience. Accordingly, these accreditation programs have an influence on the health of the total patient population as well as nursing's role in the experience. TJC is often designated by state licensure for hospital review. TJC holds deemed status for the Centers for Medicare & Medicaid (CMS); hospitals seeking to achieve or maintain provider status must be both accredited and licensed. Find more information about TJC at www.jointcommission.org.

The National Committee for Quality Assurance (NCQA) offers numerous recognition, accreditation, and certification programs, including, but not limited to, health plans, utilization management (UM) programs, disease management (DM) programs, healthcare effectiveness data and information set (HEDIS) auditing, and many other types. Information regarding the programs offered by this organization can be found at www.ncqa.org.

The Utilization Review Accreditation Committee (URAC) formally adopted the acronym URAC in 1996. It is an organization with a long track record in offering accreditation for total population health. UM, DM, and CM programs and other types of accreditations that are related to the nursing role in total population health are among the many types offered. More information on this organization can be found at www.urac.org.

The Commission on Accreditation of Rehabilitation Facilities (CARF) is yet another organization with a focus on evaluating the quality of various programs, including behavioral health services across the rehabilitation continuum, durable medical equipment providers, aging programs, and other program types. The CARF website provides a wealth of useful information (www.carf.org/Accreditation).

DNV NIAHO provides an accreditation based on the International Organization for Standardization (ISO) 9000 (www.asq.org/learn-about-quality/iso-9000/overview/overview.html) and achieved deemed status from the CMS in September 2008 (www.dnv.com/industry/healthcare). Although this organization specializes in managing risk for many types of industries, a recent focus on healthcare and the CMS deemed status has opened a new option for accreditation. This organization has focused on accrediting hospitals, primary stroke centers, and critical access hospitals. More information can be sought at https://www.dnvgl.us/assurance/healthcare/ac.html.

The Healthcare Facilities Accreditation Program (HFAP) was originally created in 1945 to conduct an objective review of services provided by osteopathic hospitals, HFAP has maintained its deeming authority continuously since the inception of the CMS in 1965 and meets or exceeds the standards required by the CMS/Medicare to provide accreditation to all hospitals, ambulatory care/surgical facilities, mental health facilities, physical rehabilitation facilities, clinical

(continued)

EXHIBIT 9.1

laboratories and critical access hospitals. HFAP also provides certification reviews for Primary Stroke Centers. Find more information about HFAP at https://www.hfap.org/about/overview.aspx

The Public Health Accreditation Board (PHAB) accredits tribal, state, local, and territorial public health departments. PHAB is a non-profit entity created in 2007 to accredit public health departments following a Robert Wood Johnson Foundation initiative *Exploring Accreditation*. PHAB has created standards and measures as a framework for evaluating the performance of public health departments. More information on PHAB can be found at http://www.phaboard.org/accreditation-overview/what-is-accreditation.

Community Health Accreditation Partner (CHAP) has the CMS deeming authority for home health, hospice, and home care medical equipment. CHAP standards are designed for home and community-based care and helpful for new and developing programs. Information about CHAP can be found at https://chapinc.org.

GOVERNMENTAL PROGRAMS

Centers for Medicare & Medicaid Services

Reimbursement is a critical element for any program. CMS is the largest payer in most adult populations, and its role will continue to grow as the population in the United States ages. In order to receive payment from Medicare and Medicaid, healthcare programs/organizations must meet the Conditions of Participation (CoP) and Conditions for Coverage (CfCs) identified by CMS. The intent of these conditions is to protect patient health and safety and to insure quality. The list of programs requiring certification of the CoPs is found in Box 9.1. Certifying that the CoPs and CfCs are met is achieved via a survey conducted by an organization on behalf of the federal government. Typically the applicable State Department of Health or a national accrediting organization approved by CMS carries out this function. These CMS approved accrediting organizations are identified as having *deeming authority*. In effect, when a healthcare entity is successfully accredited by a deeming body it is granted deemed status, which certifies that the organization has met the CMS conditions.

Organizations seeking CMS approval may choose to be surveyed either by an approved accrediting organization such as TJC, Das Norsk Veritas Healthcare (DNV), and Healthcare Facilities Accreditation Program (HFAP), or by state surveyors on behalf of CMS. About 90% of hospitals in the United States are accredited by private organizations (Castellucci, 2018). TJC alone accredits 88% of all accredited hospitals in the United States (TJC, 2017, ¶1). A TJC, DNV or HFAP survey may be followed by a random state validation survey. These validation surveys are used to evaluate the effectiveness of the accrediting organization's review process, and are carried out by the applicable State Department of Health on behalf of CMS. A list and description of organizations that are

BOX 9.1

CONDITIONS FOR COVERAGE (CFCS) & CONDITIONS OF PARTICIPATIONS (COPS)

Ambulatory Surgical Centers (ASCs)

Community Mental Health Centers (CMHCs)

Comprehensive Outpatient Rehabilitation Facilities (CORFs)

Critical Access Hospitals (CAHs)

End-Stage Renal Disease Facilities

Federally Qualified Health Centers

Home Health Agencies

Hospices

Hospitals

Hospital Swing Beds

Intermediate Care Facilities for Individuals with Intellectual Disabilities (ICF/IID)

Organ Procurement Organizations (OPOs)

Portable X-Ray Suppliers

Programs for All-Inclusive Care for the Elderly Organizations (PACE)

Clinics, Rehabilitation Agencies, and Public Health Agencies as Providers of Outpatient Physical Therapy and Speech-Language Pathology Services

Psychiatric Hospitals

Religious Nonmedical Health Care Institutions

- Rural Health Clinics
- Long Term Care Facilities
- Transplant Centers

Specific information about each of these categories can be found at CMS.gov using the following address/link:

https://www.cms.gov/Regulations-and-Guidance/Legislation/CFCsAndCoPs/index.html?redirect=/CFCsAndCoPs

Source: From Centers for Medicare and Medicaid Services (CMS). (2018a). *Conditions for coverage (CfCs) & Conditions of participations (CoPs).* Retrieved from https://www.cms.gov/Regulations-and-Guidance/Legislation/CFCsAndCoPs/index.html?redirect=/CFCsAndCoPs

approved to provide deemed status can be found in Chapter 8, Evaluation of Practice at the Population Level.

In addition to facility accreditation CMS requires organizations to be certified as Medicare approved in order to perform certain procedures such as carotid artery stenting, VAD destination therapy, certain oncologic PET scans in Medicare-specified studies, and lung volume reduction surgery. Information on Medicare approved facilities/trials/ registries can be found at www.cms.gov/Medicare/Medicare-General-Information/ MedicareApprovedFacilitie/index.html

Early clinical program planning should include a review of the National Coverage Determination in order to identify the criteria for certification by CMS (go to www.cms .gov/medicare-coverage-database/indexes/ncd-alphabetical-index.aspx).

Controlling the growth of healthcare spending is a major focus of the federal government. Pay for performance (P4P) or value-based purchasing (VBP) is an initiative instituted by CMS whereby reimbursement is based on performance that results in quality patient outcomes. Hospital-acquired conditions (HACs) is one example of a P4P focus. Post-op surgical site infections (SSI), central line-associated bloodstream infections (CLABSI), catheter-associated urinary tract infections (CAUTI), methicillin-resistant staphylococcus aureus (MRSA), and clostridium difficile (C. diff) are several examples of HACs. To fund the program, each year CMS withholds a percentage of inpatient payments from hospitals. For 2018, the withholding percentage was 2%. A hospital can earn back more than the withheld amount (effectively earning a bonus) if it performs well with VBP metrics (Advisory Board, 2017). Accordingly, VBP continues to expand to include more indicators annually across the continuum of care. Private payers frequently use CMS guidelines as a basis for their protocols, and as a result value-based care and reimbursement has expanded outside of CMS. Following the lead set by CMS, private insurance companies such as AETNA, Blue Cross, and United, to name just a few, have implemented value based purchasing contracts with providers. The Triple Aim model developed by the Institute for Healthcare Improvement (IHI) is consistent with trends in VBP. For more on Triple Aim, see Chapter 2, Identifying Outcomes in Population-Based Nursing and Chapter 8, Evaluation of Practice at the Population Level.

The focus of VBP is not just on acute care hospitals. The Medicare Access and CHIP Reauthorization Act (MACRA) is a piece of legislation that created merit-based incentive payments (MIPS) and advanced alternative payment models for other clinical settings. One such alternative payment model is the oncology care model (OCM). It serves as a good example for APRNs who practice outside of acute care hospitals. Practices that participate in the OCM have agreed to a payment model that includes financial and performance accountability related to chemotherapy administration for cancer patients (CMS, 2018b). The model essentially rewards high quality evidenced based coordinated care. Performance accountability includes data from quality measures, claims data, and patient satisfaction surveys. The Oncology Nurses Society (ONS) has identified the need for oncology APRNs to be familiar with MIPS and OCM, and to take leadership roles in participating in these programs (Galioto, 2017). More information on these CMS programs can be found at www.cms.gov/Medicare/Quality-Initiatives-Patient-Assessment-Instruments/ Value-Based-Programs/MACRA-MIPS-and-APMs/MACRA-MIPS-and-APMs.html.

Home health agencies provide skilled care to homebound patients. TJC and Community Health Accreditation Partner (CHAP) have CMS deeming authority for accrediting home health, hospice and home care medical equipment. CHAP *Standards of Excellence* (education.chaplinq.org/products/2018-chap-standards-of-excellence-for -home-health-providers) are designed for home and community-based care and provide a useful guide for developing and implementing new programs. Likewise, TJC has the *Comprehensive Accreditation Manual for Homecare* (www.jcrinc.com/2019-comprehensive -accreditation-manual-for-home-care-camhc-/cahc19), which provides standards and measures for homecare programs.

State Designations

It is important for APRNs who are developing clinical programs to review state (as well as federal) requirements for licensure of organizations, which may include requirements for accreditation and/or certification. APRNs should be knowledgeable about the corresponding state regulations for their clinical practice location (acute care, ambulatory care, long term care, etc.). Like federal designations, state designations are also premised on the concepts of patient safety and quality. Many states, for example, have formal requirements for licensing and certification of trauma, cardiac, and perinatal care to name just a few. An example of a clinical area that has been in the spotlight recently and that has evolved in many states into one of the most formalized processes for approval is stroke care. In 2004, New Jersey and Florida became the first states to legislate stroke care. Massachusetts and New York subsequently also developed regulations for care (Center for Disease Control and Prevention [CDC], 2011). Other states quickly followed suit and there is much discussion on the national level for universal standards adoption. The focus has not been limited to the hospital care of stroke patients. Stroke prevention programs as well as follow-up care are also addressed in many of the more formalized stroke continuum of care regulations.

The process for providing stroke care varies from state to state. In some states there are no requirements for providing stroke care, and in others the requirements are prescriptive and can require state licensing. In some states the requirements for licensing include achieving some level of Joint Commission Stroke Accreditation. States such as Massachusetts have developed and implemented a state-designed and state-administered Stroke Designation Program. A CDC (2011) report notes that as of July 2010 of the 18 states with enacted primary stroke center legislation or non-legislative policy three states accept TJC accreditation as the sole criterion for state designation as a primary stroke center. The other 15 states have a state-based process for primary stroke center criteria development and designation, often combining the state-based authority or identified criteria with TJC or the brain attack coalition (BAC) standards. In most of these cases, legislation or administrative policy give a state agency, typically the state's Department of Health or Emergency Management Services (EMS), the authority to develop designation criteria. Many stroke programs voluntarily choose program certification for stroke to validate the quality of their program even without a state requirement. Hospitals can achieve stroke certification from a number of national organizations including TJC, DNV, HFAP, and the American Heart Association (AHA).

One of the major features of formalized stroke care is data collection and analysis. Depending on the state or designating organization, program data may be submitted to a national database such as the American Heart Association's *Get with the Guidelines®-Stroke* or a state database. Gorelick (2013) notes that a formalized evidence-based approach to stroke care has resulted in the improvement of important stroke care metrics such as the use of imaging, time to intervention, blood pressure management, and death and dependency to name a few. In many states formalized evidence-based stroke care with certification may become the basic requirement for providing care.

Accountable Care Organizations (ACOs)

Credentialing as an Accountable Care Organization (ACO) is not a traditional accreditation or certification program but there are similarities that make a review of the program noteworthy to include here. Although ACOs started as a mechanism for reducing the cost of healthcare, the basis for achieving reduced costs is a focus on quality patient care that results in optimal outcomes. According to CMS (2017), as of January 2017 participating ACOs in all 50 states, the District of Columbia, and Puerto Rico serve over 9 million Medicare fee-for-service (FFS) beneficiaries. ACOs were designed under the Affordable Care Act (ACA) as a strategy to reduce overall Medicare costs. Under the fee-for-service Medicare payment system providers are rewarded based on the tests that are ordered. This is an area with a high potential for waste and abuse. Patients often seek care from multiple providers and this can result in repeated testing due to a lack of coordinated care. Under the traditional fee-for-service payment system providers are compensated based on the care and services provided, which can result in double billing for duplicate services. It is easy to find examples of fee-for-service abuse. Newspapers often publish articles that report on providers or facilities being investigated for Medicare/Medicaid fraud for over testing or for providing and billing for unnecessary care. A 2018 article published online reported on a national healthcare fraud takedown carried out by the Department of Justice (DOJ). This investigation resulted in charges against more than 600 defendants, including 165 doctors, nurses and other licensed medical professionals in districts across the United States (Stewart, 2018). Charges included fraud related to unnecessary testing, billing and medication prescribing. The goals of the ACO model are to monitor and coordinate care to prevent such abuse while maintaining quality of care.

The ACO model is of particular interest to APRNs as it is largely focused on wellness and preventive care. The goal of an ACO is to coordinate care to ensure that patients get the right care at the right time, prevent medical errors and at the same time avoid duplication of services (CMS, 2018c).

Technology is a key feature of ACOs because coordination and tracking of care is critical to success. The primary care provider is the one essential member of an ACO. Other members of the ACO can include specialists, hospitals, post-acute care providers, federally qualified health centers (FQHC), joint venture partners, insurers, and drug stores to name a few. To become an ACO the applicant must meet the following requirements:

1. Be a legal entity formed under state, federal or tribal law

2. Handle a minimum of 5,000 Medicare lives annually

3. Have an organizational structure with clinical and administrative effectiveness

4. Demonstrate evidence-based medicine and coordination of care, with data reporting tied to performance and cost

5. Have a legal structure to receive and distribute payments, and

6. Make a three year commitment to the program.

(CMS, 2017)

There are also a number of shared saving tracks for which the ACO applicant can apply. Details on such tracks can be found at www.cms.gov/Medicare/Medicare-Fee-for-Service-Payment/sharedsavingsprogram/about.html. Shared savings payments are based on financial performance and quality outcomes separately. The ACO model is complex with a detailed application process, and significant reporting requirements that require a knowledgeable coordinator. APRNs working with populations covered by Medicare and Medicaid should become familiar with ACOs in their geographic area, as well as opportunities for participating in ACOs. The advantage of an ACO for patients is improved outcomes as the result of coordinated evidence-based care.

NON-GOVERNMENTAL PROGRAMS

There are a host of non-governmental population-based programmatic certifications. It is generally accepted that program certification by professional organizations and accrediting organizations improves the functioning and outcomes of clinical programs. Numerous studies have been conducted over the years to qualify and quantify the value of accreditation (Melo, 2017; Procaccini, Curley, & Goldman, 2018). Even the process of preparing for and achieving accreditation is believed to improve performance. This is likely because accrediting organizations generally focus on organizational structure and processes, the environment in which care is provided, the qualifications of staff, evidence-based best practice, policies for care, and high quality patient outcomes (Lin et al., 2017). Patient outcomes are typically evaluated in the context of benchmarking, which includes analyzing performance against peer organizations. The following is a sampling of the types of clinical programmatic accreditations/certifications in existence.

Joint Commission Disease Specific Certifications

TJC has perhaps the most diverse opportunities for programmatic certifications. In 2002, TJC started the Disease-Specific Care Certification Program, which is designed to evaluate and certify the care of patients with any chronic disease or condition across the continuum (TJC, 2018). Although TJC has the ability to certify any clinical program based on a condition-based model certification format there are 13 procedural or clinical areas for which TJC offers advanced certification (see Box 9.2). TJC cites many benefits to disease specific certification (DSC) with the most important being the improvement of quality patient care by reducing clinical variation through a standardized approach. Best practice protocols and data-driven performance are the foundation of DSC.

BOX 9.2

TJC DISEASE-SPECIFIC CARE CERTIFICATION

Acute Stroke Ready Hospital

Chronic kidney disease

Chronic obstructive pulmonary disease

Comprehensive cardiac center

Comprehensive stroke center

Heart failure

Inpatient diabetes

Lung volume reduction surgery*

Palliative care

Perinatal care

Primary stroke center

Total hip and total knee replacement

Ventricular assist device*

*These are required by Centers for Medicare & Medicaid Services.

Source: With permission from The Joint Commission. (2018). *Disease specific care.* Retrieved from https://www.jointcommission.org/mobile/certification/diseasespecific_care.aspx

Community Health

Community healthcare is an important component of population health, with a long history of providing crucial services (primary, secondary, and tertiary care) to vulnerable groups. Public health is an essential element of the healthcare system. The focus of public health is in the community where people work, live and play. Public health agencies can be state, local, territorial, or tribal, and are accredited by the Public Health Accreditation Board (PHAB). PHAB is a nonprofit organization that was created specifically to accredit public health departments. The goal of PHAB is to measure the performance of health departments against national practice-focused, evidence-based standards (PHAB, 2018). Accreditation of Health Departments by PHAB is voluntary.

Professional Organizations

American College of Surgeons

The American College of Surgeons (ACoS) has a long history of validating the quality of clinical programs. The ACoS first issued minimum standards for hospitals in 1917.The creation of these standards led to the program now known as The Joint Commission (TJC). Additional achievements include the creation of the Commission on Cancer (CoC) in 1922 and the Committee on Trauma (COT) in 1950. More recently in 2005 the ACoS initiated programs for breast care (National Accreditation

Program for Breast Centers—NAPBC) and bariatric surgery. The bariatric surgery certification known as Metabolic and Bariatric Surgery Accreditation is run jointly by the American College of Surgeons (ACoS) and the American Society for Metabolic and Bariatric Surgery (ASMBS) (American College of Surgeons [ACoS], 2018). Although these programs appear to be focused exclusively on hospitals, they are all concerned with the continuum of care including pre- and post-hospital care. These programs also have comprehensive data registries that focus on the continuum of care. Patient outcomes are evaluated against benchmark data. APRNs need to be knowledgeable about these programs and specifically how their patient populations can benefit by following best practice recommendations. According to the ACoS (2018), facilities that have implemented these programs have improved surgical quality, prevented complications, reduced costs, and saved lives. The ACoS principles for quality are found on their web site (www.facs.org/quality-programs/about). These principles are similar to the foundations of many accreditation and certification processes.

American Nurses Credentialing Center

Magnet® designation by the American Nurses Credentialing Center is considered by many to be the highest recognition for nursing excellence. The term *Magnet hospital* dates back to 1983 when the American Academy of Nursing (AAN) Task Force on Nursing Practice in Hospitals conducted a study of 163 hospitals to identify work environments that attract and retain well-qualified nurses. These organizations were also evaluated on their quality of care. Of the 163 hospitals in the initial study, 41 were identified as having qualities that attracted and retained nurses, and were therefore described as Magnet Hospitals (Nursing World, 2018).

In 1990 the American Nurses Association (ANA) incorporated the American Nurses Credentialing Center (ANCC) as a subsidiary nonprofit organization. The ANCC was created to provide a body responsible for credentialing clinical nursing programs and services. Later that same year the ANA Board of Directors approved a proposal to recognize excellence in hospital-based nursing services known as the Magnet Hospital Recognition Program. This program built upon the earlier work of the 1983 ANA Task Force. In 1994 the University of Washington Medical Center, Seattle, WA, became the first ANCC Magnet-designated organization (Nursing World, 2018).

Over the years the Magnet Recognition Program® has continued to evolve and expand to include long-term care facilities, home health agencies and healthcare organizations outside of the United States. Shared governance is a critical feature of Magnet organizations. There is no 'one size fits all' model for shared governance. In addition to unit-based councils (UBCs) typically there are a number of other councils in shared governance models. These might include Professional Practice, Nursing Research, Quality and Safety, Education, Peer Review, and Collaborative Practice (among others). As clinical practice leaders, APRNs can play a significant role in the Magnet process as active members of these various Councils. The academic preparation of the DNP which includes skills in evidence-based practice, biostatistics, translational science, systems management, technology, and healthcare economics (Sanson, 2013) makes DNP graduates uniquely qualified to support the important activities of shared governance.

The 2019 Magnet Application Manual includes some changes in standards which further support the need for APRN leadership in organizations seeking Magnet recognition. There is an emphasis on nursing research and evidence-based practice. Organizations must be able to provide documentation of two completed studies and one ongoing study in their applications (Graystone, 2018). According to Jones (2016), nursing practice is often more tradition-based than evidence-based. The recognition of this lack of evidence-based practice has resulted in multiple professional nursing initiatives to increase nursing research (especially outcomes research) and evidence based practice. In recent years, research, and evidence to support the impact of nursing care on patient outcomes has become increasingly available. For example, a retrospective multiyear study of Medicare data on surgical patients comparing Magnet to non-Magnet facilities demonstrated improved mortality measures in Magnet hospitals (Friese, Xia, Ghaferi, Birkmeyer, & Banerjee, 2015). An interesting finding of this study suggests that organizations did not improve outcomes after achieving Magnet designation but rather Magnet designation recognized existing nursing excellence and outcomes.

Specialty Organizations

Many professional organizations offer certification for clinical programs. The following is a brief sampling of specialty organizations and the programs that they certify.

- American Heart Association (AHA)—Cardiovascular Care and Stroke
- American College of Cardiology/Society of Cardiovascular Patient Care—Cardiovascular Care and Chest Pain
- National Committee of Quality Assurance (NCQA)—many certifications including Patient-Centered Specialty Practice (PCSP) Recognition, Diabetes Care, Oncology Care and Behavioral Healthcare
- National Hospice and Palliative Care Organization—Community Palliative Care
- The American Society for Gastrointestinal Endoscopy (ASGE)—Gastrointestinal and Endoscopy Care
- American Academy of Pediatrics (AAP)—Pediatric Medical Home
- American Congress of Obstetricians and Gynecologists (ACOG)—Safety Certification in Outpatient Practice Excellence(SCOPE)
- Alzheimer's Association—Dementia Care

World Health Organization (WHO)—Baby Friendly Hospital Initiative (BFHI)

In addition to professional organizations, national and international organizations offer certifications/designations for specific health initiatives. One such designation is the WHO—BFHI, which was created to protect, promote, and support breastfeeding and to reduce world-wide malnutrition. BFHI designation is based on the *Ten Steps to Successful Breastfeeding* and the International Code of Marketing of Breast-milk Substitutes. Currently 152 countries have BFHI designated facilities (World Health Organization

[WHO], 2018). As of 2018 there are 539 BFHI designated facilities in the U.S. (Baby Friendly—USA, 2018). For more information on BFHI go to www.who.int/nutrition/topics/bfhi/en and www.babyfriendlyusa.org.

PLANNING FOR ACCREDITATION

APRN Role in Program Accreditation

APRNs need to be aware of the opportunities to obtain program credentialing for their population-based area of practice. They should identify such opportunities by reviewing programs offered by governmental and nongovernmental agencies. An essential first step is knowledge about the state of your clinical program. Does your organization measure critical programmatic outcomes? Does it enter data into a national database as a means to track performance? Many organizations, such as the American Heart Association and the American College of Surgeons, have databases that allow organizations and programs to participate and benchmark performance against other programs. The vast majority of Magnet recognized facilities (95%) use the National Database of Nursing Quality Indicators® (NDNQI) to assess performance on nurse-sensitive indicators (Press Ganey, 2018). Information on nurse sensitive indicators (NSI) can be found in Chapter 2, Identifying Outcomes in Population-Based Nursing. It is critically important to know how well your organization performs in comparison to others on a broader (particularly national) level and not just within your local area.

As mentioned previously, clinical program accreditation/certification frequently rests on the documentation of the prioritization of evidence-based practice (EBP) within an organization. APRNs are academically prepared to serve as champions for the use of EBP. Best practices in nursing are evidenced by measureable outcomes. An important element of implementing EBP is to measure outcomes before and after any changes in practice in order to evaluate the impact of the change.

DNP-educated APRNs performing in a variety of roles and settings may become the standard for leading organizational efforts towards accreditation. Using Magnet designation as an example, agencies applying for designation are required to have a Magnet Program Director (MPD). Although qualifications for the MPD are not specified, nor is there a specified educational requirement, the academic preparation of the DNP educated APRN includes the competencies necessary for leading efforts to achieve Magnet designation. DNP programs that are designed using the *Essentials for DNP Education* provide the APRN with the academic preparation and skills that are critical for the MPD. Specific essentials that prepare the APRN for the MPD role include: scientific underpinning for practice, organizational and systems leadership for quality improvement and systems thinking, clinical scholarship and analytical methods, and interpersonal collaboration for improving patient and population health outcomes. Findings by the American Association of Critical Care Nurses' (AACN) Advanced Practice Workgroup in 2005 identified APRN skills that are consistent with Magnet characteristics. They include:

- Being able to collaborate with other disciplines, including physicians, to improve patient care

- Advocating for evidence-based practice

- Being able to identify issues with workflow and facilitating the identification of changes to improve nursing satisfaction

- Providing education and orientation to clinical nursing staff to promote excellence in nursing practice

- Encouraging nurses to join professional organizations, obtain specialty certification, and continue their education (Bynum & Whitcomb, 2005).

Finally, APRNs are well recognized by members of the healthcare team as internal consultants and a resource for nursing staff and other members of the care team as clinical experts.

Creating the Plan

A major part of program development in preparation for accreditation is planning and creating an action plan. Program design and the development process is discussed in detail in Chapter 7, Concepts in Program Design and Development. The goal of every clinical program should be to benefit the population to be served. If the program under development requires accreditation then the requirements of such designation should be an early consideration in the planning process. Ideally the planning team should include at least one member who has expertise in the requirements for accreditation. Teams need to include members that have strong writing skills. In some cases an outside expert/consultant may be of value if there is no internal team member with significant experience and knowledge of the accreditation program. There are often resources at the accreditation organization that can be of assistance. For example, both TJC and Magnet assign liaisons to participating organizations. Many healthcare entities have contracts with best practice consulting firms, which often have clinical content experts that are available to member organizations. These companies typically have teams for the prominent clinical foci in the marketplace, such as cardiovascular, oncology, post-acute, orthopedics, neuroscience and new and emerging areas of focus.

During the earliest stages of planning for accreditation, accreditation standards need to be identified and understood. Gap analysis is another critical first step. An action plan with goals, timelines and accountabilities should be created. This plan needs to be integrated into the overall program design and development plan to insure success. In larger organizations it is imperative to have an executive sponsor, who is a senior member of administration and who will serve as a champion for the initiative. This role can be extremely useful in maintaining focus and eliminating barriers. When preparing to submit an application applicants should be sure to provide only the information that is specifically required; more is not always better. Once the document has been accepted and a site visit is imminent it is essential to prepare for the visit. Who will escort the surveyors? Who should surveyors meet with? What should surveyors see? What space will be dedicated for use by the surveyors? Remember that the site visit is used to validate the information presented in the application. Plan carefully. A detailed schedule is essential for a successful site visit. Mock site visits can be a useful tool in preparing for the visit. Once accreditation is achieved organizations should formally celebrate the accomplishment.

SUMMARY

The healthcare marketplace is extremely competitive. Achieving good rankings from external agencies such as Leapfrog, CMS Star ratings, and *US News and World Report*, to name a few, have become a desired and necessary goal for healthcare organizations. Administrators are constantly on the look out to identify opportunities to differentiate and validate their organization. Achieving accreditation helps to validate program and organizations in the context of national and professional standards. Consumers are becoming savvier in assessing programs, and often look to external rankings for help in deciding where to seek care. Payers, both private and governmental, are looking for value based care in their efforts to reduce healthcare costs. Accreditation offers healthcare providers an opportunity to qualify and quantify the quality of clinical programs.

Accreditation is recognized as a means to assess, build, and validate clinical programs and it requires extensive preparation and dedication. The process itself provides an opportunity to develop a framework for quality improvement, and to create a culture which focuses on outstanding care that requires staff engagement.

In the past, accreditation was viewed as a process separate from the everyday functioning of an organization, but organizations cannot not be successful with standards compliance when such compliance is only reviewed in cycles prior to the application for accreditation. The current paradigm requires a continuous, on-going focus on meeting standards of excellent clinical practice, analyzing performance, achieving optimal outcomes, and producing sustainable change. Accreditation provides APRNs with the opportunity to be leaders in clinical care and champions for validation of clinical practice.

EXERCISE AND DISCUSSION QUESTIONS

Exercise 9.1 Identify an accreditation and/or certification designation applicable to your area of practice/population-based program. Conduct a gap analysis to identify areas requiring additional focus/changes to achieve the accreditation. Create an action plan for each matter that is identified as an impediment to accreditation/certification.

Exercise 9.2 Imagine you are going to lead a team to obtain accreditation and/or certification for your population based program. Identify the team members you would select and provide an explanation for each selection. Identify where you may need external resources to supplement the team? Why do you need these external resources? What are your goals for these consultants?

Exercise 9.3 Identify two evidence-based nursing protocols that you want to implement at your organization. What are the performance metrics you will measure? What is your current performance? What national benchmarks can you use to measure your performance?

REFERENCES

Advisory Board. (2017). *Your hospital's VBP penalty or bonus for 2018, mapped.* Retrieved from https://www.advisory.com/daily-briefing/2017/11/08/value-based-payments-18

American Association of Colleges of Nursing. (2006). *The essentials of doctoral education for advanced practice nursing.* Retrieved from http://www.aacnnursing.org/Portals/42/Publications/DNPEssentials.pdf

American College of Surgeons. (2018). *American College of Surgeons: 100-year history of leading quality improvement.* Retrieved from https://www.facs.org/quality-programs/about

Baby Friendly USA. (2018). *Baby Friendly Initiative.* Retrieved from https://www.babyfriendlyusa.org/about

Bynum, C., & Whitcomb, J. (2005). Beacon and Magnet®: What is the APN's role in meeting criteria. *AACN News, 22*(3), p. 4.

Castellucci, M. (2018). Hospitals stand behind Joint Commission standards as House investigates. *Modern Healthcare, 48(12)*, 11.

Centers for Disease Control and Prevention. (2011). *A summary of primary stroke center policy in the United States.* Atlanta: U.S. Department of Health and Human Services. Retrieved from https://www.cdc.gov/dhdsp/pubs/docs/primary_stroke_center_report.pdf

Centers for Medicare and Medicaid Services. (2017). *Medicare shared savings program ACO: Preparing to apply for the 2018 program year.* Retrieved from https://www.cms.gov/Outreach-and-Education/Outreach/NPC/Downloads/2017-04-06-SSP-Presentation.pdf

Centers for Medicare and Medicaid Services. (2018a). *Conditions for coverage (CfCs) & Conditions of participations (CoPs).* Retrieved from https://www.cms.gov/Regulations-and-Guidance/Legislation/CFCsAndCoPs/index.html?redirect=/CFCsAndCoPs

Centers for Medicare and Medicaid Services. (2018b). *Oncology care model.* Retrieved from https://innovation.cms.gov/initiatives/Oncology-Care

Centers for Medicare and Medicaid Services. (2018c). *Accountable care organizations (ACOs).* Retrieved from https://www.cms.gov/Medicare/Medicare-Fee-for-Service-Payment/ACO/index.html

Friese, C. R., Xia, R., Ghaferi, A. A., Birkmeyer, J. D., & Banerjee, M. (2015). Hospitals in "Magnet®" program show better patient outcomes on mortality measures compared to non-"Magnet®" hospitals. *Health Affairs (Project Hope), 34*(6), 986–992. doi:10.1377/hlthaff.2014.0793

Galioto, M. (2017). APRNs have a role in leading value based care. *Oncology Nursing Society - ONS Voice.* Retrieved from https://voice.ons.org/news-and-views/apns-have-a-role-in-leading-value-based-care

Gorelick, P. (2013). Primary and comprehensive stroke centers: History, value and certification criteria. *Journal of Stroke, 15(2)*, 78–89.

Graystone, R. (2018). 2019 Magnet® Application Manual raises the bar for nursing excellence. *American Nurse Today, 13*(1), 48–49. Retrieved from www.americannursetoday.com

Institute of Medicine. (2010). *Future of nursing leading change, advancing health: Report recommendations.* Retrieved from http://www.nationalacademies.org/hmd/~/media/Files/Report%20Files/2010/The-Future-of-Nursing/Future%20of%20Nursing%202010%20Recommendations.pdf

Jones, T. (2016). Outcomes measurement in nursing: imperatives, ideals, history and challenges. *OJIN, 21*(2), 1. *ANA Periodicals.* Retrieved from http://ojin.nursingworld.org/MainMenuCategories/ANAMarketplace/ANAPeriodicals/OJIN/TableofContents/Vol-21-2016/No2-May-2016/Outcome-Measurement-in-Nursing.html?css=print

Lin, P., Chandra, F., Shapiro, F., Osman, B. M., Urman, R. D., & Ahn, S. S. (2017). The need for accreditation of office-based interventional vascular centers. *Annals of Vascular Surgery 38*, 332–338. doi:10.1016/j.avsg.2016.06.010

Melo, S. (2017). The impact of accreditation on healthcare quality improvement: A qualitative case study. *Journal of Health Organization and Management, 30(8)*, 1242–1258. doi:10.1108/JHOM-01-2016-0021

Nursing World. (2018). *Magnet Recognition Program®.* Retrieved from https://www.nursingworld.org/organizational-programs/Magnet/history

Press Ganey. (2018). *Nursing quality – NDNQI.* Retrieved from http://www.pressganey.com/solutions/clinical-quality/nursing-quality

Procaccini, D., Curley, A. L. C., & Goldman, M. (2018). Baby-Friendly practices minimize newborn infants weight loss. *Breastfeeding Medicine: The Official Journal of the Academy of Breastfeeding Medicine, 13*(3), 189–194. doi:10.1089/bfm.2017.0182

Public Health Accreditation Board. (2018). *What is public health accreditation?* Retrieved from http://www .phaboard.org/accreditation-overview/what-is-accreditation

Sanson, S. (2013). DNP-prepared APRNs: Leading the Magnet® charge. *Nursing Management, 44*, 49–52. doi:10.1097/01.numa.0000431425.39076.81

Stewart, A. (2018). *Providers from 35 states charged in healthcare fraud crackdown: Here's the breakdown.* Retrieved from https://www.beckersasc.com/asc-coding-billing-and-collections/providers-from-35-states-charged-in-healthcare-fraud-crackdown-here-s-the-breakdown.html

The Joint Commission. (2017). *Facts about Joint Commission.* Retrieved from https://www.jointcommission .org/facts_about_hospital_accreditation

The Joint Commission. (2018). *Disease specific care.* Retrieved from https://www.jointcommission.org/ mobile/certification/diseasespecific_care.aspx

World Health Organization. (2018). *Baby Friendly Hospital Initiative.* Retrieved from http://www.who.int/ nutrition/topics/bfhi/en

INTERNET RESOURCES

Baby-Friendly USA: https://www.babyfriendlyusa.org

Center for Medicare & Medicaid Services (CMS): https://www.cms.gov/Regulations-and-Guidance/ Legislation/CFCsAndCoPs/index.html?redirect=/CFCsAndCoPs

CHAP, 2018 *Standards of Excellence* for Home Health Providers: https://education.chaplinq.org/ products/2018-chap-standards-of-excellence-for-home-health-providers

CMS, MACRA: https://www.cms.gov/Medicare/Quality-Initiatives-Patient-Assessment-Instruments/ Value-Based-Programs/MACRA-MIPS-and-APMs/MACRA-MIPS-and-APMs.html

CMS, Medicare Approved Facilities/Trials/Registries: https://www.cms.gov/Medicare/Medicare-General -Information/MedicareApprovedFacilitie/index.html

CMS, National Coverage Determinations (NCD) Alphabetical Index: https://www.cms.gov/medicare -coverage-database/indexes/ncd-alphabetical-index.aspx

CMS, National Coverage Determinations (NCDs): https://www.cms.gov/medicare-coverage-database/ indexes/ncd-alphabetical-index.aspx

CMS, Shared Savings Program: https://www.cms.gov/Medicare/Medicare-Fee-for-Service-Payment /sharedsavingsprogram/about.html

CMS. What is MACRA? (Medicare Access and CHIP Reauthorization Act of 2015): https://www.cms.gov/ Medicare/Quality-Initiatives-Patient-Assessment-Instruments/Value-Based-Programs/MACRA-MIPS -and-APMs/MACRA-MIPS-and-APMs.html

Community Health Accreditation Partner (CHAP): at https://chapinc.org

DNV NIAHO: www.dnvaccreditation.com/pr/dnv/default.aspx

The Commission on Accreditation of Rehabilitation Facilities (CARF): www.carf.org/Accreditation

The Healthcare Facilities Accreditation Program (HFAP): https://www.hfap.org/about/overview.aspx

The Joint Commission (TJC): www.jointcommission.org

The National Committee for Quality Assurance (NCQA): www.ncqa.org

The Public Health Accreditation Board (PHAB): http://www.phaboard.org/accreditation-overview/ what-is-accreditation

TJC, 2019 *Comprehensive Accreditation Manual for Homecare*: https://www.jcrinc.com/2019-comprehensive-accreditation-manual-for-home-care-camhc-/cahc19

URAC (formerly The Utilization Review Accreditation Committee): www.urac.org

World Health Organization (WHO), Baby-friendly Hospital Initiative: http://www.who.int/nutrition/topics/ bfhi/en

CHAPTER 10

BUILDING RELATIONSHIPS AND ENGAGING COMMUNITIES THROUGH COLLABORATION

SONDA M. OPPEWAL | BARBARA A. BENJAMIN

One silver bracelet does not make much jingle.

—African proverb

INTRODUCTION

Let us consider this adage when we think community health assessment (CHA). The primary purpose of building relationships and engaging communities through collaboration is to facilitate a dialogue to aid in the assessment, planning, action, and evaluation of challenging care-based issues through program design and development. By working with the community, healthcare professionals have the opportunity to collaborate on issues relevant to the community to ensure sustainability and long-term success of community-based programs. This type of collaboration fosters bidirectional communication, understanding, and knowledge in the quest to ensure compassionate, quality, and culturally sensitive interventions. For collaboration to be successful, advanced practice registered nurses (APRNs) need specialized knowledge and skills to build rapport, foster trust, respect differences, and involve diverse community partners on an ongoing basis through all phases of the CHA.

FOUNDATION FOR POPULATION-FOCUSED PRACTICE

All APRNs are charged with improving the health of communities, improving population health, and decreasing health disparities and inequities. The foundation for this work is grounded in the work of numerous professional nursing organizations and legislation; four are highlighted in this chapter. They include: the American Association of Colleges of Nursing (AACN) Doctorate of Nursing Practice (DNP) curriculum; the Patient Protection and Affordable Care Act (ACA); competencies from APRN organizations; and the Quad Council Coalition Community/Public Health Nursing Competencies.

American Association of Colleges of Nursing

The AACN published *The Essentials of Doctoral Education for Advanced Practice Nurses* in 2006. This seminal curricular framework provides guidance to faculty of DNP programs by outlining eight DNP essentials that are considered critical for DNP graduate practice. The AACN defines *advanced nursing practice* as

> any form of nursing intervention that influences healthcare outcomes for individuals or populations, including the direct care of individual patients, management of care for individuals and populations, administration of nursing and healthcare organizations and the development and implementation of health policy. (AACN, 2006, p. 3)

Building relationships and engaging communities through collaborations are skills that are clearly needed for DNP *Essentials II, V, and VII. Essential II, Organizational and Systems Leadership for Quality Improvement and Systems Thinking,* calls for DNP graduates to be able to "use advanced communication skills/processes to lead quality improvement and patient safety initiatives in healthcare" and "demonstrate sensitivity to diverse organizational cultures and populations, including patients and providers" (AACN, 2006, p. 11). *Essential V, Interprofessional Collaboration for Improving Patient and Population Health Outcomes* includes competencies that require DNP graduates to demonstrate collaborative skills. And, *Essential VII, Clinical Prevention and Population Health for Improving the Nation's Health,* includes competencies related to community, individuals, aggregates, and populations, which all require effective skills for working with others (AACN, 2006). The AACN further states that DNP programs prepare graduates to: "[1] Conduct a comprehensive and systematic assessment of health and illness parameters in complex situations, incorporating diverse and culturally sensitive approaches"; ... and "[3] Develop and sustain therapeutic relationships and partnerships with patients (individuals, family or group) and other professionals to facilitate optimal care and patient outcomes" (AACN, 2006, pp. 16–17). Specialty-focused competencies required of DNP graduates with an aggregate/systems/organizational focus call for competence in "community assessment techniques" (AACN, 2006, p. 18).

The terms CHA and community health needs assessment (CHNA) may be used interchangeably, however, a CHNA must meet certain requirements specific for tax-exempt hospitals as outlined by the ACA and internal revenue service (IRS) regulations. The purpose of a CHA is to identify health problems, needs, gaps, strengths, and assets, and to be used as a stimulus for action to improve health by addressing priority needs based on community input.

The Patient Protection and Affordable Care Act

The ACA was the first comprehensive health reform legislation passed by Congress in more than 50 years. It was signed into law by President Barack Obama on March 23, 2010. The purpose of this Act was to expand access to health insurance coverage, improve systems delivering healthcare, and keep healthcare costs controlled. Key provisions included requiring that most U.S. citizens and legal residents have health insurance and barring health insurance companies from denying coverage of people with pre-existing health conditions (Kaiser Family Foundation, 2013). The ACA was designed to reduce healthcare costs by placing a cap on out-of-pocket expenses and by encouraging a shift in the healthcare system from a focus on illness to a focus on wellness and prevention. All health insurance companies in the ACA marketplace were required to have essential preventive services provided to beneficiaries without any out-of-pocket expense. Americans without insurance coverage had the opportunity to choose the insurance coverage that worked best for them (Kaiser Family Foundation, 2013).

There were several attempts by the Trump administration to repeal and weaken the ACA between 2016 and 2018. These attempts are evidenced by a decline in enrollment from the 9.2 million who enrolled through the ACA's individual health insurance marketplace in 2017 to the 8.7 million who enrolled in 2018 (Craig, 2018). The American Nurses Association (ANA), beginning in 2016 and in concert with other professional nursing organizations, has been instrumental in stopping the passage of several pieces of legislation that would have undermined the ACA. These groups continue to advocate for key health system changes including one to "Ensure universal access to a standard package of essential healthcare services for all citizens and residents" (ANA, n.d., Health System Reform, para. 4). Professional nursing organizations have joined the ANA and the American Public Health Association (APHA) in protesting healthcare reform that would endanger American health, weaken or eliminate the Prevention and Public Health Fund of the ACA, and cause a detrimental impact on healthcare quality.

One requirement of the ACA specifically applies to hospitals wishing to maintain or achieve 501(c) (3) tax-exempt status. A 501(c) (3) hospital is one that qualifies for exemption from federal income tax because it is organized and operated exclusively as a charitable organization (National Association of County and City Health Officials, 2014). The IRS is responsible for the tax provisions of the ACA. The IRS Section 501(r) requires that hospital organizations conduct a CHNA every 3 years and adopt and implement strategies to meet the community health needs identified through the assessment. The CHNA must include input from persons who represent the broad interests of the community/communities served by healthcare facilities, including those with special knowledge of, or expertise in, public health. Collaboration among healthcare agencies and public health agencies is vital. The IRS defines persons who represent the broad interests of the community/communities as: (a) persons with special knowledge of or expertise in public health; (b) federal, tribal, regional, state, or local health or other departments or agencies, with current data or other information relevant to the health needs of the community served by the hospital facility;

and (c) leaders, representatives, or medically underserved, low-income, and minority populations, and populations with chronic disease needs, in the community served by the hospital facility (IRS, n.d.).

Compliance with the ACA

In many states, nonprofit hospitals have joined with local health departments to fulfill the requirement to conduct a CHNA. Health departments are also required to conduct community assessments on a regular basis and have the expertise to do so. In urban Wake County, North Carolina (where the capital of the state, Raleigh, is located), more than 80 agencies and community partners collaborated to complete the 2016 CHNA. One intent of this large collaborative was to avoid duplication of efforts (Gintzig & West, 2016). Key players in this collaborative CHNA included Wake County Health and Human Services, WakeMed Health and Hospitals, UNC Rex Healthcare, Duke Raleigh Hospital, United Way of the Greater Triangle, Advance Community Health, and the Wake County Medical Society Community Health Foundation. Also participating were other non-profit, faith-based, educational, government, and business organizations as well as Wake County residents. The 2016 CHNA Steering Committee included 80 people from various organizations including Gale Adcock who is a family nurse practitioner and an elected member of the North Carolina House of Representative (Gintzig & West, 2016).

Advance Community Health is a federally qualified health center (FQHC) that like other FQHCs receives grants under Section 330 of the Public Health Service (PHS) Act. These safety net providers provide comprehensive outpatient care in medically underserved areas or populations and must meet specific requirements for enhanced reimbursement from Medicare and Medicaid, as well as other benefits. FQHCs must serve an underserved area or population, offer a sliding-fee scale, provide comprehensive services, have an ongoing quality-assurance program, and a governing board of directors with the majority of members receiving client care at the FQHC (Centers for Medicare and Medicaid Services [CMS], 2018).

Collaborative efforts for conducting CHNAs in rural areas may occur on a regional level across several counties. For example, in western North Carolina, the Western North Carolina (WNC) Health Network is an alliance of 17 hospitals whose mission is to improve health and healthcare across their region (WNC Health Network, 2018). One of its components, the WNC Healthy Impact, is a partnership of coordinated efforts between hospitals, public health agencies, and key community partners in the western part of the state. The WNC Healthy Impact collaborative works on a CHNA to assess community needs, develop plans collaboratively, coordinate action, and evaluate the impact and progress of the action plans (WNC Health Network, 2018).

In many places health department, hospital, and healthcare agency professionals can collaborate to assess and address health issues relevant to their community. Such efforts help to ensure sustainability and the long-term success of both hospital and community-based programs. Not only is collaboration needed for IRS compliance for 501(c) (3) hospitals under the ACA, but it makes sense to work together to avoid duplicate efforts. Successful collaborative efforts between community partners, agencies, stakeholders, and residents reflect the active involvement of diverse partners. Such CHNAs are more likely to be relevant, culturally responsive, and successful in achieving high quality healthcare and reducing health disparities and inequities than those developed by less diverse working groups.

Competencies from APRN Organizations

After the AACN published *The Essentials of Doctoral Education for Advanced Nursing Practice* with the recommendation to establish the DNP as the highest practice degree in nursing, advanced practice nursing organizations started developing practice doctorate competencies. The National Organization of Nurse Practitioner Faculties (NOPNF) was the first to publish competencies for doctorate nursing practice in 2009. The NONPF's most recent *Nurse Practitioner Core Competencies* were published in 2017. NONPF identifies specific competencies for such nurses related to leadership and collaboration (Nurse Practitioner Core Competencies Content Work Group, 2017).

The National Association of Clinical Nurse Specialists (NACNS) is the only national nursing organization dedicated to nurses who are clinical nurse specialists (CNSs). During the time period from 2006 to 2008 the National CNS Competency Task Force identified and validated core competencies for CNSs. Collaboration is one of the core competencies (defined as "Working jointly with others to optimize clinical outcomes. The CNS collaborates at an advanced level by committing to authentic engagement and constructive patient, family, system, and population-focused problem solving") (National CNS Competency Task Force, 2010, p. 21).

Like NONPF and NACNS, the professional organizations for nurse midwives and nurse anesthetists recognize the need for competency in collaboration. Collaboration is important through the entire process of conducting a CHA, from planning, data collection, analysis, and priority setting, to community validation. While conducting a CHA, APRNs may work with various community partners in hospitals, health departments, faith-based organizations, and social services, as well as first responders, and stakeholders from various community groups and members of different disciplines. Leadership requires the ability to collaborate with individuals and leaders from different groups and agencies. These people often have different perspectives about health and healthcare needs. Community-based participatory research (CBPR) is built on trusting relationships among researchers and community members and mutually identified goals. It also requires collaboration to be successful. It may take years for researchers and community members to build the trusting relationships needed to identify mutually identified goals and to conduct community-based participatory research (Fitzpatrick, 2016).

Quad Council Coalition of Public Health Nursing Organizations Community/Public Health Nursing [C/PHN] Competencies

The Quad Council Coalition of Public Health Nursing Organizations (Quad Council Coalition [QCC]) is a coalition of four nursing organizations that work together to speak collectively and visibly for public health nursing education, practice, leadership, and research. The QCC includes the American Public Health Association Public Health Nursing Section (APHA PHN), the Association of Community Health Nursing Educators (ACHNE), the Alliance of Nurses for Health Environments (AHNE), and the Association of Public Health Nurses (APHN; QCC, 2018).

The *QCC C/PHN Competencies* were initially based on the core competencies for public health professionals developed by the Council on Linkages between Academia and Public Health Practice, a collaborative established in 1992 (Public Health Foundation [PHF], 2018). In 2011 the competencies were revised to incorporate three levels of practice: generalist, supervisory, and senior management or leadership. The most recent revisions were approved in April 2018 to respond to the need to "rebrand" the competencies to improve inclusiveness and participation in Public Health 3.0, and to better reflect the definition of public health nursing (Public Health Nursing Definition Document Task Force, 2013; QCC Competency Review Task Force, 2018). Public Health 3.0 refers to efforts to improve health by providing services outside of clinical settings and implementing interventions that can reach entire populations (DeSalvo et al., 2017). The 2018 QCC competencies were revised for use in various practice settings and by all levels of public health nursing professionals (QCC Competency Review Task Force, 2018).

The QCC identifies eight practice domains for public health nursing: (1) assessment and analytic skills; (2) policy development/program planning skills; (3) communication skills; (4) cultural competency skills; (5) community dimensions of practice skills; (6) public health sciences skills; (7) financial planning, evaluation, and management skills; and (8) leadership and systems thinking skills. Each domain or skill area articulates specific core competencies for three tiers that reflect practice by generalists, supervisors, and senior managers or leaders. A copy of the *C/PHN Competencies* can be found on the Quad Council's website (quadcouncilphn.org). Table 10.1 provides specific examples of core competencies related to collaboration that exist in each domain.

In summary, the essential or core competency work of the AACN, NONPF, NACNS, and the QCC represent a comprehensive foundation for APRN practice in population-based nursing. Federal legislation enacted by the ACA supports CHNAs carried out by hospitals and public health departments with the engagement or active involvement of diverse community partners. To build relationships with communities and to be successful in population health endeavors, APRNs require skills in leadership, collaboration, research, and policy making. APRNs are educated to engage communities in activities to assess and improve health. These efforts require time, trust, teamwork, and active collaboration with community leaders, members, and stakeholders.

COMMUNITY HEALTH ASSESSMENT

Why Assess the Community?

CHA and analysis is a cornerstone of effective population-based nursing care and is the first step in improving community health. For many healthcare organizations it is also

TABLE 10.1 Select Community/Public Health Nursing Competencies related to Collaboration by Domain

DOMAIN	CORE COMPETENCIES
1: Assessment and Analytic Skills	1A9. Use varied approaches in the identification of community needs (i.e., focus groups, multisector collaboration, SWOT analysis)
2: Policy Development/ Program Planning Skills	2A9. Use program planning skills and CBPR (i.e., collaboration, reflection, capacity building) to implement strategies to engage marginalized/disadvantaged population groups in making decisions that affect their health and well-being.
3: Communication Skills	3A6. Use communication models to communicate with individuals, families, and groups effectively and as a member of the interprofessional team(s) or interdisciplinary partnerships.
4: Cultural Competency Skills	4C2b. Support the use of CBPR and other methods to measure and evaluate the effectiveness of population-level health services and programs, strategies for reducing the impact of determinants of health.
5: Community Dimensions of Practice Skills	5A3b. Function effectively with key stakeholders in activities that facilitate community involvement and delivery of services to individuals, families, and groups. 5C3a. Create strategies that enhance collaboration within and across systems and organizations to address *population health* issues. 55Cb. Maximize collaboration with key stakeholders and groups within and across systems and organizations to enhance the health of a population. 5C3c. Evaluate the effectiveness of collaborative relationships and partnerships within organizations and systems.
6: Public Health Sciences Skills	6C6a. Plan with academic partners, internal and external stakeholders, and other public health professionals to address limitations of research findings.
7: Financial Planning, Evaluation, and Management Skills	7B1c. Develop collaborations with relevant public and private systems for managing programs in public health.
8: Leadership and Systems Thinking Skills	8C3a. Create meaningful opportunities for partnerships with stakeholders to determine key values and shared vision as guiding principles for community action.

Note: Core competencies designated with A apply to generalist C/PHNs, the B designation applies to supervisors, and the C designation to leaders.

CBPR, community-based participatory research; SWOT, strengths, weaknesses, opportunities, and threats.

Source: Adapted from Quad Council Coalition Competency Review Task Force. (2018). Community/Public Health Nursing Competencies. Retrieved from http://www.quadcouncilphn.org/documents-3/2018-qcc-competencies

a legislative requirement. The end product of a CHA is the identification of community assets and needs that are congruent with the cultural diversity of the community. It involves community member participation throughout the process, particularly when validating community priorities. CHAs can reveal critical information about what works and what does not work for a community.

Any plan to meet the needs of a community that is derived from data synthesized into a CHA may truly be considered an evidence-based practice plan. According to the Centers for Disease Control and Prevention (CDC), addressing health improvement is a shared responsibility of federal, state, and local governments as well as policy makers, businesses, healthcare providers, professionals, educators, community leaders, and the American public (2014). If health improvement is the goal, many segments of the community must be involved in a CHA. A CHA may focus on a community as defined by its geopolitical boundaries (e.g., towns, cities, counties) or on an aggregate of a community (Gibson & Thatcher, 2016). CHAs are most often conducted for communities with specific geographic boundaries. These assessments can be used to identify populations that need more intensive study of specific problems or of subpopulations that require an aggregate assessment. While some CHAs have a narrow focus based on specific questions, other CHAs are more comprehensive. A comprehensive CHA addresses the characteristics of the community's physical environment, infrastructure, and population characteristics. Regardless of the scope and breadth of a CHA, APRNs need to work with community members to identify community strengths, weaknesses, and priorities. Such cooperation leads to mutually agreed-upon goals for improvement, targeted outcomes, and "buy in" by communities.

Conducting the Assessment

CHAs are not done in isolation; no one should attempt a CHA alone. The APRN may lead a CHA, serve as a member of the CHA team by representing her or his practice organization, or by providing expert information or other assistance. A key function of the planning committee of the CHA is to work collaboratively with a diverse group of community partners, solicit input from multiple sources, and agree on the choice of assessment methods best suited for the specific community. APRNs can mobilize community partners and stakeholders within the community to assist with the CHA by "thinking out of the box." The CHA team should consider soliciting input from representatives of businesses, schools, agencies who work with youth, faith-based organizations, health and social service agencies, emergency services, environmental agencies, and others. Ultimately CHA team members should represent diverse ages, interests, and points of view, so that different perspectives about health and community issues will be obtained and considered. Community members have valuable contributions to make to the CHA and are concerned and interested in the community where they live and/or work.

Assessment methods include the analysis of primary data and secondary data obtained from online databases and websites. A literature review can be done to help identify current information on health topics. CHA team members can obtain primary data from participant observation, windshield and walking surveys, key informant interviews, surveys, and focus groups. Each method has advantages and disadvantages that must be considered along with available resources such as personnel, budget, and time. Fortunately, there is a plethora of information available at one's fingertips on the Internet. Tools exist that quickly provide data for communities, counties, states, and nations. Information that is available on online databases and various websites such as county and municipal home pages provide important data elements for consideration. APRNs are well positioned to help find data from a variety of sources given their experience and education. A comprehensive discussion for locating population data is presented in Chapter 2, Identifying Outcomes in Population-Based Nursing.

Data collected from CHAs may be organized in different ways to facilitate analysis and synthesis. One comprehensive framework is the community assessment wheel. CHA data can be organized into nine components represented by a wheel with an inner circle and eight hubs (Anderson & McFarlane, 2019). The community core is the inner circle that is surrounded by eight hubs or components that together form a larger circle. The community core includes data that describes the people in the community in terms of their history, demographics, ethnicity, vital statistics, values, beliefs, and religion. The hubs of the community assessment wheel include the categories of physical environment, health and social services, safety and transportation, communication, politics and government, education, recreation, and economics (Anderson & McFarlane, 2019).

CHA team members can use the nine components of the wheel to identify questions that need to be answered about the community and to organize data in a systematic and comprehensive manner. This type of CHA can provide insight into the root causes of community health problems as well as community resources and strengths. Anderson and McFarlane (2019) recommend that assessments be conducted in incremental fashion to better manage the enormity of the task. For example, CHA team members can stop at predetermined intervals to analyze and synthesize the data as they are collected. While the process of conducting a CHA is ongoing, concurrent generation and analysis of data will identify recurrent themes that may signal that sufficient data are collected. Alternately the APRN may discover that further information is needed because of the appearance of inconsistencies within the data and gaps needing additional clarification. Qualitative or contextual information derived from participant observation, focus groups, key informant interviews, and windshield surveys provides rich and valuable information that can bring clarity to the information gleaned from surveys, literature reviews, and secondary data analyses. For example, parents and caregivers who are interviewed about childhood obesity may offer insight into family and community values and beliefs about eating and physical activity. This is important contextual information. In addition, parents may be able to describe why some strategies are not helpful and identify alternate strategies that align better with the characteristics of the family, neighborhood, or community.

An example of another framework to guide CHAs is based on a set of core measures proposed in 2015 by the Institute of Medicine (IOM) Committee on Core Metrics for Better Health at Lower Cost. Designed to increase efficiency, reduce burden, focus on the most important health outcomes, and develop a standard set of measures, the *Vital Signs: Core Metrics for Health and Health Care Progress Report Brief* proposes 15 national measures that are meaningful and have use at various levels of the U.S. healthcare system. These core metric indicators specify how to measure the indicators so that the results can be used for comparison with other communities and health systems. They include life expectancy, well-being, overweight and obesity, addictive behavior, unintended pregnancy, healthy communities, preventive services, care access, patient safety, evidence-based care, care match with patient goals, personal spending burden, population spending burden, individual engagement, and community engagement (IOM, 2015).

While the initial core measures identified by the IOM Committee focused primarily on clinical issues, they were later pilot tested in two communities, Monterey County and Fresno County, California, to determine their feasibility at the local (community) level. Findings demonstrated that the core measures were useful at the local level when the indicator set was adapted to meet the unique characteristics of the specific community. Another finding was the importance of incorporating indicators of the social determinants of health (Public Health Institute, 2018).

ASSESSMENT TOOLS AND METHODS

Assessment Tools

Numerous community health assessment resources exist to help guide CHAs and to make the process efficient. They provide useful information on how to build relationships and trust with communities, work through the community health assessment process, gather data, and design evidence-based interventions. This chapter highlights five such CHA resources: (a) the *Healthy People 2020* website, (b) the Community Toolbox, (c) the Community Health Assessment Toolkit, (d) the County Health Rankings & Roadmaps, and (e) the CDC Community Health Improvement Navigator.

Healthy People 2020

Developed by the Office of Disease Prevention and Health Promotion (ODPHP), the *Healthy People* website outlines America's roadmap for achieving good health (see Chapter 2, Identifying Outcomes in Population-Based Nursing). It also includes a treasure trove of data and resources for APRNs who are charged with working on a CHA. *Healthy People* Tools and Resources includes a program planning tool using the MAP-IT framework that is designed to guide the planning and evaluation of public health interventions to achieve *Healthy People 2020* objectives. The framework is designed to help: (a) mobilize community partners; (b) assess community needs; (c) create and implement a plan for reaching *Healthy People 2020* objectives; and (d) track a community's progress. The acronym of MAP-IT is from the framework's steps: **M**obilize, **A**ssess, **P**lan, **I**mplement, **T**rack (ODPHP, 2018a). Each step of the framework provides questions to ask and answer along with tips and resources. For example, the section on **M**obilize includes four key questions and answers. They are: What is the vision and mission of the coalition? Why do I want to bring people together? Who should be represented? Who are the potential partners (organizations and businesses) in my community? Resources such as a list of potential partners to consider and approaches for organizing a coalition are included as well as links to other valuable tools and resources.

In addition to the above, the *Healthy People 2020* website provides current data from a variety of data sources for each of 1,200 objectives that are organized by 42 topic areas. APRNs can use the interactive DATA2020 tool to quickly explore national data associated with *Healthy People 2020* and the *Healthy People 2010* objectives. Moreover, using DATA2020, APRNs can conduct searches of national data by population groups based on race and ethnicity, sex, education, income, disability, family type, country of birth, geographic orientation, gender identity, sexual orientation, and health insurance status. Users can easily create visual displays using charts or maps to show progress over time for some of the *Healthy People* objectives in each topic area (ODPHP, 2018b). Revised every 10 years, *Healthy People 2030* will be released by 2020. MAP-IT is located at www .healthypeople.gov/2020/tools-and-resources/Program-Planning.

Community Tool Box

Initiated in 1994, the Community Tool Box is an online resource for people working to improve community health. This free public service was developed by the Center for Community Health and Development at the University of Kansas along with both national and international partners. It includes more than 300 educational modules and numerous free tools to provide guidance for community assessment and other components of community practice such as planning, intervention, evaluation, and advocacy. Its resources have been widely used not only in the United States but in more than 230 countries around the world (Center for Community Health and Development, 2018a). The Community Tool Box includes 46 chapters in 13 focus areas. One of the focus areas is community assessment. Some examples from chapters in this section include *Assessing Community Needs and Resources* and *Getting Issues on the Public Agenda*. A related toolkit for the community assessment focus is entitled *Assessing Community Needs and Resources* (Center for Community Health and Development, 2018b). The Community Tool Box can be accessed at https://ctb.ku.edu/en.

Community Health Assessment Toolkit

The Association for Community Health Improvement (ACHI) is a national association for healthcare professionals interested in community health, community benefit, and population health. It is an affiliate of the American Hospital Association (AHA) and the Health Research & Educational Trust. ACHI's mission is to advance community health by providing education, resources, professional development, and other opportunities for engagement and growth (ACHI, 2017a). The *Community Health Assessment Toolkit* outlines nine steps (and includes resources) for conducting CHNAs. Its purpose is to help nonprofit hospitals meet the ACA requirement to conduct a CHNA every 3 years. The nine steps in the framework are meant to be cyclical and include: (a) reflect and strategize; (b) identify and engage stakeholders; (c) define the community; (d) collect and analyze data; (e) prioritize community health issues; (f) document and communicate results; (g) plan implementation strategies; (h) implement strategies; and (i) evaluate progress. Each step has a brief purpose and key components that are succinctly outlined and includes resources to help conduct the CHNA (ACHI, 2017b). The Community Health Assessment Toolkit can be accessed at www.healthycommunities.org/Resources/toolkit.shtml#.XArAwGhKjIU.

County Health Rankings & Roadmaps

This online tool is a free resource that provides a large amount of county-level data on important health factors, allowing for easy comparisons with other counties and states. APRNs can quickly find population-based data on education, income, the quality of air and water, smoking, obesity, healthy food access, teen births, and much more. Thirty data measures are presented in a similar format for each county in each state from various national sources. The County Health Rankings started in 2010 when the University of Wisconsin Population Health Institute collaborated with the Robert Wood Johnson Foundation to release county level data about health outcomes and associated health indices such as environmental, economic, and social risk factors. It also provides information on clinical care factors. Each year these data are updated and released to the public. APRNs can use these data to quickly identify the community needs, problems, strengths, and assets of a county. In addition to locating comprehensive data easily, the roadmaps component of the website provides resources to help understand the county data and suggests evidence-based strategies for action that will lead to healthier change (Remington, Catlin, & Gennuso, 2015; University of Wisconsin Population Health Institute, 2018). County Health Rankings & Roadmaps can be accessed at www.countyhealthrankings.org.

CDC Community Health Improvement Navigator

The CDC Community Health Improvement (CHI) Navigator is a particularly good resource for CHA teams that are comprised of numerous agencies and stakeholders. The underlying assumptions of the CHI Navigator are that it is important to work together with diverse and numerous partners, engage communities in the CHA process, keep lines of communication open, and sustain results. Tools and resources are organized into four key areas: (a) the who, what, where of improving community health; (b) collaborative approaches to CHI; (c) establishing and maintaining effective collaborations; and (d) finding interventions that are effective (CDC, 2016). Numerous tools and resources are available that explain the steps for successful CHA efforts. These include: assess needs and resources; focus on what is important; choose effective policies and programs; act on what is important; and evaluate action (CDC, 2016). APRNs will discover that this resource provides a "one-stop-shop" with expert tools and resources to refer to when leading or participating in CHA and improvement efforts. The CHI Navigator can be accessed at www.cdc.gov/chinav/index.html.

Assessment Methods

Focus Groups

CHA teams can use focus groups to obtain valuable contextual data about communities. Through the focus group format, community members can provide input about what they feel their community needs. Sometimes specific stakeholders in a community such as members of government, designees from police or fire departments, clergy, and representatives from senior or youth groups form the focus group. More often the focus groups are open meetings to which all members of a community are invited. Several community destinations such as churches or public libraries provide appropriate settings, and a variety of meeting times optimize the opportunities for community members to participate.

A well-trained and prepared moderator leads the focus group. The moderator should guide the group so that it does not stray from the issues or topics being addressed, and the moderator should ask explicit questions that are specifically worded to elicit public input. Without an experienced moderator, group member focus can vacillate or become lost and the discussion may become tangential and too diffuse to extract useful information. An experienced moderator will prompt or cue the members in a way that elicits descriptions of the problem and its root causes, as well as innovative and constructive ideas and creative solutions. Many focus groups are recorded for transcription or later review to avoid missing any thoughts and ideas or nuances from the discussion.

During focus group discussions it may become apparent that projects under consideration are not important or viewed as a high priority by the community members in the meeting. Subsequently the focus of the assessment may shift. This should be considered a successful outcome of the focus group and not a negative outcome. It is critically important for community members to prioritize their own assets and needs so they will be more likely to "buy into" agreed upon projects and assist with long-term sustainability efforts (Center for Community Health and Development, 2018d).

A team working with the Center for Healthy African American Men through Partnerships used focus groups to generate information to guide the development of prevention programs to reduce disparities in education, violence, and premature mortality experienced by African American males (Phillips, Branch, Brady, & Simpson, 2018). Parents of African American male children enrolled in a middle school received a letter of invitation to participate in discussion groups about risk-taking behaviors. Experienced African American moderators facilitated the groups. An example of one script topic is: "What are the most important issues affecting the well-being and future success of young people in the African Americancommunity?" A total of nine related topics were covered (Phillips et al., 2018, p. S84).

Those who participated in the focus groups revealed that a lack of social support and male parental presence in homes, anger among their sons, and insufficient licensed counselors to assist their sons in school were major factors impacting the health and success of their children. The parents cited a need for young males to assume more leadership roles. Information elicited from the parents provided insight into the needs of this aggregate group. The study team planned to combine focus group data with key informant interviews of community stakeholders and data from a school-wide youth survey to select and "refine" an evidence-based intervention to support the future academic success and healthy development of young African American males in the community (Phillips et al., 2018).

Key Informant Interviews

Key informant interviews are useful for obtaining information from people who are well acquainted with a topic or subject that is being explored by the CHA team. Key informant interviews can provide useful contextual data and insight about community issues, problems, and assets. Key informants are most often selected from people representing different sectors of the community and who have the knowledge and experience to fill in gaps from data collected using other methods. Depending on time and resources, interviews may be conducted face-to-face, via telephone, through email, or in a focus group format. CHA team members are tasked with identifying what information is needed for the CHA and compiling the questions to ask informants. Key informant interviews can be highly to loosely structured depending on the type of information that is being sought. The most common interview format type for eliciting information from key informants is semi-structured. In a semi-structured interview the interviewer does not follow a formalized list of questions but asks open-ended questions to allow more flexibility with the discussion. This is a more common method than a straight-forward question-and-answer format because informants can digress and elaborate on answers. An additional bonus of a more loosely structured format is that informants have the freedom to raise issues of concern that CHA team members may not yet have become aware of (Center for Community Health and Development, 2018e).

In 1992, this author participated in a CHA of a rural county in Tennessee. CHA data were derived using several methods including 48 key informant interviews with people who were well acquainted with the county. These key informants were recommended by community members. They included beauticians, country store owners, teachers, pastors, and law enforcement personnel. These initial informants led the CHA team members to other people who had additional information and knowledge of the community. A semi-structured interview format was used. While the CHA was completed many years ago, the consequences of that CHA are still felt today in the form of two school-based health centers. Both outpatient clinics are part of a faculty practice network of nurse-managed health centers operated by East Tennessee State University's College of Nursing (www.etsu.edu/nursing/clinics/aboutus.php). The need for the school-based health centers was identified through the key informant interviews (Oppewal & Shuman, 1992).

Surveys

Surveys offer another assessment method for generating data for a CHA. Surveys are not always used by CHA teams because they are expensive to carry out, and it can be difficult to find a reliable and valid survey tool related to the topic of interest. When surveys are used in a CHA they are most often employed to survey either a subgroup of a population or the entire community to reach people who might not otherwise have the opportunity to provide input. For example, part of the Hancock County CHA included the administration of the CDC Youth Risk Behavior Survey (YRBS) to students who attended the one high school in the county. It allowed high school students to have a voice in the CHA. Data from the YRBS provided compelling rationale to develop a school-based health center.

CHA surveys can be conducted using different sampling approaches from a convenience sample carried out in various locations of the community, to one that is randomized and clustered. They can be used to elicit both quantitative and qualitative data related to community concerns, resources, and strengths. Often numerous methods for distributing surveys are used depending on the resources available to the CHA team and the characteristics of the community. Surveys can be conducted at different community locations like faith-based organizations, grocery stores, or other places where people gather. They may be distributed via email, postal mail, or newspaper. They can also be carried out through telephone interviews or using social media. Surveys are most often completed by individuals, but assistance can be offered to people who may, for one reason or the other, not be able to complete surveys independently. The point of a survey is to include information from as many community members as possible in the CHA (Center for Community Health and Development, 2018c). Please refer to more specific information about how to conduct surveys in Section 13 of the Community Tool Box (Center for Community Health and Development, 2018f, 2018g).

Windshield and Walking Surveys and Participant Observation

A windshield survey refers to information gleaned from purposeful observations made from a moving vehicle; a walking survey has the same purpose, but data are obtained by walking. These collection methods can help CHA teams to obtain an overall feel or impression of a community and they also aid in the identification of community challenges, problems, assets, and strengths. The APRN can use windshield and walking surveys (WWS) to make observations about the physical environment, the amount of green space, the type and condition of available housing, public spaces, and businesses (including both retail stores and commercial developments), as well as other details that can reveal information about a community (Stanhope & Lancaster, 2016). Before implementing a WWS, CHA team members should first identify the purpose of the WWS and then decide on questions that will guide the scope and structure of the WWS. For example, the survey may be guided by a broad question about the nature of a community or by narrower questions such as types and conditions of physical activity options, including sidewalks (Center for Community Health and Development, 2018h).

One CHA windshield survey that undergraduate students conducted in a small industrial town revealed a large number of taverns. The students discovered that many of the men who patronized them smoked cigarettes. Students learned that it was the usual custom for the men in this community to stop on their way home after work to enjoy some socialization. A review of local health department data also revealed a high incidence of oral cancer in this town. This is an example of how a windshield survey, combined with health-related data, can be used to identify potential areas for intervention in a community. The interventions that ensued included an oral screening clinic and a smoking-cessation program that targeted the tavern patrons.

Participant observation is a research method used to obtain purposeful observations indirectly (or passively) or more directly by participating in community activities. CHAs may include participant observation as a data collection method when there is a need for direct observation or participation in community activities. A CHA team might decide to use participant observation to better understand information gleaned from surveys, key informant interviews, or focus groups. For example, the APRN may use participant observation to purposely observe a town hall meeting after key informants describe the meetings as tense and contentious. Observations can help CHA team members better understand community conflict or to follow up on information obtained from focus group discussions or key informant interviews.

Secondary Data Analysis and Literature Reviews

Secondary data sources and literature reviews are often used for CHAs because they are relatively inexpensive, efficient, and easy to use. Secondary data are data that are collected by someone other than the user. Common sources of secondary data used for CHAs include censuses, information collected by government departments (such as the CDC), and organizational records (e.g., from churches, schools, or local government records). Such data can be used to describe demographic and socioeconomic characteristics of communities as well as the health of a community. A general recommendation is for CHA teams to determine local assets and needs by using data and indicators at the smallest geographic level for counties such as census blocks or zip codes (CDC, 2017). Analyses of existing data from various sources or from literature located for the purpose of better understanding a community or its problems should be done systematically. The CHA Toolkit has many online resources to help CHA team members find relevant and meaningful community health data and indicators. Other sources of community-level indicators and benchmarking information are briefly highlighted in Table 10.2.

Census Data

As required by the U.S. Constitution, the U.S. Census Bureau conducts a census of the entire population every 10 years. While basic data are collected on everyone, a selected sample of the population is surveyed in greater detail using the "long form." Those data provide a plethora of community characteristics (e.g., age, sex, race, education, employment, income) to better describe the makeup of communities. The information gathered is compiled and analyzed and reported to the nation. It is used by the government to make planning decisions, including the allocation of funds to government agencies (U.S. Census Bureau, 2018). It should be noted that despite the efforts of census workers to be as inclusive as possible, low-income and migratory populations are often underrepresented

TABLE 10.2 **Sources of Community-Level Indicators**

SOURCE OF COMMUNITY-LEVEL INDICATORS	BRIEF DESCRIPTION	WEBSITE
Behavioral Risk Factor Surveillance System (BRFSS)	Telephone survey of health conditions and risk factors	https://www.cdc.gov/brfss
CDC Wonder	Online databases to analyze public health data	https://wonder.cdc.gov
Community Commons	Data, tools, and stories for promoting community change	https://www.communitycommons.org
Dartmouth Atlas of Health Care	Data on distribution of medical resources using Medicare data	http://www.dartmouthatlas.org
Disability and Health Data System (DHDS)	State-level adult disability-specific data	https://www.cdc.gov/ncbddd/disabilityandhealth/dhds/index.html
National Health Indicators Warehouse	Searchable datasets of government data on a wide range of topics	https://healthdata.gov/dataset/health-indicators-warehouse Healthdata.gov

(continued)

TABLE 10.2 Sources of Community-Level Indicators (*continued*)

SOURCE OF COMMUNITY-LEVEL INDICATORS	BRIEF DESCRIPTION	WEBSITE
U.S. Census Bureau	Population, housing, economic and geographic information	https://www.census.gov
U.S. Food Environment Atlas	Food environment indicators that influence food choices and diet quality	https://www.ers.usda.gov/data-products/food-environment-atlas.aspx
Centers for Medicare &Medicaid Services (CMS) DataNavigator	Search tool of data and information resources of CMS programs, health topics, settings of care	https://dnav.cms.gov
National Environmental Public Health Tracking Network (Tracking Network)	Environmental data and health data from city, state, and national sources	https://ephtracking.cdc.gov/showHome.action
Health Research and Services Administration (HRSA)Warehouse	Data and maps on HRSA's Health Care Programs	https://data.hrsa.gov
Healthy People 2020 Leading Health Indicators	High-priority health objectives, issues and actions	https://www.healthypeople.gov/2020/leading-health-indicators/2020-LHI-Topics
Kids Count (Annie E. Casey Foundation)	Data about children, policy recommendations and tools	https://www.aecf.org/work/kids-count
National Center for Health Statistics	Statistical information to guide actions and policies to improve health	https://www.cdc.gov/nchs/index.htm
Pregnancy Risk Assessment and Monitoring System (PRAMS)	State-specific, population-based data on maternal attitudes and experiences before, during and shortly after pregnancy	https://www.cdc.gov/prams/index.htm
Web-Based Injury Statistics Query and Reporting System (WISQARS)	Interactive, online database of injury statistics	https://www.cdc.gov/injury/wisqars/index.html
Youth Risk Behavior Surveillance System (YRBSS)	Youth risk behavior surveillance for leading causes of death and disability	https://www.cdc.gov/healthyyouth/data/yrbs/index.htm

Source: From Centers for Disease Control and Prevention. (2017). Public health professionals gateway. Data and benchmarks. Retrieved from https://www.cdc.gov/stltpublichealth/cha/data.html

in the data. Census data as a source of information are invaluable. They are a rich source of information and can provide details that will help identify important community characteristics (e.g., culture, socioeconomic characteristics). Census information is available at www.census.gov.

Health Department Vital Statistics and Disease and Health Reports

Vital statistics are an excellent source of information about a community and are easily obtainable. Although considered "dry" by many community assessors, data on births, deaths, marriages, and divorces are vital statistics within a community and are collected on an ongoing basis. There is also a wide spectrum of quantitative information on populations available on the Internet. Information from health departments, in combination with information gleaned from other sources such as surveys or focus groups, can help provide valuable data to consider for improving the health of communities.

The CDC publishes data in the *Morbidity and Mortality Weekly Report* (www.cdc.gov/mmwr/index.html) that are not often available elsewhere; these reports are valuable sources of health information for APRNs. Morbidity and mortality data are also available from other DHHS and CDC websites. Information on notifiable diseases, adverse drug reactions, injuries, occupational health, and birth defects are some examples of the wide range of information that is available from these two government agencies.

Another useful resource is the public-use data files available through the CDC's National Center for Health Statistics (NCHS). Public-use data files include downloadable data sets and questionnaires from the National Health and Nutrition Examination Survey (NHANES), National Health Care Surveys, National Vital Statistics System (NVSS), National Survey of Family Growth, National Health Interview Survey (NHIS), National Immunization Survey, Longitudinal Studies of Aging (LSOA), State and Local Area Integrated Telephone Survey (SLAITS), NCHS Data Linkage, and Compressed Mortality File (CDC, 2018). The NCHS can be accessed at www.cdc.gov/nchs/index.htm.

BUILDING RELATIONSHIPS

Collaboration/Community Partnership

A community is comprised of many people, and the APRN needs to have a comprehensive understanding of those people in order to build a trusting relationship. Understanding a community's culture is essential to program success. The APRN should expect this process to take time, patience, commitment, and persistence. Moreover, understanding the makeup of a community and its cultural norms, and being sensitive and respectful of differences, is essential for successful collaboration and community partnership.

Community involvement is the foundation of a successful CHA. The members of the community, including the people, the government, the health department, the churches, the local businesses, to name a few, all need to be involved. Who are the leaders in the community? APRNs can identify the people who are respected and trusted and who encourage other community members to participate in activities. This is not always a political leader but can be a church member, a parent, a community advocate, or someone else. Many communities do not have an inherent trust in "outsiders" who come into their community. There may be a history in the county of well-intentioned CHA teams providing assessments and starting needed programs only to leave without providing community members with the tools (financial or otherwise) to sustain programs after they are gone. The APRN will have the most success with planning, conducting, and evaluating a CHA by working with and being guided by trusted members of the community rather than doing these activities without active community partnership.

It is also imperative that communities are not viewed as having a "problem" that needs to be fixed. Communities want to feel they are productive and cohesive and do not want someone to tell them how to fix their problems. They want partnership and understanding of who they are and what they stand for. When approaching a community, it is essential that you identify both the community's assets and weaknesses. By identifying the assets (or strengths), you can elicit more trust from community members because they do not want to be defined only by their problems. This mutual understanding can build trust and cooperation. It requires listening by both parties involved; education and learning should be bidirectional. Program leaders such as the APRN should provide the community and its members with the tools to sustain programs on their own. A sense of independence and self-sufficiency is important for long-term success. This is the ultimate form of partnership—one that is built upon trust, cooperation, and communication.

Building Relationships and Engaging Communities Through Collaboration: An Example

The concept of community collaboration can be illustrated by discussing a CHA in Lee County, North Carolina. Lee County is a rural county located in the center of the state. It is one of the smallest counties in North Carolina, encompassing just over 227 square miles. It is comprised of eight townships and its population increased steadily to 60,430 as of July 1, 2017 (U.S. Census Bureau, 2017). The population is approximately 58% White, 20% African American, and 19% Hispanic or Latino. Slightly over 11% of the population was born outside of the United States. Most recent reports indicate a median household income of $46,402. The percent of people living in poverty is 16.9%. About 81% of the county residents have a high school diploma and 21% have earned a bachelor's degree or higher (U.S. Census Bureau, 2017).

Lee County Public Health Department leads the county in a CHA every 4 years using a variety of data collection methods. One of its first tasks was to form a CHA Task Force. Members who were selected include representatives from the Health Department, a Board of Health Commissioner who also served as the supervisor of school nurses for Lee County, and members of the Healthy Carolinians Partnership in Lee County, known as the Community Action Network (LeeCAN). LeeCAN is a partnership with representation from government agencies, civic groups, citizen groups, and members from the faith-based communities. The mission of the LeeCAN is to use collaborative community effort to improve awareness of and resources to effectively deal with health and safety issues in the county (Lee County, North Carolina Government, 2018). One of the many strengths of Lee County is due to its rural nature. People know each other and work well with each other.

The CHA Task Force decided to use a survey to optimize community member participation. Members of the CHA team looked for an appropriate instrument for collecting information that would measure variables of interest consistently, dependably, and accurately. They selected a survey that had been originally used in three other rural North Carolina counties and that was previously validated for use as a health-focused data collection tool. The survey was made available in both hard copy and electronically via Facebook and on a publicized website. It was distributed and made available in the local newspaper, through "open house" and "community forum" events, local churches, volunteer fire departments, and local businesses.

The data were analyzed and reviewed by an advisory team from the Lee County Public Health Department and members of LeeCAN. Data analysis revealed the top three health priorities identified by community members as obesity, teen pregnancy, and mental health/substance abuse (Lee County Public Health Assessment Team & LeeCAN, 2014). These findings were similar to the needs identified in the 2010 CHA.

After analyzing the initial survey data, the CHA team noted that two areas in Lee County had a poor rate of survey returns. One location was in the incorporated town of Broadway, which has just over 1,000 residents. The second location, Lemon Springs, is a small community outside of these two areas; however, it is not incorporated into a town. Very few surveys (fewer than 10) were received from Broadway and Lemon Springs. The team thought that literacy or language barriers, distrust of government agencies, and general complacency were potential factors associated with the poor survey response rate.

Given the concern with the low input from community members in Broadway and Lemon Springs, the assessment team decided to conduct focus groups in each of the areas. Topics were preselected from the previous surveys, and a moderator familiar with the CHA process but not actively involved in the earlier data collection efforts was chosen. The meetings were held on a weekday in a central location during midday. Food and door prizes were incentives to attend; a record of attendees was not kept so that anonymity could be maintained.

The focus groups unearthed valuable information. Common themes were affordability of health insurance, lack of specialty care in Lee County, and the need to educate residents about public health services. Specific concerns included drugs and the subsequent negative impact on their communities. In addition, more activities or community facilities were requested to cater to older adults and children. In general the focus group participants felt that their community was a good place to live and to raise a family. Participants stated that they wanted to know how to teach children about avoiding drug use and to provide parents who have problems in this area with help. They also commented about the need for the unemployed to have access to training that matched available employment in the area. Additionally, transportation was noted as "always an issue." More public transportation to access healthcare services in the community was identified as one of their priority needs.

The qualitative data collected from the focus groups provided rich information that confirmed and built on results from the previously completed surveys. Data obtained from surveys and focus groups were used to develop action plans to target the issues identified by community members. The CHA survey and the focus groups were helpful in revealing residents' perceptions about health and quality-of-life issues in Lee County.

The CHA team used secondary data analysis to validate findings from the surveys and to fill in gaps in information. Data sources included:

- Statistical data from the North Carolina State Center for Health Statistics
- North Carolina Department of Health and Human Services

- North Carolina Division of Public Health: Office of Minority Health and Health Disparities

- North Carolina Department of Public Instruction

- 2010 Census Data

- Sanford/Lee County Strategic Services

- Center for Health Services Research, University of North Carolina

- Kids Count data from the Annie E. Casey Foundation

- Employment Security Commission of North Carolina

- North Carolina Office of the Governor

- North Carolina Child Advocacy Institute

- North Carolina Crime Statistics: North Carolina State Bureau of Investigation

The 2014 Lee County CHA team included numerous community partners and leaders. It engaged community members by providing a wide range of opportunities for community participation. The information garnered from the CHA helped community agencies in formulating program goals and objectives. Data obtained during the CHA process also supplied necessary information for grant proposals, and documentation for the need for resources and funding for priority county issues. An additional benefit was the addition of a list of community resources available to the public on the Health Department's website (List of Health Resources by the Lee County Health Department, 2018).

SUMMARY

The CHA process extends beyond collecting community data; it includes establishing trust and rapport with community partners and involving community members actively throughout the entire assessment process. Community programs are most successful when community members participate in the planning, implementation, and evaluation of programs that address local health concerns. Building relationships and engaging communities through collaboration is a rewarding experience for the APRN. The CHA must be totally inclusive and reflect the collaboration necessary to create an accurate and comprehensive depiction of the community. It is also a dynamic process and should incorporate multiple methods to assess and address a community's needs.

The CHA should be readdressed at regular intervals to identify changing needs. With the information obtained through a well-designed CHA, the APRN has the data needed to develop evidence-based projects that meet the needs of the community. Working with community leaders is critical for success, especially in engaging community members in the process. Only then can community programs be developed and integrated into a successful healthcare plan for the community. These strategies are not always easy but they allow community members to become empowered and creative in their own approach to improving their community.

Building relationships and engaging communities through collaboration requires time, persistence, and patience. It does not happen quickly but is a process that builds over time and may involve years. The information collected in a CHA can be used to inform policies, develop new programs, and design health promotion activities.

EXERCISES AND DISCUSSION QUESTIONS

Exercise 10.1 APRNs should recognize the value of collaboration and make it a regular part of their practice regardless of whether they will lead a CHA process or participate as a team member in a CHA.

- Describe ways that you anticipate using collaboration as an APRN.
- What are barriers to collaboration?
- What are potential facilitators of collaboration?

Exercise 10.2 The APRN who practices in the only primary care center in Tyrrell County, North Carolina, is asked to participate on the CHA team. The APRN takes a quick look at the U.S. Census Data for Tyrrell County and then County Health Rankings to quickly obtain general information about the county. Next is a review of the *2014 Martin-Tyrrell-Washington District Health Department Tyrrell County Community Health Assessment* to learn more about how the CHA was previously conducted. Search the Internet using the title *2014 Martin-Tyrrell-Washington District Health Department Tyrrell County Community Health Assessment* to help you to answer the following questions.

1. What information can be found from the U.S. Census Bureau to help the team understand the demographic makeup of the county?

2. What information does County Health Rankings provide related to health outcomes and the social determinants of health for Tyrrell County, North Carolina? (The website is www.countyhealthrankings.org.)

3. What county strengths were identified in the 2014 CHA report?

4. What five priority health areas and three recommendations were identified by the CHA planning committee for 2015 to 2018 based on the 2014 CHA data? Find this information in the *2014 Martin-Tyrrell-Washington District Health Department Tyrrell County Community Health Assessment.*

Exercise 10.3 A CHA team sets the goal of increasing a community survey response rate by 15% in an upcoming CHA.

1. What strategies might be considered for reaching more respondents and achieving the survey response rate goal?

2. CHA team members used educational data as a proxy for literacy when reviewing the survey for appropriate reading level. According to the 2010 census data, 55% of county residents have a high school education; 42% have a bachelor's degree; and 8% have a graduate degree. How can health literacy be considered when selecting or adapting the survey?

3. How can CHA planning members identify additional distribution sites for the community survey?

REFERENCES

American Association of Colleges of Nursing. (2006). *The essentials of doctoral education for advanced nursing practice*. Washington, DC: Author. Retrieved from http://www.aacnnursing.org/Portals/42/Publications/DNPEssentials.pdf

American Nurses Association. (n.d.) Health system reform. Retrieved from https://www.nursingworld.org/practice-policy/health-policy/health-system-reform

Anderson, E. T., & McFarlane, J. (2019). *Community as partner: Theory and practice in nursing* (8th ed.). Philadelphia, PA: Wolters Kluwer Health.

Association for Community Health Improvement. (2017a). About who we are. Retrieved from http://www.healthycommunities.org/About/index.shtml

Association for Community Health Improvement. (2017b). Community health assessment toolkit. Retrieved from http://www.healthycommunities.org/Resources/toolkit.shtml#.W7L2nfYpCwU

Center for Community Health and Development. (2018a). About the Tool Box. Retrieved from the Community Tool Box https://ctb.ku.edu/en/about-the-tool-box

Center for Community Health and Development. (2018b). [Toolkit 2] Assessing community needs and resources. Retrieved from the Community Tool Box https://ctb.ku.edu/en/assessing-community-needs-and-resources

Center for Community Health and Development. (2018c). Chapter 3, Section 7: Conducting needs assessment surveys. Lawrence, KS: University of Kansas. Retrieved from the Community Tool Box https://ctb.ku.edu/en/table-of-contents/assessment/assessing-community-needs-and-resources/conducting-needs-assessment-surveys/main

Center for Community Health and Development. (2018d). Chapter 3, Section 6: Conducting focus groups. Lawrence, KS: University of Kansas. Retrieved from the Community Tool Box https://ctb.ku.edu/en/table-of-contents/assessment/assessing-community-needs-and-resources/conduct-focus-groups/main

Center for Community Health and Development. (2018e). Chapter 3, Section 12: Conducting interviews. Lawrence, KS: University of Kansas. Retrieved from https://ctb.ku.edu/en/table-of-contents/assessment/assessing-community-needs-and-resources/conduct-interviews/main

Center for Community Health and Development. (2018f). Chapter 3, Section 10: Conducting concerns surveys. Lawrence, KS: University of Kansas. Retrieved from the Community Tool Box https://ctb.ku.edu/en/table-of-contents/assessment/assessing-community-needs-and-resources/conduct-concerns-surveys/main

Center for Community Health and Development. (2018g). Chapter 3, Section 13: Conducting surveys. Lawrence, KS: University of Kansas. Retrieved from the Community Tool Box https://ctb.ku.edu/en/table-of-contents/assessment/assessing-community-needs-and-resources/conduct-surveys/main

Center for Community Health and Development. (2018h). Chapter 3, Section 21: Windshield and walking surveys. Lawrence, KS: University of Kansas. Retrieved from the Community Tool Box https://ctb.ku.edu/en/table-of-contents/assessment/assessing-community-needs-and-resources/windshield-walking-surveys/main

Centers for Disease Control and Prevention. (2016). CDC Community Health Improvement (CHI) Navigator. CHI Navigator Resources. Retrieved from https://www.cdc.gov/chinav/resources/index.html

Centers for Disease Control and Prevention. (2017). Public health professionals gateway. Data and benchmarks. Retrieved from https://www.cdc.gov/stltpublichealth/cha/data.html

Centers for Disease Control and Prevention. (2018). National Center for Health Statistics. Public-use data files and documentation. Retrieved from https://www.cdc.gov/nchs/data_access/ftp_data.htm

Centers for Medicare & Medicaid Services. (2018). Federally qualified health center. Medicare Learning Network (MLN) booklet published January 2018. Retrieved from https://www.cms.gov/Outreach-and-Education/Medicare-Learning-Network-MLN/MLNProducts/Downloads/fqhcfactsheet.pdf

Craig, G. (2018, August 29). States and Trump administration push to roll back health care gains. [Email] American Nurses Association (ANA) *Capitol Beat*. Retrieved from https://anacapitolbeat.org/2018/08/29/states-and-trump-administration-push-to-roll-back-health-care-gains/

DeSalvo, K. B., Wang, Y. C., Harris, A., Auerbach, J., Koo, D., & O'Carroll, P. (2017). Public Health 3.0: A call to action for public health to meet the challenges of the 21st century. *Prevention of Chronic Diseases, 14*, 170017. doi:10.5888/pcd14.170017

Fitzpatrick, J. (2016). Community-based participatory research: Challenges and opportunities. *Applied Nursing Research, 31*, 187. doi:10.1016/j.apnr.2016.06.005

Gibson, M. E., & Thatcher, E. J. (2016). Community as client: Assessment and analysis. In M. Stanhope & J. Lancaster (Eds.), *Public health nursing: Population-centered health care in the community* (9th ed., pp. 396–421). St. Louis, MO: Elsevier.

Gintzig, D., & West, J. (2016). *2016 Wake County community health needs assessment: Opportunities & challenges*. Retrieved from http://www.wakegov.com/wellbeing/Documents/2016%20Wake%20County%20CHNA%20Full%20Document%20Final.pdf

Internal Revenue Service (n.d.). *Requirements for 501(c)(3) hospitals under the Affordable Care Act-Section 501(r)*. Retrieved from https://www.irs.gov/charities-non-profits/charitable-organizations/requirements-for-501c3-hospitals-under-the-affordable-care-act-section-501r

Institute of Medicine of the National Academies. (2015). Vital signs: Core metrics for health and health care progress. [Report Brief]. Retrieved from https://www.nap.edu/resource/19402/VitalSigns_RB.pdf

Kaiser Family Foundation. (2013). Summary of the Affordable Care Act. Retrieved from https://www.kff.org/health-reform/fact-sheet/summary-of-the-affordable-care-act

Lee County, NC Government. (2018). Retrieved from https://leecountync.gov/Departments/PublicHealth/LeeCAN

Lee County Public Health Assessment Team and LeeCAN. (2014). Lee County community health assessment. Retrieved from https://leecountync.gov/Portals/0/Content/files/state-of-the-county-health-report-2014-finalize.pdf

List of Health Resources by the Lee County Health Department. (2018). Appendix C. Retrieved from https://leecountync.gov/Portals/0/Content/Departments/uploads/Health/List%20of%20Statistical%20Resources%202018.pdf

National Association of Clinical Nurse Specialists Press Room. (2018, August 6). Esteemed panel composed of leading nursing, health experts met to revise, validate clinical nurse specialist statement. Retrieved from https://nacns.org/2018/08/esteemed-panel-composed-of-leading-nursing-health-experts-met-to-revise-validate-clinical-nurse-specialist-statement

National Association of County and City Health Officials. (2014). *Public health infrastructure and systems*. Retrieved from http://www.naccho.org/topics/infrastructure/mapp/chahealthreform.cfm

National CNS Competency Task Force. (2010). Clinical nurse specialist core competencies: Executive summary 2006–2008. Retrieved from http://nacns.org/wp-content/uploads/2017/01/CNSCoreCompetenciesBroch.pdf

Nurse Practitioner Core Competencies Content Work Group. (2017). Nurse practitioner core competencies content. Retrieved from https://cdn.ymaws.com/www.nonpf.org/resource/resmgr/competencies/2017_NPCoreComps_with_Curric.pdf

Office of Disease Prevention and Health Promotion. (2018a). Program planning. In *Healthy People 2020*. Retrieved from https://www.healthypeople.gov/2020/tools-and-resources/Program-Planning

Office of Disease Prevention and Health Promotion. (2018b). How to use DATA2020. In *Healthy People 2020*. Retrieved from https://www.healthypeople.gov/2020/How-to-Use-DATA2020

Oppewal, S., & Shuman, P. (1992). *Community needs assessment of Hancock County*. Report prepared for the First Tennessee Community Health Agency, East Tennessee State University, School of Nursing, Department of Family/Community Nursing, Tennessee.

Phillips, J. M., Branch, C. J., Brady, S. S., & Simpson, T. (2018). Parents speak: A needs assessment for community programming for Black male youth. *American Journal of Preventive Medicine, 55*(5), S82–S87. doi:10.1016/j.amepre.2018.05.014

Public Health Foundation. (2018). [Website] About PHF. Retrieved from www.phf.org

Public Health Institute. (2018). Core metrics pilot project: Final report. Retrieved from http://www.phi.org/uploads/application/files/ojxskqfes39tcd33bpxflw8kmelezjff4oevqo93rmzf4yu214.pdf

Public Health Nursing Definition Document Task Force. (2013). The definition and practice of public health nursing. American Public Health Association, Public Health Nursing Section. Retrieved from https://www.apha.org/~/media/files/pdf/membergroups/phn/nursingdefinition.ashx

Quad Council Coalition. (2018). [Website] Retrieved from http://www.quadcouncilphn.org

Quad Council Coalition Competency Review Task Force. (2018). Community/public health nursing competencies. Retrieved from http://www.quadcouncilphn.org/documents-3/2018-qcc-competencies

Remington, P. L., Catlin, B. B., & Gennuso, K. P. (2015). The County Health Rankings: Rationale and methods. *Population Health Metrics, 13*, 11. doi:10.1186/s12963-015-0044-2

Stanhope, M., & Lancaster, J. (2016). *Public health nursing: Population-centered health care in the community* (9th ed.). St Louis, MO: Mosby Elsevier.

U.S. Census Bureau. (2017). QuickFacts: Lee County, NC. Retrieved from https://www.census.gov/quickfacts/fact/table/leecountynorthcarolina/SBO040212#viewtop

U.S. Census Bureau. (2018). About the Bureau. Retrieved from https://www.census.gov/about/what.html

University of Wisconsin Population Health Institute. (2018). About us. County Health Rankings & Roadmaps. Retrieved from http://www.countyhealthrankings.org/about-us

WNC Health Network. (2018). [Website]. Retrieved from https://www.wnchn.org

INTERNET RESOURCES

Association for Community Health Improvement, Community Health Assessment Toolkit: http://www.healthycommunities.org/Resources/toolkit.shtml#.XArAwGhKjIU

CDC Community Health Improvement Navigator: https://www.cdc.gov/chinav/index.html

CDC, *Morbidity and Mortality Weekly Report*: https://www.cdc.gov/mmwr/index.html

CDC, National Center for Health Statistics: https://www.cdc.gov/mmwr/index.html

Community Tool Box: https://ctb.ku.edu/en

County Health Rankings and Roadmaps: http://www.countyhealthrankings.org

MAP-IT: www.healthypeople.gov/2020/tools-and-resources/Program-Planning

Office of Disease Prevention an Health Promotion, *Healthy People 2020*, MAP-IT: https://www.healthypeople.gov/2020/tools-and-resources/Program-Planning

Quad Council Coalition, C/PHN Competencies: www.quadcouncilphn.org

U.S. Census Bureau: www.census.gov

Also refer to Internet sites listed in Table 10.2

CHAPTER 11

CHALLENGES IN PROGRAM IMPLEMENTATION

JANNA L. DIECKMANN

INTRODUCTION

The role of the nurse includes compassionate and quality care not only for the individual but also for the family and the community. Advanced practice registered nurses (APRNs) seek to improve the circumstances that contribute to poor population health by working with community members to modify or change the behaviors that may contribute to poor health outcomes. This type of collaboration has the potential to make or facilitate changes that improve health and reduce morbidity and mortality.

The APRN should approach communities with an open mind and a focus on a comprehensive community health assessment (CHA). A CHA helps the APRN to gain an understanding of the community, its residents, their diversity, their goals, their aspirations for healthier lives, and the barriers to achieving these goals (see Chapter 10, Building Relationships and Engaging Communities Through Collaboration). People want a better life. They want to be healthier and they want to live longer, happier, and more productive lives. The challenge lies in changing the behaviors and attitudes of individuals and communities. For many, change is uncomfortable or difficult, but it is a necessary process for communities that want to make improvements. But a process of change is unlikely to be smooth if community members do not buy into this change and are not willing to take a risk. Like Chapter 10, Building Relationships and Engaging Communities Through Collaboration, the focus of this chapter is on *Essential V, Interprofessional Collaboration for Improving Patient and Population Health Outcomes* and *Essential VII, Clinical Prevention and Population Health for Improving the Nation's Health*. It continues with and builds on the discussion of those skills and strategies that are effective when working with others (American Association of Colleges of Nursing [AACN], 2006).

LEWIN'S STAGES OF CHANGE

Lewin's Three-Stage Model of Change provides a brief but profound approach to change at the aggregate or community level (Allender, Rector, & Warner, 2013). In the role of a change agent, the APRN begins by destabilizing the group or community by asking questions to generate hope and visions of something different, something possibly better. Perhaps the group or community is already experiencing a desire for something different. Disequilibrium in the current moment underscores the relevance and potential of change and of moving out of the current comfort zone.

Unfreezing

The first stage of change is *unfreezing*, and may arise from the community's own self-assessment or it may be activated by the APRN through motivation, health education, advocacy, or other strategies (Allender et al., 2013; Connelly, 2016). An APRN may initiate unfreezing during the course of usual practice. For example, as part of a primary care practice, an APRN may find that many adult patients want to increase their physical activity, but the lack of designated walking or biking trails is a barrier that prevents this change. The APRN initiates a conversation with the head of the local farmers' cooperative and with the director of the county's agricultural extension office. A community meeting is planned, with broad attendance by local residents and representatives of other community organizations. Many express interest in increased physical activity, but doubt their ability to make changes to their community that will make it more "walker friendly." This meeting is the first of many opportunities to present the problem to the community and address possible solutions, and begin to build a bridge of confidence between the community and the healthcare provider. Focus groups (see Chapter 10, Building Relationships and Engaging Communities Through Collaboration) can also further this goal and provide more individual attention to potential barriers while proposing possible solutions to address those concerns.

Changing, Moving, or Transition

The second stage in Lewin's model reflects an understanding that change is not a timed event but an ongoing process that can be facilitated by the actions of the APRN. This stage is known variously as *changing*, *moving*, or *transition* (Allender et al., 2013; Connelly, 2016). Community members begin as individuals and as a group to transition to new attitudes and behaviors as they acquire new skills and perspectives.

The combination of destabilizing the present state and the challenge of questioning the status quo of behaviors and attitudes can make the second stage the most difficult. The support role of the APRN is very important, as the nurse must accept the community's attempts at change against the risk of early failures. The APRN cannot necessarily direct community change, as community residents benefit from developing their own new patterns of behavior as these emerge from who they are and their past experiences. The APRN can motivate and guide community members and help them build on their experiences to make the changes necessary for success. Using the earlier example, the

APRN should provide encouragement about the value of change (e.g., an improvement in residents' physical activity levels leads to improved health and less need for medications), implement strategies to reduce fears (e.g., educate residents about other successful programs), develop skills to unlock new behaviors (e.g., encourage residents to work together as peer support), provide prompts underscoring the importance of change attempts (e.g., use simple outcome measures for residents [i.e., step counters] to track progress and set goals), and remind residents about the benefits of the community's goal (e.g., a healthier community is a more productive community; Allender et al., 2013; Connelly, 2016). As a result of regular community meetings, the rural community raises funds and constructs new walking trails on public land. A park with a picnic shelter is also built to provide families and groups a place to gather after walking.

Refreezing

The third stage of change is *refreezing* (or *freezing*), which reflects the restabilization of the community that follows after making a change. This stage can require a period of time, as the change or transition that community members experience can lead to a change in their relationships and in their daily lives as they internalize what is now different. The system adapts to the impact of the change, and the community integrates the change into a newly stable and rebalanced present state. For example, the walking trails that were once seen as improbable are now embraced and accepted by the community. The APRN can provide the community with additional tools to stabilize the change and to reinforce and maintain new community behaviors. Families are encouraged to try out the new walking trail and to use the new picnic area for a healthy meal. Neighborhood events can center on the use of the park so as to introduce other community members to the benefits of the community space. Periodic reminders to area residents about the walking trails can be included in local print and social media outlets.

The success of the change process can lead to an enhanced partnership between the nurse and the community with the potential for further collaboration. Ideally, over time, the rural community will increase its physical activity and may seek additional consultation, for example, on how to select and prepare nutritious meals. Two-way communication can identify and address resistance or barriers to change. The APRN needs to identify potential problems or doubts and reinforce the benefits and values of the changed behaviors. The emergence of a new equilibrium signals a potential exit point for the APRN's engagement with the community (Allender et al., 2013; Connelly, 2016).

COMMUNITY ENGAGEMENT

Engagement

APRNs are more likely to succeed in addressing community concerns when communities are prepared to engage in the process of change. *Engagement* is different from wishing or acknowledging that "something" needs to change in order to improve. According to the Centers for Disease Control and Prevention (CDC), community engagement is "the process of working collaboratively with and through groups of people affiliated by geographic proximity, special interest, or similar situations to address issues affecting the well-being of those people" (McCloskey et al., 2011a, p. 7). Before beginning a community engagement effort, the APRN must carefully consider the target community/ population. What are the results of the CHA, and what is known about the community? What has been the history of this community during and following previous change and engagement efforts? How will the community and its various groups likely perceive the APRN, and what is the potential for a successful engagement of community members (McCloskey et al., 2011b)? Is the community prepared to engage in change? Would the community's social or physical environment facilitate or impede change? During this assessment and initial contact, the APRN needs to recognize the core principle of community self-determination and the limits of professional action. It is critical that the APRN clearly recognize the principle that "[n]o external entity should assume it can bestow to a community the power to act in its own self-interest" (McCloskey et al., 2011a, p. 16). Community members will find their own power when they seek it in themselves and take action for themselves, their families, and their community.

Involving the community is a second important and necessary step in assessing the potential for engagement. The APRN needs to establish relationships and build trust through contacts with community leaders and community organizations. As mentioned in earlier chapters, the community leaders are not always the political leaders, but rather can include leaders in the church, schools, charitable foundations, or any member of the community who is trusted as a leader. The successful engagement with the community will depend on developing relationships with these community leaders. Each community is distinctively unique; engaging with a community will require acknowledgment and inclusion of the cultures and diversity of that community in all steps of the engagement. Only by taking these steps can the APRN fully identify and mobilize community assets and resources and lay the groundwork for building long-term change in the community. With that said, healthcare professionals must recognize the limits of professional control and the need and/or cost of making a long-term commitment with the community and its residents (Hatcher, Warner, & Hornbrook, 2011; see Box 11.1).

Gaining the Trust of the Community

When working with a community, population, or aggregate, the APRN must include strategies to initiate, develop, and sustain trust among the APRN and community leaders, community members, and stakeholders. Trust requires mutual intention and is characterized by reciprocity (Lynn-McHale & Deatrick, 2000). As a key element in social interaction, trust facilitates communication and mutual understanding. Trust is a basis for change, a constant connection that provides support when the change process destabilizes a known situation in favor of an unknown outcome. A focus on developing trust begins with the initial contact with community members (Macali, Galanowsky, Wagner, & Truglio-Londrigan, 2011). The resulting nurse–community relationship is a critical prerequisite to population intervention. Through a trusting relationship, the community member gains the security of the APRN's stable presence as a prerequisite to risking the unknown.

BOX 11.1

PRINCIPLES OF COMMUNITY ENGAGEMENT

Before starting a community engagement effort:

- Be clear about the purposes or goals of the engagement effort and the populations and/or communities you want to engage.

- Become knowledgeable about the community in terms of its economic conditions, political structures, norms and values, demographic trends, history, and experience with engagement efforts. Learn about the community's perceptions of those initiating the engagement activities.

For engagement to occur, it is necessary to:

- Go into the community, establish relationships, build trust, work with the formal and informal leadership, and seek commitment from community organizations and leaders to create processes for mobilizing the community.

- Remember and accept that community self-determination is the responsibility and right of all people who constitute a community. No external entity should assume it can bestow to a community the power to act in its own self-interest.

For engagement to succeed:

- Partnering with the community is necessary to create change and improve health.

- All aspects of community engagement must recognize and respect community diversity. Awareness of the various cultures and other factors of diversity must be paramount in designing and implementing community engagement approaches.

- Community engagement can only be sustained by identifying and mobilizing community assets and by developing capacities and resources for community health decisions and actions.

- An engaging organization or individual change agent must be prepared to release control of actions or interventions to the community and be flexible enough to meet the changing needs of the community.

- Community collaboration requires long-term commitment by the engaging organization and its partners.

Source: From Clinical and Translational Science Awards Consortium Community Engagement Key Function Committee Task Force on the Principles of Community Engagement. (2011). Principles of community engagement (NIH Publication No. 11-7782). Retrieved from https://www.atsdr.cdc.gov/communityengagement/pdf/PCE_Report_508_FINAL.pdf

Four categories of trust have been described: calculative, competence, relational, and integrated. In *calculative trust*, potential members of the community initiative estimate the balance of benefits and costs to be derived from a potential collaboration as well as each member's assets and linkages. *Competence trust* hinges on whether group members are capable of doing what they commit to do; this type of trust also underlies the development of mutual respect among the participants. *Relational trust* reflects the personal relationships that quickly arise among members of any group. Members may express the value of mutual exchanges and develop a sense of commitment to mutual goals. Taken together, these three categories of trust constitute *integrated trust*, the foundation of an ongoing partnership (Logan, Davis, & Parker, 2010).

Initiating trust is an essential first step in building a bond between the nurse and the community. The nurse's *presence* in the community is qualitative evidence of the intent to develop a professional relationship with the community and its members. The community's willingness to view this presence positively will hinge on the APRN's clear communication of his or her role with the community. The APRN should seek to frame his or her presence within the broader outlines of the consensus needs or goals of the community, to the extent that these are known.

On the basis of knowledge obtained from a CHA, the APRN should interact appropriately with community members, for example, in relation to personal demeanor, communication patterns, cultural sensitivity, expressions of interest, and communication of knowledge about the community. Being "liked" by community members can be indefinable in its intent or as a goal, but either way it is nearly essential in practice. The APRN should always review and consider what the community needs or wants first. The nurse's expressions of interest in the community and its members are concrete indications of commitment and, to a certain extent, obligate the APRN to the community and to assisting with the community members' priorities. If there is a specified time frame or funding for the program, the APRN needs to share this limitation with the community and provide the community with the tools needed to sustain or build the program on its own.

Processes of Developing and Sustaining Trust

The process of developing trust between the APRN and the community will likely emerge from early collaborative efforts. In most cases, selecting small, achievable goals that can be met swiftly is recommended. The success of early visible outcomes enhances the nurse's credibility and increases the community's willingness and openness to trust. Increasing the breadth and depth of community participation with these goals will also increase the proportion of community members who have had contact with the APRN and will be an advantage as the nurse–community collaboration continues. It is likely that the community will embark on testing or probing the nurse's knowledge, behavior, and character for the sake of better understanding and will withhold open trust until the community's needs begin to be met. As the nature of the nurse–community relationship is constructed and evolves during this period of role negotiation, the APRN must maintain commitment to the initial shared goals, demonstrate professional openness to engagement with the community, and continue visible and concrete participation in the community. As APRNs share a community presence with the public health nurse, it is relevant to consider that "[t]he less experience people have with trusting relationships and the less sense of personal power and control they have, the more time public health nurses must spend developing trust and strength" (Zerwekh, 1993, p. 1676).

Sustaining the community's trust is built on a record of commitment and ongoing interaction with the community and its members. The nurse's continuing presence within the community establishes a sort of continuity that is reinforced by reliable actions.

Decisions by APRNs that become predictable to the community build the community's independence in self-management. When community members can predict "what the nurse would do," they are well on their way to independent decision-making for their health. As community members gain independence, the importance of the APRN's leadership becomes less necessary. With increased community competence, the APRN may face new challenges in sustaining the community's trust, and the APRN's role as a leader will change. As a community gains self-efficacy and confidence in self-determination and in its individual perspectives, conflicts become more likely. Mutual participation in thoughtful resolution is essential. Sustaining the community's continued trust will depend on the APRN's personal and professional skills and willingness to modify relationships with the community and its members and accept a new role as defined by a strengthened community.

Building Partnerships

If trust is an essential prerequisite for change, then partnerships are the essential underpinning for negotiating, planning, and implementing change. The long-lasting relationships that characterize some partnerships build on existing strengths even as new capacities are forged and developed. Themes of engagement, autonomy, and self-determination have shaped contemporary ideas of partnership since the mid-20th century. The Alma-Ata Declaration (1978) proposed a social model of health that underscored the need for "citizen's greater self-reliance and decisional control over their own health" (Gallant, Beaulieu, & Carnevale, 2002, p. 152), and alerted national health systems to more formally involve citizens in healthcare decisions (Gallant et al., 2002). This is even more salient when addressing 21st-century healthcare demands that require individual and community initiatives to address and improve health promotion and disease prevention (Courtney, Ballard, Fauver, Gariota, & Holland, 1996).

Agency–Academic Partnerships

One long-standing approach to partnership is the bridging of health agencies and academic institutions through joint ventures. An early example occurred in Ohio in which the University Public Health Nursing District (in Cleveland, Ohio, 1917–1962) linked local schools of nursing with an independent nursing agency that provided clinic services, public health services, and nurse home visiting (Farnham, 1964). Nursing students were assigned to the district for their public health nursing experiences. Assignments for diploma school students tended more to observation of activities during a brief few weeks, compared to collegiate nursing students, who became fully engaged over a semester in the breadth of public health nursing work. The key structural element was the public health nursing staff of the district, who served as clinical educators for students as well as direct care providers.

As effective and contributory as such programs are, the agency–academic partnership model of collaboration between a health agency or primary care practice and an academic institution has a limited impact when community residents and the wider service-resource network remain uninvolved, and when services are delivered outside of a collaborative planning process that includes community participants at the table from the beginning. Agency–academic partnership programs that focus on delivering services and improving health, but do not address the critical underlying barriers to improving health, are too limited in scope. Changes in the community—both change that benefits community members and change that transforms the community's health—are more likely to occur successfully with the participation of community representatives, both community members and leaders. One promising approach for successful academic–community partnerships uses the community-oriented primary care model to address the structural inequalities underpinning these challenges by placing a community-based organization in the central coordinating role for the partnership (Cherry & Shefner, 2004). An example of one such partnership is the one between Rush University and a community located in Chicago. The Rush University Colleges of Nursing, Medicine, and Health Sciences formed an academic partnership with Marillac House, an existing and trusted social service agency. The goal of the partnership was to provide interdisciplinary and primary health-care services to a medically underserved neighborhood in Chicago. This partnership benefits both the community and the university as it provides much needed medical services to community residents, and the university uses the clinical site for its students, who gain valuable experience working with a diverse and underserved population (McCann, 2010). The university fostered engagement with the community by partnering with an established agency within the neighborhood and working with community members.

This discussion of agency–academic partnerships highlights the contrast between the APRN as advocate or as catalyst when engaging with a community for health changes. In both the advocate and catalyst roles, the APRN respects the community and its self-determination as a basis for developing strategies to assist or complement the community's efforts for improved health. The *advocate* understands "the world view, life circumstances, and priorities of those requesting or receiving care and exploring the possible options with them in light of their preferences" (Walker, 2011, p. 75). While recognizing the community partner's individuality and self-determination, the nurse advocate takes action on behalf of a community to raise awareness in community members or make change in policy, economic, or social systems affecting the community (Walker, 2011). This advocate approach is closest to the APRN role in the agency–academic partnership. In contrast, the APRN as *catalyst* understands the community as containing "all the necessary qualities and resources for change" and focuses on providing "the spark that will initiate change, as desired by the community and on its terms" (Walker, 2011, p. 75). The "nurse as advocate" role provides the framework for APRN practice in sustainable partnerships and coalitions.

Sustainable Partnerships

Developing long-term relationships between the APRN and community representatives and organizations is a necessary component for preparing communities for long-term change. Sustainable partnerships are characterized by a relationship process through which the nurse and partners "work and interact together" (Gallant et al., 2002, p. 153). Power is shared in a "power with" approach "emphasizing the positive force created between partners and how this force sustains and propels a relationship forward" (Gallant et al., 2002, p. 154). Win–win negotiation models are recommended in the clinical nursing context (Roberts & Krouse, 1990), and have value in the APRN's collaborations with community leaders and members. Not only are all parties' views heard and valued, but also the power to make decisions is shared, leading to "a sense of responsibility and power" (Roberts & Krouse, 1990, p. 33). This is particularly important when establishing a context for the emergence of an empowered community.

Sustainable partnerships are supported by public participation that enhances decision-making by reflecting the interests and concerns of partnership members and by highlighting the underlying values guiding partnership operation. The community that is affected by a decision should be able to participate in influencing the decision and should be included in a way that enables their full participation. Including community members in decision-making committees is an important part of community engagement. Decisions are likely to be more sustainable when the needs, concerns, and interests of all parties are communicated. Communication strategies themselves should be open and negotiated to accommodate representative styles and approaches. Finally, feedback must be provided to all participants and the public about how the decision was made and the role of their input in making the decision (International Association for Public Participation, 2017; Rippke, Briske, Keller, & Strohschein, 2001).

Partnerships can only be characterized as such when certain conditions exist: Each partner must be recognized as having his or her own power and legitimacy, own purpose and goals, and own connection to that locale or community. At the same time, the work of the partnership itself must be or become more than any one partner's own goals. This is reflected in clear partnership objectives and mutual expectations. Regular patterns of feedback from and among all parties should be planned and shared. And finally, all partners should strive for open-mindedness, patience, and respect for others' views (Labonte, 2012).

Working With Community Leaders and Members: Building Coalitions

A coalition-building strategy can establish the groundwork and/or initiate intracommunity relationships that contribute to an effective, sustained effort to identify and respond to community challenges and needs. Coalition building "promotes and develops alliances among organizations or constituencies for a common purpose. It builds linkages, solves problems, and/or enhances local leadership to address health concerns" (Keller, Strohschein, & Briske, 2008, p. 204). Coalitions bridge sectors, organizations, and constituencies to provide a benefit to the wider community.

Coalitions are used widely in community interventions because of their flexibility and their "democratic appeal" (Parker et al., 1999, p. 182). For example, *Healthy People* coalitions at the county or city level study their community and develop several health-promotion or disease-prevention objectives. As these coalitions include health and social service professionals, business people, and religious and social organizations, they contain the expertise and connections that have an impact on a community's health. Coalitions are useful for many reasons. First, involving a broad range of community groups provides a diverse basis to address local problems and change community expectations. Second, health professionals believe that coalitions develop the capacity of local organizations; skills gained in one effort lead to organizational abilities that will later be applied to solve other problems. Third, coalitions can improve service coordination among community agencies, resulting in less duplication and more effective use of resources (Parker et al., 1999). For example, when organizations exchange information as part of the coalition's work, organizational leaders may identify overlapping programs. The cost of duplicate efforts can then be reduced through cooperation across agencies or consolidation at one host agency. Coalitions can also provide a springboard for community empowerment, "an enabling process through which individuals and communities take control of their lives and their environment" (Rippke et al., 2001, p. 212).

The APRN should consider the use of a coalition as it can bring diverse resources together and assist in the community's recognition and response to health concerns. Even though coalitions have many important characteristics, the APRN should consider whether devoting existing resources (such as time, energy, and commitment) to coalition building will lead to the best outcome. The decision also depends on the availability and willingness of the right members for the coalition. Candidate members for the coalition should represent an organization or constituency, and they should have access to the members and resources of the groups they represent. Coalitions can include 12 to 18 members, but smaller groups are able to address more specialized interests or more easily gain sufficient trust to permit mutual collaboration (Rippke et al., 2001). Many coalitions may need to add additional members as the coalition's focus broadens. Depending on the coalition's program, additional groups may need to be added and additional resources may need to be requested from new partners. For example, a coalition meeting to address head injuries among children might refine its focus to promote safety-helmet usage in activities such as bicycling and skateboarding. This coalition might add the expertise of emergency department representatives and the resources of local store owners who sell bicycles or safety helmets.

The intent of a coalition is to assemble around a common interest in which each coalition member has a stake in the outcomes. As in any organization, coalitions require both structure and resources to achieve goals. As coalitions incorporate representatives of diverse organizations who hold diverse perspectives, it is important to facilitate good interpersonal dynamics and to develop reliable group processes for decision-making (Rippke et al., 2001). A community coalition should be able to work together on a broad vision of what needs to be accomplished. A mission statement can be useful in providing formal guidance to the coalition effort, especially when a variety or range of perspectives exist among members. When developed collaboratively, this "common vision" can assist with formalization of the next steps (Wald, 2011).

The Process of Establishing Community Priorities

Most community leaders and members can easily identify a wide range of concerns or issues that reflect their wants or needs to improve their community's health. In strained economic times, such lists are likely to become even longer. During prioritization, the available data and community information are reviewed by the coalition and community members to decide what to address and where resources should be targeted (Issel, 2013). The process of setting priorities includes selecting the most important concerns for attention by the coalition. Making this selection can be difficult or frustrating, because in many cases there are multiple problems that need to be addressed in the community. Some community leaders and members will approach this by advocating critical priorities affecting the community, whereas other coalition members will advocate their own personal priorities. Identifying a consensus priority will facilitate the coalition's purpose of finding a common vision or goal.

When considering what actions should receive high-priority attention, how can *wants* and *needs* be differentiated? Needs reflect an objective assessment or conform to a set of expected requirements, as compared to wants, which may be personal wishes or aspirations that fail to rise to the level of necessity. But it may be that the dividing line between wants and needs has more to do with *who* sorts wants from needs, rather than *how* the sorting is done. Wishes and needs for the same target community may differ based on the perspective of the viewer: Insiders and outsiders to the community may propose quite different lists. Rather than asking how to separate needs and wants, the better question may be: Should needs and wants be separated? Perhaps it is more constructive to view both as important and critical to address. For example, a group of health professionals concluded that the priority intervention for a neighborhood in a small, rural community in North Carolina should be to reduce infant mortality based on significant epidemiological evidence. However, when neighborhood residents heard about the professionals' proposal, they insisted that their priority was a safe playground for their children—and it was built. This should not be considered a failure but rather a success. Although one priority solution was sought, another priority was identified and addressed, leading to a positive outcome for the community.

The practice of priority setting is not purely quantitative; the highest ranking items do not have to be selected over lower ranked items. The process of decision-making is interactive, perhaps even political. For example, an APRN may believe that funding and personnel resources should be directed toward the most common diseases in a community. But what if the most frequent disease in a community is sinusitis? Should sinusitis receive attention above all other chronic diseases? Perhaps severity of illness should be an additional criterion. How should duration of illness be factored in? What about considering the possibility of recovery or rehabilitation as a criterion? And what about the actual cost of illness care? Perhaps immunizations are cost-effective because they prevent morbidity and mortality at a very low price. Through questions such as these and related community and partnership discussions, priority-setting discussions reveal much about the values and beliefs of the community and the coalition members.

Ordinarily, several priorities are selected by a coalition. Several of the selected priorities may require different resources, and some priorities may separately seek external grant funding. Priority setting can be helpful in suggesting which items should be addressed first and which should be discarded from the list because of lack of coalition interest or lack of confidence that the problem is solvable given existing resources (Blum, 1981). On the other hand, the availability of external resources or funding may justify selecting a priority, as it is most likely to be viable. In practice, the availability of funding often guides program decisions.

If a coalition priority requires financial support that is not immediately available, the coalition could make a decision (a) to wait for a specified period of time until a funding source is willing to provide financial support, (b) to raise local funding specifically to support the coalition priority, or (c) to downsize the magnitude of the coalition's planned program by implementing a small pilot program or by initially implementing only a portion of the program. For example, if a community seeks to address the low immunization rates among preschool children, then the coalition's priority might be to improve access to and parental education on immunizations for all preschool children in their community. However, no funding is available for their larger goal. Because the coalition has some resources, they decide to develop a pilot program that focuses on improving MMR (measles, mumps, and rubella) immunization rates in preschoolers. The coalition can begin their program immediately, which reinforces the success of the coalition's common goals and actions. The coalition will also gain a lot of information as well as organizing and technical skills through implementing the pilot program. Additionally, information on cost savings and health benefit should be obtained to further justify continuing and/or expanding the program. In some cases, coalitions can work with insurance providers to fund programs such as these to prevent or reduce costs incurred with emergency and hospital admissions for preventable diseases. This skill acquisition, as well as the pilot program experiences and outcomes, will provide a strong foundation and justification when applying to fund a broader program to improve childhood immunizations rates.

Priority-Setting Approaches

The process of setting priorities is best conducted through a combination of qualitative and quantitative methods. Statistics about the frequency, duration, severity, disability, and mortality of certain health problems tell one story. Social understandings of health concerns and qualitative estimations of these health problems tell a different story. By making the community aware of the current state of health in their community, discussions can commence and goals for the community can be set. Priority setting allows for open discussion about perceptions, judgments, and understandings that can be the most valuable part of conducting a priority-setting session. When the coalition discusses the community and its priorities, this furthers the coalition's work.

Criteria that are used to rate priorities can vary. A coalition's discussion is best served if it first decides which criteria are important to the group, and, second, applies these criteria to rank the community's issues and concerns. Coalition members will learn much about each other's preferences from both the first and second parts of the discussion, and subsequent decision making will be enhanced. Community members' viewpoints should also be incorporated; community forums or focus groups can be an effective means for involving community members. Those unable to attend a forum because of family obligations, work-shift timing, or disability can be contacted directly and their perspectives and opinions can still be included as input. For example, Dallas County, Texas, initiatives directed by Parkland Hospital's Community-Oriented Primary Care program employed a community prioritization approach that focused on "(1) leadership forums and (2) community advisory boards associated with each health center" (Pickens, Boumbulian, Anderson, Ross, & Phillips, 2002, p. 1729).

Priority Chart

As mentioned earlier, several priority-setting approaches use a combination of quantitative and qualitative methods to provide comparative rankings that can highlight community concerns and issues that should receive attention. Tarimo (1991) includes a priority chart that incorporates several variables in a brief format suitable for discussion by nonprofessionals. Small groups are formed to evaluate the health problems (preferably no more than seven) or risk factors of concern in a population. The problems or factors are then listed and should relate to a single target population. Ranking is simplified when the list includes either health problems (heart disease, asthma, arthritis, adolescent pregnancy, etc.) or risk factors (tobacco use, high-fat diets, sedentary lifestyles, poor access to birth control methods, etc.). Small-group members discuss and rank each health problem or risk factor using the following variables: frequency in the population, mortality in years of potential life lost, morbidity in years of reduced health, costs of solutions, and effectiveness of solutions (Tarimo, 1991, pp. 20–21). The priorities selected by the small groups are reported back to the larger group, tallied, and discussed. This approach can be powerful and instructive in the priority-setting process.

Problem Priority Criteria

Shuster and Goeppinger (2004) propose a more complex, mathematical system that shares some of Tarimo's Priority Chart assumptions. Their *Problem Priority Criteria* include the following:

> (1) community awareness of the problem, (2) community motivation to resolve or better manage the problem, (3) nurse's ability to influence problem solution, (4) availability of expertise to solve the problem, (5) severity of the outcomes if the problems are unresolved, and (6) speed with which the problem can be solved. (p. 362)

Each criterion is independently rated on a 1 (low) to 10 (high) scale based on two questions: (a) How important is the criterion to problem solution? (b) Does the partnership have the ability to resolve the problem? In addition, a rationale for rating each parameter is documented. The two resulting numeric ratings (for problem importance and for ability to resolve) are multiplied to yield a problem-ranking number (variable from 0 to 600). These steps are repeated for each separate problem that the group seeks to address (Shuster & Goeppinger, 2004). The community problems are then ranked from highest to lowest score. As this system requires detailed knowledge about each separate problem, it works best if those involved are very familiar with the issues or concerns being prioritized, such as coalition leaders.

A "Skilled Planner" Approach

For setting priorities, Green and Kreuter (2004) recommend a series of key questions for use by "skilled planners" in "a process that balances the perceptions of stakeholder [*sic*] with objectively constructed descriptions of prevailing health problems and how these are distributed in the target population" (p. 99). Green and Kreuter's key questions reflect many of the themes of the two previous priority approaches, including comparison of relative mortality, morbidity, costs, and ease of solution. For example, one key question asks: "Which problems are most amenable to intervention?" (p. 99). Added themes include a concern for higher risk subpopulations (such as children, mothers, or ethnic minorities), and the disproportionate burden of the problem on the focus community compared to other communities. For example, a key question here is: "Which problem is not being addressed by other organizations in the community?" (Green & Kreuter, 2004, p. 99). This approach works well when professionals (the "skilled planners") conduct prioritization comparisons. Although this approach is less helpful in the APRN's work with community coalitions, the "key questions" have the potential to add to or help guide discussions or reflections by coalition members or community residents.

The Hanlon Method and PEARL

The *Hanlon Method,* also referred to as the *Basic Priority Rating System* (Pickett & Hanlon, 1990, pp. 226–228), is a complex method of prioritization "which objectively takes into consideration explicitly defined criteria and feasibility factors" (National Association of County & City Health Officials [NACCHO], n.d., p.7).

Three main components are independently rated on a scale for each candidate priority: (a) size of the problem, (b) seriousness of the problem, and (c) estimated effectiveness of the solution. The numerical results for each of the three variables are placed into an equation, and the results multiplied by the *PEARL factor* score to obtain the comparative rating (NACCHO, n.d.).

The PEARL factors are interpreted as strongly influencing whether or not a particular goal can be addressed in a specific community, even though the factors are not directly related to the health problem. The PEARL factors are broken down as follows: *Propriety* (P) asks whether a proposed problem or program is consistent with the overall mission of the sponsoring organization. *Economic feasibility* (E) balances the costs of intervening or not intervening, including the economic outcomes of not intervening. *Acceptability* (A) addresses whether the community or program recipients will accept any intervention to address the goal. *Resources* (R) are assessed to determine whether sufficient resources are available to address this goal. And last, *Legality* (L) poses the question of whether current laws will permit addressing this goal (Vilnius & Dandoy, 1990).

The PEARL factors are scored individually as "possible" or "not possible" (e.g., each is rated as "one" or "zero," respectively); given the mathematical formula, if even one of these qualifying factors is rated as "not possible" (e.g., as zero), then the Basic Priority Rating is zero, which indicates that the particular candidate priority should not be considered. When this occurs, a planning coalition may decide that their first step is to modify the PEARL factor that is rated as "not possible." For example, if an intervention is currently not *acceptable* to the population, steps might be taken to educate the population on the potential benefits of the intervention. If population opinion shifts and becomes more accepting of the intervention, it could be reconsidered and implemented (Vilnius & Dandoy, 1990). Incorporating the PEARL factors into priority setting provides a stronger and more comprehensive perspective, as part of the process is deciding which goal or program to select. The PEARL factors may also lead to additional analyses in combination with any priority-setting approach, especially as it addresses each individual component (e.g., PEARL) of a proposed need or program.

Selecting Goals to Address Prioritized Issues and Concerns

As a result of the priority-setting process, the community coalition identifies a ranked group of issues and concerns. The next question is: Should the coalition focus on a single goal or on multiple goals? Single goals do have an appeal of simplicity and require fewer resources. When a coalition focuses on multiple linked goals, it has more of an impact on the underlying causes of the problem and more opportunity to draw community members into understanding these linkages. In the earlier example of creating walking trails, the combination of increasing physical activity and improving healthy food choices both address achieving an appropriate weight to prevent chronic disease. By linking two disease prevention behaviors through the walking trails intervention, the need for community members to combine several related actions to reduce the risk of poor health outcomes is underscored.

In fact, most community health issues and concerns are complex, multifaceted, and challenging to address. Based on the multicausation model (see Chapters 3 and 4, both on Epidemiological Methods and Measurements in Population-Based Nursing Practice), multilevel planning models underscore the numerous sources of health problems. The *Multilevel Approach to Community Health* (MATCH) suggests that health problems will be resolved only when they are addressed simultaneously at the individual/family, organization, community, and government levels. This allows for a more effective modification of policy, practice, and behavior. Although this approach requires a potentially vast skill set, it can offer more efficient use of resources at a faster speed (Simons-Morton, Greene, & Gottlieb, 1995; Simons-Morton, Simons-Morton, Parcel, & Bunker, 1988). For example, it is not sufficient for the APRN to convince a patient and his or her family that sodium intake should be reduced. A broader approach should be taken to address the barriers in the community that make it difficult for an individual to make long-term changes. As in this case, the best patient teaching cannot easily overcome the barriers if local food stores carry only high-sodium food choices. The APRN could participate in a community coalition to advocate local food stores to stock healthier, low-sodium foods. County or state policy changes could persuade food stores that stocking low-sodium foods is to their advantage if, for example, they received a tax credit for the amount of healthier foods they carried and sold. Multilevel approaches provide more effective and sustainable changes, as these modify the underlying causes of current health problems and address the issues at a community and policy level.

The *Transtheoretical Model of Change* suggests that in any given population, individuals are at different points or stages in considering or implementing personal change. Ten stages are included in this model. The first five are experimental stages and begin with consciousness raising (increasing awareness), and the last five are behavioral, ending with self-liberation (committing) (Prochaska, Redding, & Evers, 2008). This model suggests that patients prescribed a lower sodium diet will undergo a personal change process in deciding and acting on reducing dietary sodium. When a community coalition plans to modify personal health choices among community members, it should consider designing interventions that simultaneously target residents at each of the stages of change. The intervention design will also support individuals and families in moving stepwise through the stages of change and in assisting backsliders to recommit to engaging in change.

In the *Diffusion of Innovations* model, the members of a population adopt new behaviors, new technologies, and so on, at predictable but very different rates and for very different reasons (Oldenburg & Glanz, 2008). In this case, to reach all members of the community, the coalition should target strategies at early, middle, and late points in the campaign to reduce dietary sodium. Those who are early adopters of the innovation respond to different approaches than those who are late adopters, and specific targeted approaches are employed based on their ability to change and the stage of change.

Both *Lewin's 3-Stage Model of Change* and the Diffusion of Innovations models underscore the importance of using multiple methods in modifying health-promoting behaviors among diverse community members. As with many learning theories, APRNs must recognize that individuals learn differently and change their behaviors at different rates. By recognizing this early on in the change process, more success is likely to occur and sustainable success is also more likely as approaches are adaptable and targeted. As a means to understand these complex relationships and to identify possible interventions, *The Community Guide* provides intensive, highly developed recommendations for community-targeted health promotion and disease prevention programs (Community Preventive Services Task Force, 2019). Given the complex nature of contemporary health promotion and disease prevention, theoretical and evidence-based approaches are critical in properly addressing individual and community issues and concerns. For example, if an APRN is planning a program to reduce dietary fat, *The Dietary Guidelines for Americans, 2015-20* (Office of Disease Prevention and Health Promotion [ODPHP], 2019) is a useful and evidence-based resource to assist in guiding this process.

Sustaining New Programs: Identifying Barriers in the Program-Planning and Implementation Process

One challenge to sustaining new programs is not addressing existing or potential problems at the time the goal or program was selected as a focus by the coalition. Thorough, objective assessment of proposed community goals/programs will often yield doubts about implementation of a program or whether the implementation effort risks serious obstacles. The APRN and the coalition's intervention team must be both carefully analytic and thoroughly honest. When potential problems are revealed, they must be acknowledged and addressed because a "wait-and-see" approach is not effective. Barriers to program success can also emerge during implementation. Symptoms of potential problems include the following: delays in the implementation timeline, waning resources, disaffected partnerships, or recurring communication difficulties during coalition meetings. These challenges can be detected early by conducting an ongoing program review or formative evaluation. Both symptoms of problems and problems detected during program evaluation require the community intervention team to be honest about the presence of and need to address the barriers, and the importance of taking prompt action to address threats to the coalition's work. The APRN brings problem-solving experience to these situations and should remind the coalition of the normative nature of the challenges to implementing a health-promotion/disease prevention program.

Regardless of when in the process a barrier is identified, the characteristics of barriers can be grouped as follows: (a) characteristics of the goal/program; (b) characteristics of needed resources; (c) characteristics of community members, coalition members, and coalition leadership; (d) characteristics of the APRN; or (e) a mismatch between community or coalition partners and the APRN.

Barriers Caused by Program Characteristics

Certain types of programs or goals may not be feasible to study in certain communities. Some goals may receive community support and have the weight of evidence behind their use, but are a violation of law (or illegal). For example, needle-exchange programs are effective in preventing the spread of blood-borne pathogens (Arkin, 2011), but are illegal in some areas. In the United States current federal law prohibits the use of *federal* funds to purchase sterile needles or syringes for the purposes of illegal use of drugs by injection.

In another case, the timeline necessary to achieve the stated program or goal may not match community expectations. For example, would the community's support wane before program goals are achieved? Will the community demand program outcomes immediately, but lack the means or resources to quickly achieve the goals? Air quality is an important quality-of-life issue, and poor air quality is a short- and long-term health problem; however, modifying the sources of air pollution is time-consuming and challenging (Yip, Pearcy, Garbe, & Truman, 2011). The community might not have patience to wait for change during successive law suits and environmental policy interventions over a prolonged period of time.

Barriers Due to Unavailable Resources

Another barrier that is commonly encountered occurs when goals/programs lack sufficient resources to succeed, perhaps because of inadequate financing or because of insufficient, inadequate, or poorly trained leadership. Some groups may proceed to develop programs or goals even after the lack of resources has been recognized in the hope that sufficient personnel or financial resources will be secured. Not only are such programs initiated on unstable foundations, but existing resources that could be dedicated to program development are instead lost to failed attempts to explore and acquire needed resources.

Barriers Due to Human Factors

The leadership involved in the coalition can often be a barrier to its success. Community or coalition partners, who participate in the development of community goals, may be unenthusiastic or disaffected in relation to the focus that was actually selected for implementation. Community partners may simply lack interest in the current priority and may wish to terminate their involvement in the coalition. Partners can also become disengaged or separated from coalition communications; they may disengage in working meetings or miss meetings altogether. Given the contrasting possibilities, the APRN and other coalition members need to assess the reasons these coalition members appear to be disaffected.

Partners can also become distracted by what is to them a more salient goal or concern, leaving little time and attention for coalition priorities. Reassessment of the goal or program should be carried out if it is deemed unlikely that these partners will change their minds. If they do change their minds, then one of the coalition's interventions should address recruitment and community awareness about program/goal benefits.

Apparent disinterest in coalition activities may also quietly signal that two or more subgroups in the coalition are unable to collaborate, even though both are necessary to the project's success. The APRN and other coalition leadership should reach out to these subgroups to have a more complete picture of the difficulties and to support and counsel reinclusion of the subgroups. In this serious situation, negotiation among the conflicted subgroups may be possible, but the APRN must be extremely diplomatic to avoid the appearance of siding with one group and further damaging the potential for collaboration.

The APRN may also experience a lack of sustained interest in the program focus, perhaps because the selected program is only indirectly related to health concerns. Similar to community members or other coalition partners, the APRN may find another goal more salient. It is difficult to consider, but important to acknowledge, if the nurse has become disengaged from the community and the coalition, whether because of circumstances in the nurse's personal life or because working with the community and/or the coalition has become difficult, that the APRN may find herself/himself overwhelmed with responsibilities that compete with other obligations. It may be difficult for the nurse to agree to a realistic timeline for goal or program implementation if it appears that there may be a prolonged timeline or the potential for a significant time commitment. The APRN should acknowledge these personal challenges and seek support from within the coalition, or from elsewhere, to identify the barriers to participation and make a plan to reconstruct linkages with the coalition, or to make a decision to acknowledge the barriers and formally withdraw.

Barriers Due to the Nurse–Coalition Interface

Last, it may emerge that the community/coalition lacks the skills to partner with the APRN. One appropriate step is to delay immediate programmatic work and focus efforts on skill building. This challenge is more likely to be revealed and addressed early if program implementation begins in an incremental way that permits skill and confidence building. In fact, incorporating these necessary elements as a first, planned stage of a larger program implementation is advantageous.

Preventing Problems in Collaborative Efforts

In the midst of hard work and complex organizing, some would suggest that some of these barriers could *not* have been anticipated or prevented. But on the whole, these problems should be foreseen by the coalition leadership and actions taken to prevent a negative impact on developing collaborative efforts. Three steps must be included in any initiative: First, during the planning stage, a coalition should dedicate time to honest refection, anticipation, and identification of potential problems and barriers to any identified goals. Are coalition members genuinely "buying into" group plans? Is the coalition's road map realistic in its timeline and requirements for community participation? Second, every coalition should periodically reassess its goals and plans. Depending on the nature and composition of the coalition, this reassessment can be conducted by the leadership (in its broadest, most representative, and diverse sense). In addition, a community meeting will generate an even better understanding of the current status of the coalition's efforts. The community meeting provides a forum for recognizing and acknowledging successes and failures to date, celebrating the successes and focusing/refocusing on next steps. Honest reflection on symptoms and suggestions of problems should lead to specific strategies to further understand and address the issues and concerns to minimize negative consequences on the larger coalition and the initiative itself. Third, if issues and concerns are revealed, the coalition leadership should make a judgment about the nature and process of the initiative. Should the initiative continue as currently planned, or should changes be made? Would it be better to modify or eliminate a goal, or would this lead to a coalition member dropping out? Coalition leaders might decide to face a conflict and openly discuss the challenge and its many facets, and by identifying a solution, strengthen the overall initiative and the coalition itself.

In sum, "side-stepping" the problems means that the APRN and the coalition can and should be alert to potential challenges. Regular reassessment of the program and early awareness of potential problems are essential for success, as is finding a prompt solution. Early success in any effort builds the collaborative and spurs efforts forward. Conflicts and confusion that drain energy from the coalition partners should be prevented if possible or at least minimized. Facing confusion and/or conflicts can strengthen collaborative work and model problem-solving strategies that can result in increasing community capacity to address future challenges.

Developing Outcomes for Coalition Work

The priority-setting discussions should identify at least one issue or concern, but likely several, for the APRN and the coalition's project. The next step is to develop outcomes and related means to achieve these outcomes, based on the selected priorities. Identifying outcomes is essential to later work, including program evaluation. The process of defining outcomes or even revising outcomes can be daunting (see Chapter 2, Identifying Outcomes in Population-Based Nursing). This process can be a critical step in program development and can lay the groundwork for successful and sustainable programs. Even when all of the constituencies in the coalition have previously agreed on the priorities for the community's health, establishing outcomes for these priorities can lead to unforeseen barriers. First, traditional academic/professional configuration of outcomes may be unfamiliar to community members within the partnership; consideration of alternative means to present these ideas, steps to achievement, and a related timeline can facilitate the process. Outcomes should remain in a contextual format that is appropriate for the target community for the duration of the project. Second, well-defined outcomes that are clearly stated may be the first indication to coalition partners of the extensive work ahead. Presenting the outcomes with a clear timeline and delineation of the steps needed to achieve these goals are a way to demonstrate a well-thought-out plan that addresses the process that is necessary to achieve these outcomes. It can also facilitate a sense of community efficacy, as it sets up the framework to show that these goals are achievable. In addition, having well-defined outcomes can also demonstrate long-term feasibility and potential reduction in healthcare costs, which can assist in securing long-term funding.

When the APRN and coalition members have agreed on the stated outcomes, the next step is to commit to work toward improving these outcomes. As coalition members represent their constituencies, these members should take responsibility for communicating with their organizations or neighborhoods about the coalition's plans. The APRN can assist coalition members to design campaigns to involve their constituencies (see Chapter 7, Concepts in Program Design and Development). These campaigns can assist coalition members to facilitate adoption of both the outcomes and the steps to achieve the outcomes among their constituents. Focused organizational or neighborhood meetings/gatherings are useful in accomplishing this. The overall goal is to achieve a "buy-in" and commitment to work on the goals among the constituents and the coalition partners.

To support the coalition members, the APRN and the coalition as a whole should set a "launch date" for the planned program and have a celebration to develop energy and reflect the commitment of the diversity of coalition partners. Coalition efforts to recruit and retain the dedication and interest of constituency members will also validate the leadership role of each constituency's representative within the coalition. This results in strengthening the leader roles of coalition representatives in their community. APRN activities in coalitions can often include leadership development of the coalition members.

Continued work toward achieving the planned outcomes will likely have both periods of accomplishment and periods of minimal progress. The APRN can remind the coalition of the previously identified interim markers of progress toward the selected coalition outcomes. Achievement of each significant step should be recognized and celebrated. Pictures that are posted in fund-raising campaigns that show increases in donations using an oversized thermometer posted in a visible location are a good example of a way to mark progress. Visible indicators or a giant "checklist" can convey to community members the status and growing impact of the coalition's efforts. Small rewards or giveaways, such as a celebratory balloon or a coalition-emblazoned key chain, can also be used to signal progress toward outcomes.

The APRN and the coalition members should plan periodic formative evaluations of the progress in attaining outcomes, as well as summative evaluations of those elements of the overall plan that have been completed. Marking success and progress is important for the coalition efforts as well, and offers possibilities for events that build the coalition team and the interpersonal relationships among coalition representatives. When the APRN breaks down the program into doable steps, the efficacy of community members and retention of coalition partners is enhanced.

Sustaining Programs and Initiatives

As programs and initiatives gain strength and the coalition members see their planning lead to better health outcomes in the community, the APRN should consider ways to keep the work going and to establish it as a permanent element of that community. To do this, the APRN and the coalition must take steps to institutionalize the initiative. These plans will ensure the continuity of the work and, with increased duration of the program, will increase the potential for achieving the identified outcomes. The APRN should introduce and guide the coalition first through a careful strategic plan for institutionalization. This will focus the coalition on what is needed. In fact, consideration of sustaining or institutionalizing an initiative should begin when it is first conceptualized, or at least when clear outcomes have been identified and are beginning to be implemented (Community Toolbox, 2018a). The importance of the institutionalization plan underscores the APRN's key role in guiding program development and in guiding the team to an understanding about what steps are necessary at which phase in the program planning and implementation.

Planning for Institutionalization

How should the APRN guide the coalition in planning for institutionalization? A first step is to acknowledge that what it does is important and that the coalition's program is worth continuing. In that light, it will make sense to ensure that the program's mission, staffing, and resources are adequate. Given continued confidence in its planned outcomes, noting program accomplishments will provide the coalition with motivation to continue to build. Publicizing the coalition's successes will solidify both the coalition and its constituencies and, more important, can draw the public into the coalition's mission and work. Community members are key players in long-term sustainability and can assist in the institutionalization process. When programs involve more people, their staying power increases (Community Toolbox, 2018b). Perhaps a nearby community would like to develop a similar program? Perhaps outsiders would like to learn about how the program operates and how it achieves its goals? Enhancing the connections and respect for the program and spreading the coalition's programs to new neighborhoods improve how others see the program, and this translates into more support for the program.

Funding: A Major Barrier to Sustainability

The major barrier to sustainability and to institutionalization is adequate financing. For many organizations, sustained financial support is an ongoing challenge to accomplishing the planned outcomes. As with other factors that support sustainability, planning for future financial security is best addressed from the start of program inception. A place to begin is to market the organization by letting others know what the coalition's program has accomplished. It can also be helpful to show financers what other similar programs have accomplished using similar models in different communities. Additionally, presenting the potential cost savings in the long term can also secure financial support, as funders can see the long-term benefits of financial investment in such programs. The APRN and coalition members can build their image and community relations, develop members and friends, and actively deliver the coalition's message for health and personal/community change.

Existing financial resources may go further if staff positions are shared with another compatible organization. Or the coalition's program may become so successful that a larger organization would like to support it, or perhaps even assume responsibility for the coalition, its identified outcomes, and its programs in operation. Grants, fund-raising functions, third-party funding, public funding, a fee schedule, and in-kind support may also assist with financing (Community Toolbox, 2018c). Community health programs can be particularly attractive to academic partners, such as nursing, public health, medical schools, and universities, which the APRN can assist in recruiting or in facilitating relationship building. Personnel resources may be available in the form of educational or training programs in nursing, medicine, social work, public health, and other professions.

Stabilization and Reassessment

The role of the APRN with the coalition and the change process is very active, but this role draws to an end during the step in Lewin's 3-Stage Model of Change known as *refreezing*. During this step, reassessment and stabilization are typical and expected, and this focuses "the change agent's and actor's attention and energy on progress and continuity for the change" (Kettner, Daley, & Nichols, 1985, p. 288). The APRN may or may not continue with the community coalition. But even when the APRN continues, the role of change agent is less necessary and begins to fade as the change is institutionalized or stabilized. But rather than immediately separating from a successful coalition program, the APRN should emphasize the autonomous functioning and continued survival of the program (Kettner et al., 1985).

The APRN should initiate a reassessment of the change process and the coalition's work. Input is sought from all participants about whether the impact of the coalition's changes is meeting their needs. Members of the community coalition itself give feedback, as do a sample of their constituents who are recruited to reflect on the practical consequences and the meaning of the change effort. To what extent has the change been accepted, approved, and adopted among coalition members, their constituents, stakeholders, and other community members? A careful review of whether the community coalition's goals were met should be included. Although perhaps challenging to anticipate, this step will be easier if, early in the project, the APRN guides the community coalition to accompany specification of goal outcomes with clear descriptors for outcome achievement.

The APRN will also assist and explore with the community coalition appropriate ways to share their experiences with a wider audience through oral presentations; visual and audio social media; and articles for publication in magazines, journals, community newspapers, and online postings. The APRN and coalition members may offer assistance to other community groups that are in the early stages of planning similar efforts. Coalition members may take the strengths of this coalition experience, with their new skills and abilities, and apply what they have gained to other issues in support of their own communities.

SUMMARY

The APRN's ability to employ the change process is an essential component of reaching beyond the clinical encounter to address the community context and conditions that lead to poor health in individuals, families, and aggregates. The community encounter engages the APRN and community partners in an ongoing process of increased understanding and skill/ability development.

The APRN who sets out to engage communities in change requires many skills. Foremost is the ability to strategically and successfully introduce the need for change to improve population health. At any time, the APRN may be called on to moderate a focus group, diplomatically defuse a situation, collect data in order to identify targets for intervention and to measure change, and help in the identification and construction of achievable outcomes. Although the initial role of the APRN is leader, he or she must also be prepared to step aside and allow members of the community to identify priorities for change. It is paramount that the APRN understands that it is community members who make final decisions about health priorities. An important role of the APRN is helping community members to acquire the necessary skills to make changes and to create a sustainable environment. It requires a true partnership between the APRN and the community to create meaningful changes, and by helping communities to sustain those changes and by becoming leaders themselves that those changes will become embedded in the community.

Extending APRN practice into the community improves clinical outcomes directly because, as community problems are identified and managed, this complements the APRN's efforts to reduce individual, family, and population health problems. Sustaining the coalitions and programs that develop as a result of the APRN's partnership with community members has the potential to achieve far-reaching improvements in population health.

EXERCISES AND DISCUSSION QUESTIONS

Exercise 11.1 What ethical principles apply when working with communities? Conduct a personal skills inventory. Of the ethical principles that you have identified, which ones do you have sufficient skills in to be able to work effectively with a community coalition? Are there areas in which you would like to develop stronger abilities? How would you go about developing the skills and knowledge to do so?

Exercise 11.2 Consider a community known to you. If you were working with a partnership group to set priorities for community collaboration, which priority-setting criteria would you recommend for use by your group?

Exercise 11.3 What factors would you consider before you made an implicit/explicit commitment to engage with a community or neighborhood to improve residents' health status? How would you specifically engage with the community to negotiate your role?

Exercise 11.4 Consider a community known to you. You wish to take initial steps to build a partnership with the community. What data and information should you analyze and consider before you contact community leaders/members/organizations? Which area leaders/members/organizations would you contact initially, to introduce the idea of a partnership?

Exercise 11.5 The community coalition that you are working with has set a goal to reduce the consumption of sugar by children who live in the community. What information do you need before you develop a plan? You know that a multilevel approach will be needed to achieve an effective and sustainable change. Design a plan and explain your reasons for each approach.

REFERENCES

American Association of Colleges of Nursing. (2006). *The essentials of doctoral education for advanced practice nursing.* Washington, DC: Author. Retrieved from http://www.aacn.nche.edu/DNP/pdf/Essentials.pdf

Allender, J. A., Rector, C., & Warner, K. (2013). *Community health nursing: Promoting and protecting the public's health* (8th ed.). Philadelphia, PA: Wolters Kluwer/Lippincott Williams & Wilkins.

Arkin, E. (2011). Studies confirm effectiveness of harm reduction for people who inject drugs. *HIV/AIDS Policy & Law Review, 15*(3), 29. Retrieved from http://search.ebscohost.com/login.aspx?direct=true&db=mnh&AN=22165261&site=ehost-live&scope=site

Blum, H. L. (1981). *Planning for health: Genetics for the eighties* (2nd ed.). New York, NY: Human Sciences Press.

Clinical and Translational Science Awards Consortium Community Engagement Key Function Committee Task Force on the Principles of Community Engagement. (2011). Principles of community engagement (NIH Publication No. 11-7782). Retrieved from https://www.atsdr.cdc.gov/communityengagement/pdf/PCE_Report_508_FINAL.pdf

Cherry, D. J., & Shefner, J. (2004). Addressing barriers to university-community collaboration: Organizing by experts or organizing the experts? *Journal of Community Practice, 12*(3), 219–233. doi:10.1300/J125v12n03_13

Community Preventive Services Task Force. (2019). *About the community guide.* Retrieved from https://www.thecommunityguide.org/about/about-community-guide

Community Toolbox. (2018a). *Our model of practice: Building capacity for community and system change.* Kansas University website. Retrieved from http://ctb.ku.edu/en/table-of-contents/overview/model-for-community-change-and-improvement/building-capacity/main

Community Toolbox. (2018b). *Strategies for the long-term institutionalization of an initiative: An overview.* Kansas University website. Retrieved from http://ctb.ku.edu/en/table-of-contents/sustain/long-term-institutionalization/overview/main

Community Toolbox. (2018c). *Strategies for sustaining the initiative.* Kansas University website. Retrieved from http://ctb.ku.edu/en/table-of-contents/sustain/long-term-institutionalization/sustainability-strategies/main

Connelly, M. (2016). *The Kurt Lewin change management model.* Retrieved from http://www.change-management-coach.com/kurt_lewin.html

Courtney, R., Ballard, E., Fauver, S., Gariota, M., & Holland, L. (1996). The partnership model: Working with individuals, families, and communities toward a new vision of health. *Public Health Nursing, 13,* 177–186. doi:10.1111/j.1525-1446.1996.tb00238.x

Farnham, E. (1964). *Pioneering in public health nursing education: The history of the University Public Health Nursing District, 1917–1962*. Cleveland, OH: Press of Western Reserve University.

Gallant, M. H., Beaulieu, M. C., & Carnevale, F. A. (2002). Partnership: An analysis of the concept within the nurse-client relationship. *Journal of Advanced Nursing, 40*, 149–157. doi:10.1046/j.1365-2648.2002.02357.x

Green, L. W., & Kreuter, M. W. (2004). *Health program planning: An educational and ecological approach* (4th ed.). Boston, MA: McGraw-Hill.

Hatcher, M., Warner, D., & Hornbrook, M. (2011).Managing organizational support for community engagement. In *National Institutes of Health* (NIH Publication No. 11-7782). Retrieved from http://www.atsdr .cdc.gov/communityengagement/pdf/PCE_Report_Chapter_4_SHEF.pdf

International Association for Public Participation. (2017). *IAP2 Federation's core values for public participation*. Retrieved from https://cdn.ymaws.com/www.iap2.org/resource/resmgr/pillars/2017_core_values-24x36_iap2_.pdf

Issel, L. M. (2013). *Health program planning and evaluation: A practical, systematic approach for community health* (3rd ed.). Burlington, MA: Jones & Bartlett Learning.

Keller, L. O., Strohschein, S., & Briske, L. (2008). Population-based public health nursing practice: The intervention wheel. In M. Stanhope & J. Lancaster (Eds.), *Public health nursing: Population-centered health care in the community* (7th ed., pp. 187–214). St. Louis, MO: Mosby Elsevier.

Kettner, P. M., Daley, J. M., & Nichols, A. W. (1985). *Initiating change in organizations and communities: A macro practice model*. Monterey, CA: Brooks/Cole.

Labonte, R. (2012). Community, community development, and the forming of authentic partnerships: Some critical reflections. In M. Minkler (Ed.), *Community organizing and community building for health* (3rd ed., pp. 95–109). New Brunswick, NJ: Rutgers University Press.

Logan, B. N., Davis, L., & Parker, V. G. (2010). An interinstitutional academic collaborative partnership to end health disparities. *Health Education and Behavior, 37*, 580–592. doi:10.1177/1090198110363378

Lynn-McHale, D. J., & Deatrick, J. A. (2000). Trust between family and health care provider. *Journal of Family Nursing, 6*, 210–230. doi:10.1177/107484070000600302

Macali, M., Galanowsky, K., Wagner, M., & Truglio-Londrigan. (2011). Hitting the pavement: Intervention of case finding. In M. Truglio-Londrigan & S. B. Lewenson (Eds.), *Public health nursing: Practicing population-based care* (pp. 185–219). Sudbury, MA: Jones & Bartlett.

McCann, E. (2010). Building a community-academic partnership to improve health outcomes in an underserved community. *Public Health Nursing, 27*(1), 32–40. doi:10.1111/j.1525-1446.2009.00824.x

McCloskey, D. J., McDonald, M. A., Cook, J., Heurtin-Roberts, S., Updegrove, S., Sampson, D., . . . Eder, M. (2011a). Community engagement: Definitions and organizing concepts from the literature. In *National Institutes of Health* (NIH Publication No. 11-7782). Retrieved from http://www.atsdr.cdc.gov/communityengagement/pdf/PCE_Report_Chapter_1_SHEF.pdf

McCloskey, D. J., McDonald, M. A., Cook, J., Heurtin-Roberts, S., Updegrove, S., Sampson, D., . . . Eder, M. (2011b). Principles of community engagement. In *National Institutes of Health* (NIH Publication No. 11-7782). Retrieved from http://www.atsdr.cdc.gov/communityengagement/pdf/PCE_Report_Chapter_1_SHEF.pdf

National Association of County & City Health Officials. (n.d.). Guide to prioritization techniques. Retrieved from https://www.naccho.org/uploads/downloadable-resources/Gudie-to-Prioritization-Techniques.pdf

Office of Disease Prevention and Health Promotion. (2019). The dietary guidelines for Americans 2015-2020. Retrieved from https://health.gov/dietaryguidelines/2015/guidelines/introduction/dietary-guidelines-for-americans

Oldenburg, B., & Glanz, K. (2008). Diffusion of innovations. In K. Glanz, B. K. Rimer, & K. Viswanath (Eds.), *Health behavior and health education: Theory, research, and practice* (4th ed., pp. 313–333). San Francisco, CA: Jossey-Bass.

Parker, E. A., Eng, E., Laraia, B., Ammerman, A., Dodds, J., Margolis, L., & Cross, A. (1999). Coalition building for prevention. In R. C. Brownson, E. A. Baker, & L. F. Novick (Eds.), *Community-based prevention: Programs that work* (pp. 182–198). Gaithersburg, MD: Aspen.

Pickens, S., Boumbulian, P., Anderson, R. J., Ross, S., & Phillips, S. (2002). Community-oriented primary care in action: A Dallas story. *American Journal of Public Health, 92*, 1728–1732. doi:10.2105/ajph.92.11.1728

Pickett, G., & Hanlon, J. J. (1990). *Public health: Administration and practice* (9th ed.). St. Louis, MO: Times Mirror/Mosby College Publishing.

Prochaska, J. O., Redding, C. A., & Evers, K. E. (2008). The transtheoretical model and stages of change. In K. Glanz, B. K. Rimer, & K. Viswanath (Eds.), *Health behavior and health education: Theory, research, and practice* (4th ed., pp. 97–121). San Francisco, CA: Jossey-Bass.

Rippke, M., Briske, L., Keller, L. O., & Strohschein, S. (2001). *Public health interventions: Applications for public health nursing practice*. St. Paul, MN: Minnesota Department of Health.

Roberts, S. J., & Krouse, H. J. (1990). Negotiation as a strategy to empower self-care. *Holistic Nursing Practice, 4*(2), 30–36. doi:10.1097/00004650-199002000-00007

Shuster, G. F., & Goeppinger, J. (2004). Community as client: Assessment and analysis. In M. Stanhope & J. Lancaster (Eds.), *Community and public health nursing* (6th ed., pp. 342–373). St. Louis, MO: Mosby.

Simons-Morton, B. G., Greene, W. H., & Gottlieb, N. H. (1995). *An introduction to health education and health promotion* (2nd ed.). Prospect Heights, IL: Waveland Press.

Simons-Morton, D. G., Simons-Morton, B. G., Parcel, G. S., & Bunker, J. F. (1988). Influencing personal and environmental conditions for community health: A multilevel intervention model. *Family and Community Health, 11*(2), 25–35. doi:10.1097/00003727-198808000-00006

Tarimo, E. (1991). *Towards a healthy district*. Geneva, Switzerland: World Health Organization. Retrieved from http://apps.who.int/iris/bitstream/10665/40785/1/9241544120.pdf?ua=1

Vilnius, D., & Dandoy, S. (1990). A priority rating system for public health programs. *Public Health Reports, 105*(5), 483–490.

Wald, A. (2011). Working together: Collaboration, coalition building, and community organizing. In M. Truglio-Londrigan & S. B. Lewenson (Eds.), *Public health nursing: Practicing population-based care* (pp. 267–283). Sudbury, MA: Jones & Bartlett.

Walker, S. S. (2011). Ethical quandaries in community health nursing. In E. T. Anderson & J. McFarlane (Eds.), *Community as partner: Theory and practice in nursing* (6th ed., pp. 73–85). Philadelphia, PA: Wolters Kluwer/Lippincott Williams & Wilkins.

Yip, F. Y., Pearcy, J. N., Garbe, P. L., & Truman, B. I. (2011). Unhealthy air quality—United States, 2006–2009. *Morbidity and Mortality Weekly Report, 60*(1). Retrieved from http://www.cdc.gov/mmwr/preview/mmwrhtml/su6001a5.htm?s_cid=su6001a5_w

Zerwekh, J. V. (1993). Commentary: Going to the people—Public health nursing today and tomorrow. *American Journal of Public Health, 83*, 1676–1678. doi:10.2105/ajph.83.12.1676

INTERNET RESOURCES

Community Toolbox: https://ctb.ku.edu/en

Principles of Community Engagement (NIH Publication No. 11-7782): https://www.atsdr.cdc.gov/communityengagement/pdf/PCE_Report_508_FINAL.pdf

The Community Guide: https://www.thecommunityguide.org

The Dietary Guidelines for Americans 2015–2020: https://health.gov/dietaryguidelines/2015/guidelines/introduction/dietary-guidelines-for-americans

CHAPTER 12

IMPLICATIONS OF GLOBAL HEALTH IN POPULATION-BASED NURSING

LUCILLE A. JOEL | IRINA McKEEHAN CAMPBELL

CORE COMPETENCIES IN GLOBAL HEALTH

The American Association of Colleges of Nursing (AACN) 2005 Task Force on the Essentials of Nursing Education for the Doctorate of Nursing Practice (DNP) outlined the requirements of DNP practice. Throughout this book, these essentials and core competencies are addressed for multiple advanced practice registered nurse (APRN) roles. Particularly relevant to global health issues are *Essential V: Healthcare Policy for Advocacy in Healthcare, Essential V: Interprofessional Collaboration for Improving Patient and Population Health Outcomes,* and *Essential VII: Clinical Prevention and Population Health for Improving the Nation's Health* (AACN, 2006).

There is no shortage of those speaking out on models of competency for working in global health. So that we are all proceeding from the same frame of reference, let us start with the basics. What is global competence? Global competence is the capacity and disposition to understand and act on issues of global significance. Collectively, global competence represents the knowledge, attitudes, skills, and behaviors necessary to thrive in today's interconnected world (World Health Organization [WHO], n.d.a). The AACN formed an interdisciplinary collaboration with the Association of Schools and Programs of Public Health (ASPPH) to develop global health competencies. This partnership led to the publication of the *Global Health Competency Model* in 2011. An updated version of the competencies, *Global Health Concentration Competencies for the Master of Public Health Degree,* was released in 2018. The domains in the ASPPH–AACN Global Health Model clearly demonstrate the relationship between ASPPH global health concentration competencies and the AACN DNP Essentials particularly as they both relate to community engagement, ethical practice, and social justice (ASPPH, 2018).

Healthcare delivery to individuals and populations often involves working with programs that cross political and national borders. Global health is an extension of population health. In terms of geographical scale, diseases can affect people across geographical boundaries and specific population aggregates, such as mothers and children or those who have hepatitis or are HIV positive. APRNs who implement the global health domains in practice can play a focal role in developing the models that are proposed by the Global Health Initiative (GHI), Centers for Disease Control and Prevention (CDC), and WHO as a means for linking population health with health policy, the containment of infectious diseases, and the elimination of health disparities. The core competencies in global health complement GHI projects in domestic and international programs by promoting the following strategies: capacity strengthening, collaborating and partnering, ethical reasoning and professional practice, health equity and social justice, program management, sociocultural and political awareness, and strategic analysis. To view the *Global Health Concentration Competencies for the Master of Public Health Degree* go to: s3.amazonaws.com/ASPPH_Media_Files/Docs/APPENDIX+A-Final_2018-07-16.pdf

To access the *WHO Global Competency Model* go to: www.who.int/employment/competencies/WHO_competencies_EN.pdf

This chapter explores the implications, benefits, and barriers of practicing global health for the APRN. The following areas are discussed:

- How geography, climate, and demographic factors influence the causes, transmission, and outcomes of communicable and noncommunicable diseases

- Global health competencies developed by the ASPPH and AACN

- Effects of multilevel contexts of global health, population, and individual health

- Relationships between global health competencies and interdisciplinary collaboration

- Health initiatives of pivotal international agencies, such as the United Nations (UN) and WHO

- Global health educational opportunities that exist for APRNs and doctorally prepared practitioners.

Changing American Demographic Landscape

The demographic landscape of the American population has become more culturally diversified and mobile as immigrants, migrants, and refugees seeking a higher quality of life enter the United States. The number of corporate, business, student, and academic exchanges has also increased in recent decades. The APRN, working on the front lines of primary and preventive care, will increasingly encounter people from other countries. These new arrivals have an increased likelihood of having been exposed to infectious diseases, may lack vaccinations, and may be at high risk for chronic diseases. APRNs, guided by the core competencies, can work with existing stakeholders and international programs to provide optimal health services to both citizens and noncitizens in the United States.

The United States admitted almost 3.4 million refugees between 1975 and 2018. The U.S. Immigration and Nationality Act (INA), derived from the post–World War II UN 1951 Convention, defines a refugee as "someone who: is located outside of the U.S.; is of special humanitarian concern to the U.S.; demonstrates that they were persecuted or fear persecution due to race, religion, nationality, political opinion, or membership in a particular social group" (U.S. Citizenship and Immigration Services [USCIS], 2017, p. 1). In 2018, there were more than 16.7 million refugees globally: these refugees live predominantly in the Middle East; Africa; Syria; south, east, and central Asia; the Americas; and Europe. Many will seek entry into the United States. About 3 million refugees have been resettled in the United States since Congress passed the Refugee Act of 1980, which created the Federal Refugee Resettlement Program and the current national standard for the screening and admission of refugees into the country (Pew Research Center, 2017).

On March 1, 2003, the USCIS assumed responsibility for the immigration service functions of the federal government. The Homeland Security Act of 2002 dismantled the Immigration and Naturalization Service (INS) and separated the agency into three components within the Department of Homeland Security (DHS). The Homeland Security Act created the USCIS to enhance the security and efficiency of national immigration services by focusing exclusively on the administration of benefit applications. The law also formed the Immigration and Customs Enforcement (ICE) and Customs and Border Protection (CBP) to oversee immigration enforcement and border security.

The INA has regulated immigration into the United States through a variety of laws since 1921. The Act was amended in 1965 as the Hart–Celler Act. This Act made changes to the immigration quota system based on country and nationality. It was designed to maintain the same ethnic proportion in the United States as was reflected in the 1920 Census. Asians were excluded from immigration by amendments to the Act in 1924. In 1965, immigration criteria replaced nationality or country-of-origin quotas with requirements for employable skills and reuniting families with connections in the United States. The United States has more immigrants than any other country in the world. Today almost 44 million people living in the United States were born in another country, accounting for about one fifth of the world's migrants. The population of immigrants is also very diverse, with just about every country in the world represented among U.S. immigrants. Since 1965, when U.S. immigration laws replaced a national quota system, the number of immigrants living in the United States has more than quadrupled. Immigrants today account for 13.5% of the U.S. population, nearly triple the number (4.7%) in 1970. However, today's immigrant share remains below the record 14.8% share in 1890, when 9.2 million immigrants lived in the United States (Pew Research Center, 2017).

In fiscal 2017, a total of 53,716 refugees were resettled in the United States. Since the creation of the federal Refugee Resettlement Program in 1980, about 3 million refugees have resettled in the United States—more than any other country. The largest origin group of refugees was the Democratic Republic of the Congo, followed by Iraq, Syria, Somalia, and Burma (Myanmar). Among all refugees admitted in that fiscal year, 22,861 are Muslims (43%) and 25,194 are Christians (47%). California, Texas, and New York resettled nearly a quarter of all refugees admitted in fiscal 2016. In 2016, most immigrants lived in just 20 major metropolitan areas, with the largest populations in New York, Los Angeles, and Miami. These top 20 metro areas were home to 28.3 million immigrants, or 65% of the nation's total. Most of the nation's unauthorized immigrant population lived in these top metro areas as well. The number of unauthorized immigrants in the United States fell to its lowest level in more than a decade, according to new Pew Research Center (2018) estimates based on 2016 government data. The decline is due almost entirely to a sharp decrease in the number of Mexicans entering the country without authorization. Unauthorized immigrants are increasingly likely to be long-term U.S. residents. Two thirds of adult unauthorized immigrants have lived in the country for more than 10 years.

As of August 31, 2018, nearly 700,000 young adults who came to the United States illegally as children were recipients of Deferred Action for Childhood Arrivals (DACA). DACA was created by executive order in 2012; the current presidential administration announced in 2017 that the program would end, but it has been kept alive by court challenges. An additional 317,000 people from 10 nations benefit from Temporary Protected Status, which is granted to visitors from countries where natural disaster or violence make it difficult to return. The DHS has announced plans to end protections for immigrants from six nations, including El Salvador, Honduras, and Haiti, which account for the vast majority of the total (Pew Research Center, 2018).

Immigrants in the United States as a whole have lower levels of education than the U.S.-born population. In 2016, immigrants were three times as likely as the U.S. born to have not completed high school (29% versus 9%). However, immigrants were just as likely as the U.S. born to have a college degree or more, 32% and 30%, respectively. Immigrants from Mexico (57%) and Central America (49%) are less likely to be high school graduates than the U.S. born (9%). On the other hand, immigrants from south and east Asia, Europe, Canada, the Middle East, and sub-Saharan Africa were more likely than U.S.-born residents to have a bachelor's or advanced degree. Among all immigrants, those from south and east Asia (52%) and the Middle East (47%) were the most likely to have a bachelor's degree or more. Immigrants from Mexico (6%) and Central America (9%) were the least likely to have a bachelor's degree or higher. Literacy is an important issue. Among immigrants ages 5 and older, Spanish is the most commonly spoken language. Some 43% of immigrants in the United States speak Spanish at home. The top five languages spoken at home among immigrants outside of Spanish are English only (16%), followed by Chinese (6%), Hindi (5%), Filipino/Tagalog (4%), and French (3%). In 2016, about 28 million immigrants were working or looking for work in the United States, making up some 17% of the total civilian labor force. Lawful immigrants made up the majority of the immigrant workforce at 20.6 million. An additional 7.8 million immigrant workers are unauthorized immigrants (Pew Research Center, 2018). Such diversity in the population, with an increased rate of mobility across international borders, presents challenges for the APRN.

APRNs need to be familiar with federal policies that bar hospitals from asking about citizenship before providing services. The 1986 Emergency Medical Treatment and Active Labor Act (EMTALA), which is part of the Consolidated Omnibus Budget Reconciliation Act (COBRA), stipulates that hospitals deliver emergency healthcare to everyone, regardless of national origin, legal status, or ability to pay (Title 42 – The Public Health and Welfare, 2013). Such care is uncompensated at the hospital and state level, unless Medicaid funds are appropriated for various population health programs to cover charity care.

Twenty-first-century advances in communication, trade, transportation technologies, and scientific exchanges bring health issues from other continents to the threshold of the American urban and community hospital. These advances are accompanied by national security concerns, as was acutely evident with the 2014 Ebola outbreak in West Africa. APRN population-based practice has daily relevance as people bring their national, environmental, socioeconomic, and cultural contexts with them whenever they visit their healthcare provider. APRNs, who encounter individuals from other countries, need to understand and become familiar with programs or policies addressing the complex global factors influencing the context of individual and population health.

Health as an International Phenomenon

Individual health is embedded in the larger socio-ecological context of the global community. Not only does each individual's health status affect others, but also the health of one group in a society can influence the welfare of other groups. The importance of maintaining health in populations was also exemplified in the measles outbreak of 2015. The spread of preventable disease again revealed the importance of vaccination not only nationwide but worldwide. This in turn led to an increasing awareness of the need for reinforced education regarding the evidence behind vaccination. The diffusion of medical technology and evidence-based practice can positively affect a nation's health, much as the spread of infectious diseases can affect it adversely. The reform of international health systems to better address these issues was facilitated by the recognition of healthcare as a universal human right after World War II.

Article 25 of the Universal Declaration of Human Rights (UDHR) stipulates that all people have the right to a standard of living that guarantees health (UN, n.d.a). This article was adopted by the UN Charter of 1948. In 1960, the UDHR further specified health as the highest attainable standard of physical, social, and mental well-being rather than as solely the absence of disease. Health, according to the UDHR, is achievable through the promotion of maternal and child health, reduction of mortality and morbidity, improvements in environmental sanitation, and the provision of adequate medical services (UN, n.d.a). The UN reaffirmed health as an intrinsically valuable end by emphasizing that poor health is caused primarily by poverty and environmental conditions. A 1978 WHO conference held in Alma-Ata, Kazakhstan, a republic of the now former Soviet Union, supported the global issue of equity through accessibility to health for all, by recommending the implementation of primary healthcare and disease prevention strategies in national policies (Campbell, 1995).

The human rights movement in health, which raised the issue of equity in health status, tied universal access to comprehensive medical and health services for different social groups. Universal access implies the availability of services to all individuals and groups. Evaluating the distinctions between individual medical care and public healthcare becomes important as a means of monitoring health status, measured by indicators of equity and quality of care. Equity in access does not automatically lead to equity in health status. Equity in health status among social groups is constrained by the macro social process of the delivery of healthcare, as well as by the sociocultural, economic, and political arrangements of the community in which the delivery system functions. Global health programs have initiated various strategies to resolve these social determinants of health, increase access to basic health services, and achieve equity in outcomes. Essentially, equity in outcomes is the only true measure of equity in health status.

Social Determinants of Health

The social determinants of health are the conditions in which people are born, grow, live, work, and age. These circumstances are shaped by the distribution of money, power, and resources at global, national, and local levels. The social determinants of health are mostly responsible for health inequities—the unfair and avoidable differences in health status seen within and between countries.

There are many conceptual frameworks for social determinants of health crafted by public and private entities, among them the CDC, WHO, the European Union, and more. In fact, they all contain the multifactorial components of population health that impact health outcomes; a composite is presented in Box 12.1.

Inherent in this framework are the interactions between these social determinants; their influence on inequities; and the sociopolitical and economic influences on health and well-being. The status of the health of a nation is an international phenomenon that is embedded within the larger socio-ecological, cultural, and political context of the global community. Arguably, the United States is the most technologically advanced country in the world, with internationally renowned medical centers and cutting-edge treatment modalities that are grounded in the tenets of Western medical scientific research. Yet among civilized nations, its healthcare outcomes, especially for preventable diseases and access to health services, lag far behind those of its counterparts with regard to multiple indicators, including infant mortality (the United States ranked 25th) and life expectancy (the United States ranked 23rd; WHO, 2018a).

Multilevel Model of Global Health

The growth of population-based nursing not only illustrates the need for further documentation of ethnocultural variation in health outcomes but provides an equally important mandate to translate clinical research into culturally competent programs. Population health is an emerging paradigm, differentiated from global health not only by scope but also by a focus on which groups are susceptible or at greater risk for specific diseases. Global health, on the other hand, provides a broader perspective on the extent to which

BOX 12.1

SOCIAL DETERMINANTS OF HEALTH IMPACTING POPULATIONS

Employment conditions
Measures to clarify how different types of jobs and the threat of unemployment affect workers' health.

Social exclusion
The relational processes that lead to the exclusion of particular groups of people from engaging fully in community and social life.

Public health programs and social determinants
Factors in the design and implementation of programs that increase access to healthcare for socially and economically disadvantaged groups.

Women and gender equity
Mechanisms, processes, and actions that can be taken to reduce gender-based inequities in health by examining different areas.

Early child development
Well-established evidence illustrates that opportunities provided to young children are crucial in shaping lifelong health and development status.

Globalization
How globalization's dynamics and processes affect health outcomes: trade liberalization, integration of production of goods.

Health systems
Innovative approaches that effectively incorporate action on social determinants of health.

Measurement and evidence
The development of methodologies and tools for measuring the causes, pathways and health outcomes of policy interventions.

Urbanization
Broad policy interventions related to healthy urbanization, including close examination of slum upgrading.

the complex relations of macro structural factors of health determine the distribution of population-level and individual-level health outcomes. Macrofactors of salience explain how the environment, education policy, information technology, ethnic diversity and health disparity, geographical, socioeconomic factors, and inequities affect disease transmission and the delivery of health services across national borders.

To promote a greater understanding of the links among individual health, population health, and global health, the U.S. government has developed programs that address such relationships, domestically and abroad. The best practices and lessons learned from global health programs, such as the GHI, have demonstrated that the more acute issues visible in global environments are also relevant in the domestic context. Since GHI was legislated as a national priority in 2009, government agencies have sought to address global health challenges that may compromise well-being at home and around the world. The GHI seeks to align national security interests through collaboration with global partners to strengthen aid effectiveness. However, effectiveness in health promotion and disease prevention depends on aligning the dominant models of health, from individual clinical assessment to accessing primary care, and from population attributable risk assessment to ecological and multilevel models of health.

Multilevel models of global health (Figure 12.1) take into account the emergent properties of social structure, such as cultural norms, poverty, social policies, and distribution of primary care physicians, in conjunction with microlevel properties, such as genetics, gender, ethnicity, educational level, and individual health behaviors. Context or emergent properties of structure at each level refer to those characteristics that exemplify aspects of the whole unit of analysis and not the separate components of that unit. Whole units, such as population groups or health systems, have distinct properties other than the sum of their individual parts. Contextual analysis can explain the influences that a unit has within a hierarchy, and multilevel analysis can focus on multiple hierarchies of units within the same model. The individual is part of

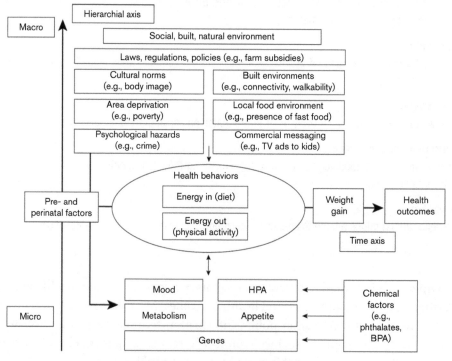

FIGURE 12.1 Micro- and macrofactors in obesity as health outcomes.

BPA, bisphenol A; HPA, hypothalamic–pituitary–adrenal axis.

Note: The life span is horizontal; factors are depicted hierarchically, individual level at the bottom of the figure to community level at top of the figure.

Source: From Glass, T. A., & McAtee, M. J. (2006). Behavioral science at the crossroads in public health: Extending horizons, envisioning the future. *Social Science & Medicine, 62*(7), 1650–1671. doi:10.1016/j.socscimed.2005.08.044

a family, ethnic group, social network, community, political group, geographical area, and country. It is a central objective in the population health perspective of healthcare to assess the context in which macro- and microunits change, given the complex nesting of individuals within social groups and cultures (Campbell, 2004; Campbell, 2006; McKeehan, 2000).

Effective population health strategies aim at identifying groups at risk and specific risk factors causing poor health. Emergent properties of social structure are often not considered as determinants of health by medical practitioners. Health-promotion policies may develop two distinct intervention strategies by which health risks can be reduced for vulnerable groups as well as for the general population: (a) high-risk interventions, such as tertiary care (e.g., specialized consultative care; medical technology or surgery), which reduce high risks for a small number of individuals; and (b) population risk interventions, such as primary prevention (e.g., prohibiting lead in consumer paints, seat belt requirements), which reduce pervasive low risks for large sectors of a population (Association of Faculties of Medicine of Canada [AFMC], n.d.).

Application of both intervention strategies is necessary to avert the "prevention paradox"; that is, individual-level interventions affect community health minimally, whereas community-level interventions have limited impact on high-risk individuals. The "prevention paradox" is paralleled by the "risk intervention paradox"; that is, the mass exposure of a large number of individuals to low levels of negligible risks, such as trans fats, may produce a larger number of disease cases than a small number of individuals exposed to high risks, such as BMI (body mass index) >35. Treating only very sick individuals leaves scarcely sick populations with minimal health treatment.

Preventing disease by shifting the population distribution of specific disease risks may be more productive than treatments directed only toward high-risk individuals.

For instance, estimates suggest that in North America a 14% decrease in the number of cerebrovascular accidents could be achieved either by decreasing the average blood pressure by 2 mmHg or by successfully treating everyone with a diastolic pressure of 95 mmHg or greater. (AFMC, n.d., para 2)

Mass prevention reduces negligible risk a little for many and not at all for some, whereas most derive at least minimal benefits.

The prevention paradox proposes the concept that population health policies are developed for sick populations rather than for sick individuals, a cost borne by the "healthier" community. Global health intervention differs from medical intervention foremost in its emphasis on the socio-environmental context of individual health status. Second, global health recognizes that a continuous distribution in health status, such as blood pressure, characterizes populations. Third, global health programs are not restricted by focusing solely on the clinical designation of individuals, as potential cases for treatment, with or without disease.

A clearer understanding of global health identifies the differences in individual health, while retaining the ethnocultural context experienced by people. The multilevel model of population and global health enables the identification of health differences among individuals and among social groups. It also identifies specific structural conditions in the community that affect the health of people living there. Last, it separates the structural and ethnocultural determinants of health from the effects of individual psychosocial and health behaviors on health outcomes. For example, health disparity is part of the community context within which people live: country of origin, ethnicity, and cultural values are group characteristics. But ethnocultural factors are almost always measured at the individual level, a misspecification of the research model. The domain of preventive strategies in community health is the at-risk population as a whole and that of clinical medicine is the at-risk individual.

A multilevel evaluation of global health, therefore, gauges negligible and high-risk factors at both the population level and the individual level. As abundant research has shown, individual lifestyle behaviors, given a specific level of socioeconomic development, account for a majority of the risk factors for general well-being. A major issue is to determine which risk factors are amenable to policy interventions. Mass levels of low exposure require a mass level of intervention even if the impact is negligible, because the community will benefit as a whole, and subsequently individual members will benefit. The risk factors, which affect individual health, are not the same at the community level. Population health policy, therefore, needs multilevel research strategies that include the *sui generis* properties of communities and their attendant risk factors. These community properties cannot be reduced to a collective aggregate of its individual members. Access to health systems and geocultural environments may be designated as structural properties of communities rather than of individuals, and as such are the community context in which individuals live. GHIs tend to emphasize structural community factors to improve health outcomes, as is discussed in the section on the UN Millennium Development Goals.

Improvements in the quality of life depend in large part on the development of a model of health that puts the individual back into the community context. Personal risks to health under control of the individual (amount of daily sugar or salt intake) and social risks to health not directly controllable by the individual (a clean water supply) are embedded in a larger community context. Effective global programs sift through such causal complexity, expanding the biomedical model of disease to an ecological multilevel model of health.

Global health programs promote information initiatives to connect systems capable of supporting a broad range of public health functions: disease detection, surveillance, analysis, interpretation, alerting, and interventions. For example, in WHO's Health Report, the term "health services" is used to include promotion, prevention, treatment, and rehabilitation. It includes services aimed at individuals (e.g., childhood immunization or treatment for tuberculosis) and services aimed at populations (e.g., mass media anti-smoking campaigns) (WHO, 2018b).

Evaluating public health risk factors at multiple levels is even more relevant in global health in which community and cultural contexts vary significantly across geographic regions. Modifiable community factors have a direct effect on health, separately and independently from the effects of nonmodifiable individual factors and modifiable individual lifestyle practices. Individual behavioral solutions may be sought for population-level issues, when attributing or generalizing individual characteristics to the group. In designing or implementing large-scale health programs, the APRN should be aware that both individual and community contextual factors, including geographic locators, should be systematically included in public health education and research, to design effective programs (Campbell, 1995).

An effective APRN-administered population health program considers several factors:

- Community context has a direct effect on individual health outcomes, controlling for individual demographic factors.

- The relative ranking of geographic areas by healthcare access, environmental quality, and socioeconomic factors are characteristics of the area and a contextual determinant of individual health, controlling for individual demographic characteristics.

- Living in areas ranked as having better healthcare access, better environmental quality, residential land use, and less poverty has a positive effect on individual health outcomes.

- Beneficial community context has a moderating effect on the individual health outcome of individuals from disadvantaged or vulnerable demographic subgroups.

- Living in higher quality-ranked areas has a greater positive effect on individual health outcomes for minority individuals than for individuals who are not characterized as being from disadvantaged or vulnerable demographic subgroups.

As part of planning a population-based program, APRNs should assess which modifiable community factors have a direct effect on health, separately and independently from the effects of modifiable individual lifestyle behaviors and nonmodifiable individual demographic factors.

National Global Health Initiatives

The U.S. administration has spent over $120 billion to increase access to health services in global programs and to ensure national security since 2006. The GHI prioritizes a three-pronged health strategy to contain infectious diseases and foster national security. This includes initiatives to protect communities from infectious diseases, eliminate AIDS in the new generation, and prevent child and maternal mortality (USAID, 2019). A poll conducted by the Henry J. Kaiser Family Foundation (KFF) found that more than half of the U.S. public believes that the United States should play a leading (13%) or major (41%) role in improving health for people in developing countries (KFF, 2016). USAID has bipartisan support in Congress, which has a longstanding tradition of working in unison for humanitarian causes. The Trump administration has been less supportive as its rhetoric of "America First" implies. President Trump has proposed a substantial cut in the 2019 USAID budget. There are some indications that the current administration has softened its stance on foreign aid as it has created the U.S. International Development Corporation (IDFC) which has bipartisan support in Congress and from the USAID.

Although infectious diseases still abound and new outbreaks of such diseases as Ebola, severe acute respiratory syndrome (SARS), and H1N1 threaten national security, vaccine-preventable diseases have been nearly eliminated in the United States. At the time of this publication, however, measles infections have reached their highest numbers (since the resurgence of 1989–1991) in the United States because of unvaccinated immigrants entering the United States, unvaccinated Americans traveling outside of the United States and returning with the disease, and because of inconsistent vaccination practices and parental refusal of vaccines in the United States. APRNs have a role in shaping public opinion and have many opportunities to improve population health through health promotion, education, and research (see www.cdc.gov/vaccines/pubs/pinkbook/meas.html for more details about measles). Public health programs and health education, for example, have successfully contained the HIV epidemic, and many preventive programs in the United States focus on chronic diseases. Until the 20th century, communicable diseases were the singular cause of mortality, but chronic diseases now top the list. The smallpox vaccine was responsible for preventing nearly 2 million annual deaths around the world by 1980. In the 1950s, polio crippled about 35,000 children in the United States annually, but was largely eradicated through vaccination by 1979. However, several other countries, such as Afghanistan, Nigeria, and Pakistan, with absent or low vaccination rates, continue to experience high polio rates. Polio is currently spreading in the war-torn countries of Syria, Djibouti, Eritrea, Ethiopia, and Somalia (CDC, 2017). Another example of a preventable infectious disease is meningitis A. Although largely controlled in the United States, over 100,000 people died of meningitis A in the 1990s across Africa, spurring the CDC, the USAID, and the National Institutes of Health (NIH) to develop an affordable vaccine, MenAfriVac, for distribution. More recently, millions of dollars have been invested in a critical search for a safe Ebola vaccine. Such quick collaboration among national groups underscores the critical role that the United States plays in global health, as well as the interconnections between national security and public health.

Healthy People 2010 outlined national health goals for America but did not include global health as an issue. Following the 2003 SARS epidemic and 2009 H1N1 flu outbreak, *Healthy People 2020* added a new global health goal "to improve public health and strengthen U.S. national security through global disease detection, response, prevention, and control strategies" (*Healthy People 2020*, 2019). The 2014 Ebola outbreak demonstrates how the *Healthy People 2020* connections between American health status and global developments are relevant. Diseases prevented with vaccinations are the cause of one of every five deaths among children younger than 5 years in underdeveloped countries. For example, measles was largely eradicated by 2000 in the United States, but in 2018 there were 349 cases, almost entirely because of people bringing the disease with them into the United States (this includes both foreign born and Americans who traveled overseas), where an increased number of American families are choosing not to vaccinate their children, reducing the strength of herd immunity (CDC, 2019). *Healthy People 2020* and the Institutes of Medicine (IOM) advocate a focal role for the United States in increasing the global capacity for establishing an infectious disease surveillance system to protect U.S. national security and to prevent the cross-border spread of diseases.

Many U.S. government agencies provide funding, human resources, and technical support to international health agencies and initiatives, including the UN's *Millennium Development Goals* (MDGs); WHO *Global Polio Eradication Initiative*; the *President's Emergency Plan for AIDS Relief* (PEPFAR); and the CDC programs to address *malaria*, neglected tropical diseases (such as Ebola), and tobacco use. The U.S. administration's health strategy in 2018 recognizes communicable diseases as a leading cause of mortality globally and the second major problem faced by the United States in health-promotion and disease prevention projects. Africa is an exception, because it must still address infectious diseases as a health priority. The GHI invested $63 billion over 6 years to help partner countries improve health outcomes through strengthened health systems, with a particular focus on improving the health of women, newborns, and children.

The Ebola outbreak of 2014 serves as an example of how important it is for the United States to work with multiple organizations to protect the health of the American people. In November 2014, there was a $6.2-billion appropriations request before Congress to fight Ebola in West Africa (U.S. Senate Committee on Appropriations, 2014), and the CDC funded $2.7 million for personal protective equipment (PPE) kits to help American hospitals and to augment the Strategic National Stockpile. The DHS issued travel restrictions in October 2014 on flights to the United States from Liberia, Sierra Leone, and Guinea. All flights from these three West African countries were directed to fly to one of only five airports with screening protocols in place: New York's JFK, Chicago's O'Hare, Atlanta's Hartsfield-Jackson, Newark's Liberty, and Washington's Dulles. Although WHO continued during this time to issue alerts for changing incidence and mortality rates attributed to Ebola by country, the U.S. Department of Health and Human Services (DHHS) instituted travel regulations to the United States, restricting entry to anyone either sick or exposed to Ebola from Guinea, Liberia, or Sierra Leone on November 12, 2014. The CDC and professional associations also invested in developing education programs for health practitioners to ensure the safety of clinicians by updating protocols on patient treatment and monitoring of Ebola patients as well as developing nationwide hospital and outpatient clinic surveillance systems (AACN, 2019; American Medical Association [AMA], 2014). The U.S. military was deployed to West Africa as part of humanitarian aid to deliver supplies and equipment and to build temporary hospitals, developing the health infrastructure required to contain the Ebola crisis (The White House, 2014). These combined efforts led to a decreased threat from Ebola in the United States, and by 2016 the CDC had revised its recommendations on travel to Guinea, Liberia, and Sierra Leone. Americans are no longer advised against nonessential travel, and recommendations for enhanced precautions when traveling to these countries have also been removed (U.S Department of State – Bureau of Consular Affairs, 2018).

The United States and the Global Health Gap

Mortality differences among nations have been associated with various theories of health disparities between populations and countries, some of which are dependent on policy. This is an extensive list that includes socioeconomic transformation, environmental pollution, lack of an adequate social safety net, relative poverty, socioeconomic deprivation, historical, and generational effects of a political heritage, regional disparities, and psychosocial stress. Other perspectives emphasize individual lifestyle such as poor health practices and violent behavior. The United States has the highest standard of living in the world, yet health indicators lag behind those of European and other high-income members of the Organization for Economic Cooperation and Development (OECD). OECD member countries control 80% of global trade and investments. The Organization for European Economic Cooperation was formed after World War II to support the reconstruction of Europe. Canada and the United States joined in 1960, establishing the OECD in 1961. Japan joined in 1964. As of 2018, there were 36 members of the OECD with one more country (Colombia) invited to join. These OECD countries participate in discussing solutions to world economic and health problems (OECD, n.d.a).

The relationship between average income, gross domestic product (GDP) or per capita, and life expectancy is attenuated after a certain standard of living is achieved, as has been the case in market economies in OECD countries. Average income is weakly related to mortality within wealthier countries, such as the United States. However, the relative distribution of income, rather than average income, is more strongly associated with differences in death rates within wealthy countries. This is due to the relative deprivation of some population sectors and not others because of an uneven distribution and concentration of resources.

Life expectancy is higher in countries with more egalitarian distributions of income, such as those of Scandinavia, where relative deprivation is less pronounced. The effect of average income on the life expectancy of men and women in Western economies of OECD countries is consistent with a relationship between wealth and health. Health disparities increase with comparative income disparities relative to various groups having different income levels (OECD, n.d.b). Health outcomes appear to be more closely related to how national health systems are organized than to the size of health expenditures, which are inflated by multiple private for-profit interests. In the United States, the growth in the cost of health services is not related to a concomitant growth in better health status of the population. A study of hospital administrative costs in eight countries found that the United States has the highest costs, with 25% of U.S. hospital spending going to salaries for staff responsible for coding and billing, among other administrative costs. The Netherlands was second highest, spending 20% on administrative costs, followed by England at 16%, and Canada at 12% (Himmelstein et al., 2014).

OECD (2018) statistics indicate that the total health expenditure of the United States in 2016 was 16.8% of the GDP and $9,536 per capita, as compared to total OECD expenditures of close to 10.0% of global GDP. The average health expenditure worldwide was $1,000 per capita, but half of the world's countries spent less than $350 per person. In 2016, life expectancy at birth for U.S. men was 76 and for men in OECD countries it was

77.3. Although the difference in life expectancy between the United States and other OECD countries is less than 2 years, health expenditures are almost double in the United States. Recent economic research (Lorenzoni, Belloni, & Sassi, 2014) indicates that most of the growth in differences of health expenditure between the United States and OECD was due to private health sector prices, particularly pharmaceuticals, and not due to growth in provider health delivery or performance (OECD, 2018).

Health sector costs are the most important component of U.S. health expenditure growth. The "staggering levels of expenditure" in the United States cannot be fully explained by higher wealth levels, the age structure of the U.S. population, or the larger prevalence of risk factors such as obesity. Instead, "high health sector prices are due to intense use of health-related technologies, low productivity, decentralized price negotiations, fragmentation in the insurance market, and a high level of provider concentration, as the main explanations for high spending" (Lorenzoni et al., 2014, p. 84). A positive relationship between health sector prices and better health outcomes has not been established for the United States, as comparative global health indicators demonstrate (Lorenzoni et al., 2014; OECD, 2017a).

An international comparison of U.S. health status with those of other high-income countries demonstrates that the United States has lower health outcomes on several indicators: infant mortality and low birth weight, injuries and homicides, adolescent pregnancy and sexually transmitted infections, HIV and AIDS, drug-related deaths, obesity and diabetes, heart disease, chronic lung disease, and disability. In 1970 U.S. life expectancy was 1 year above the average for OPEC counties. In 2017 it was 2 years below the average. These poorer health outcomes in America are attributed to several lifestyle and health system factors: a large uninsured population, barriers to accessing primary care, likelihood of having a BMI >29, and physical inactivity. The United States has the highest obesity rate of all OPEC countries, and the rate is rising. The lack of primary care practitioners in the United States is notable, given that most chronic diseases are preventable. An international OECD survey found that the United States had the lowest ratio of general practitioners out of all physicians, when compared to 15 other high-income countries. The United States also has a large sector of the population living below the federal poverty level and significant income inequality, both related to poor health status. On a more positive note, air pollution in the United States is low relative to other OPEC countries and smoking rates are also better (OECD, 2017b).

American National Security and Global Health

Although Americans have a comparatively poorer health status than peer countries, federal initiatives, such as *Healthy People 2020*, try to address these health disparities. *Healthy People 2020* includes the global health goal of strengthening U.S. national security by detecting, preventing, and controlling global diseases. The U.S. government, through the USAID and the CDC, actively collaborates with global health agencies and participates in global, regional, and country-specific public health programs. The two focal organizations are the UN and WHO. The mission of the USAID is to work with governmental and nongovernmental agencies, as well as the military, providing foreign assistance to resolve and prevent instability or active conflicts around the world. The USAID works to ensure domestic security by investing in health systems, democratic institutions, and agricultural advances (USAID, 2018).

The Foreign Assistance Act of 1961, supported by President Kennedy, formed the USAID from several post-World War II foreign assistance programs. The USAID was responsible for promoting development by administering aid to other countries. The USAID has spearheaded U.S. technical and financial aid to increase health and economic self-sufficiency in the developing world through polio eradication, family planning, and maternal and child health programs. The U.S. President's Emergency Plan for AIDS Relief and President's Malaria Initiative are successful programs that have significantly impacted the incidence and prevalence of these infectious diseases. The DHHS launched the GHI in 2009 to integrate multiple government programs with global partners, as well as to cooperate with WHO in health-promotion and disease prevention efforts.

Historically, the USAID has focused primarily on preventing hunger, promoting women's education and health, and population planning around the world as a means to curtail political conflicts. These efforts have also entailed supporting free market economic growth, nongovernmental organizations (NGOs), and antipoverty programs. The USAID, as the main government agency tasked with ending extreme poverty and building democracy abroad, was responsible for helping to rebuild Afghanistan and Iraq by building social safety nets with healthcare and education programs in the region (USAID, 2017).

APRNs should be aware that U.S. global health initiatives fluctuate over time due to differing views and political philosophies. For example, the United States is the largest donor to family planning (FP) and reproductive health (RH) in the world but funding is impacted by U.S. policies. The Mexico City Policy that was implemented during the Reagan administration stipulates that overseas nongovernmental organizations will not perform or promote abortion as a method of family planning as a condition for receiving U.S. funding. This policy was rescinded by President Clinton, reinstated by President Bush, rescinded by President Obama, and then reinstated and expanded by President Trump in 2017 (KFF, 2018).

Former Secretary of State Hillary Clinton implemented policy reforms in global health with GHI funding, including establishing a new agenda "USAID Forward." Included in the agenda are strategies that seek to establish evidence for what works and what does not work in global health programs. Box 12.2 enumerates some of the successful results the USAID has obtained with global health investments.

WHO

USAID works with WHO to promote and protect health as an essential element for human welfare, economic, and social development (USAID, 2016). WHO was created in 1946, as part of the UN, to find solutions for post-World War II Europe. Any member country of the UN can be a member of WHO. WHO, recognizing that international collaboration could control infectious diseases better than any single country, spearheaded

BOX 12.2

USAID GLOBAL HEALTH PROGRAM OUTCOMES 2017

- Provided 25 countries with support for integration of health information systems
- 21 million children under the age of five reached by nutrition-specific interventions
- 1.4 million people gained access to a basic sanitation service
- 194,000 community health workers provided family planning information, referrals, and/or services
- 202,000 individuals received HIV testing services (HTS) and received their test results
- 79,000 individuals received testing and counseling services for HIV and received their test results
- 99,000 priority populations (clients of sex workers) were reached with the standardized, evidence-based interventions required that are designed to promote the adoption of HIV prevention behaviors and service uptake
- 242,000 participants in gang prevention and education programs

Source: From USAID. (n.d.). *Dollars to results.* Retrieved from https://results.usaid.gov/results

the establishment of International Health Regulations (IHR, formulated in 1969, revised in 2005, in force 2007), which delineates the legal framework for global public health security (Prentice, Reinders, & World Health Report Team, 2007). WHO states that

> global public health security minimizes vulnerability to acute public health events that endanger the collective health of populations living across geographical regions and international boundaries, and includes the impact on economic, political stability, trade, tourism, access to goods and services, and demographic stability. (WHO, 2007, "Overview" section, para. 2)

The goals of the IHR are to promote collective defense against the international spread of disease and population health emergencies by addressing diplomatic, political, economic, trade, and business interests. The IHR lists diseases for mandatory reporting by all countries (polio, smallpox, etc.) specifies responses to radioactive, nuclear, or chemical emergencies; encourages global cooperation in science and technology; and recommends increased workforce and laboratory capacity.

As part of global health security, WHO established several international collaborations, enumerated in Box 12.3.

WHO also manages global disease registries, databases, and classification of diseases that are used by members, including the United States, to maintain comparable definitions of health indicators (WHO, 2018b). WHO, with the agreement of member countries, developed Nomenclature Regulations in 1967. The regulations standardize nomenclature (Box 12.4) with respect to morbidity and mortality, and established globally consistent coding, age groupings, territorial regions, and languages for the compilation and

BOX 12.3

WHO GLOBAL HEALTH COLLABORATIONS

- Global Outbreak Alert and Response Network (GOARN), which initiates an international disease outbreak alert, technical support, vaccines, drugs, specialists, and equipment, to prevent spread, such as the plague in India, in 1995, which had an economic cost of over $1.7 billion

- Chemical Incident Alert and Response System (ChemiNet): initiates alerts of industrial accidents and chemical, water, sanitation, radionuclear or environmental health emergencies

- Global network of national health systems

- Global Polio Eradication Initiative Network (GPEIN)

- Global Influenza Surveillance and Response System (GISRS)

- FluNet

- H5N1 Avian flu tracking

- XDR-TB drug-resistant tuberculosis tracking

- Containment of 21st-century threats of bioterrorism (anthrax, etc.), SARS, and toxic chemical waste dumping, such as the 2006 illegal dumping of 500 tons of chemical waste in Abidjan, Cote d'Ivoire

- WHO Foreign Policy and Global Health (FPGH) Initiative

- Coordination of responses to natural disasters, with concomitant infectious diseases, malnutrition, mental illness, and displacement of large numbers of people

WHO, World Health Organization.

Source: From WHO. (2019a). *Collaborations and Partnerships.* Retrieved from https://www.who.int/about/collaborations/en

publication of health information. All members of WHO have agreed to use the same nomenclature to collect and publish annual data.

The *International Classification of Diseases (ICD)* is used in the United States to code billing in order to standardize diagnostic categories and thereby to track the incidence and prevalence of disease. The 11th revision of the *ICD* was released in 2018, and can be downloaded from the WHO website at www.who.int/classifications/icd/en.

WHO included the International Classification for Nursing Practice (ICNP) in 1996. It was updated in 2017, and another update is scheduled for 2019. The ICNP is copyrighted by the International Council of Nurses (ICN), which ensures the integrity of the classification system. ICNP is translated into several languages and may be downloaded for noncommercial purposes with an authorizing agreement (ICN, 2019). The ICNP is designed to enable comparisons of nursing data across countries. It includes nursing diagnoses, nurse-sensitive patient outcomes, and nursing interventions.

The ICNP is a classification system that improves communication among nurses from different countries through standard language. It describes nursing practice in institutional and noninstitutional environments. It also facilitates international

BOX 12.4

WHO FAMILY OF INTERNATIONAL CLASSIFICATION (FIC)

I. WHO Family of International Classification

- *International Classification of Diseases* (ICD-10)
- International Classification of Diseases for Oncology (ICD-0-3)
- ICD-10 for Mental and Behavioral Disorders: Clinical Descriptions and Diagnostic Guidelines
- ICD-10 for Mental and Behavioral Disorders Diagnostic Criteria for Research
- International Classification of Functioning, Disability and Health (ICF)
- WHODAS 2.0 General Disability Factor
- International Classification of Health Interventions (ICHI)

II. Family of International Classifications Network

III. Related International Classifications

- International Classification of Primary Care, Second Edition (ICPC-2)
- International Classification of External Causes of Injury (ICECI)
- Technical aids for persons with disabilities—Classification and terminology (ISO9999)
- Anatomical Therapeutic Chemical Classification System with Defined Daily Doses (ATC/DDD)
- International Classification for Nursing Practice (ICNP)

WHO, World Health Organization.

Source: From Madden, R., Sykes, C., Ustun, T. B., National Centre for Classification in Health, Australia, Australian Institute of Health and Welfare, & WHO. (n.d.). *The WHO family of international classifications: Definitions, Scope and purpose.* Retrieved from http://www.who.int/classifications/en

nursing research and the promulgation of health policy (ICN, 2019). The ICN maintains collaboration with other systems of classification to facilitate cross-mapping of vocabularies and interoperability. The ICN indicates that it has a number of formal agreements to best represent the nursing domain and promote semantic interoperability. The ICNP is recognized as a related classification within the WHO Family of International Classifications to promote harmonization with the other WHO classifications (Box 12.4).

The International Health Terminology Standards Development Organization (IHTSDO) and the ICN have engaged in a formal Harmonization Agreement to ensure that nursing requirements are adequately captured within the Systematized Nomenclature of Medicine—Clinical Terms (SNOMED CT). In addition to harmonizing ICNP and SNOMED CT, the ICN serves as the international representation for nursing practice to the IHTSDO. The ICN also has Liaison A status with the International Organization for Standardization (ISO) Technical Committee on Health Informatics (TC215) and is represented at the International Medical Informatics Association through participation in the Nursing Special Interest Group. More recently, the ICN has collaborated with SabaCare to develop linkages between the Clinical Care Classification (CCC) and ICNP concepts. The CCC System emerged from a Research Project Contract conducted by Virginia Saba as the Principal Investigator (1988–1991) at Georgetown University School of Nursing. The research project was designed to develop a method to assess and classify patients to determine their resource requirements as well as measure their outcomes. To accomplish this goal, live patient data on actual resource use that could be objectively measured were collected and used to predict resource requirements. The CCC System offers a new approach for documenting patient care in an electronic health record (EHR) system (SabaCare, 2018).

UN Millennium Development Goals

As part of the UN, WHO follows the prescriptions of the UN MDGs, which organize global strategies and priorities in improving health status across countries. UN members committed $2.5 billion in 2013 to accelerate meeting the MDG outcomes by 2015. The MDGs are eight international development goals that were established in 2000 by the UN to reaffirm the commitment of individual nations for a collective responsibility for human dignity, equality, and equity (UNGeneral Assembly, 2000).

The MDGs (Box 12.5) and targets were articulated by the Millennium Declaration of 2000, signed by 189 countries, including 147 heads of state and governments and at least 23 international organizations. The MDGs were further confirmed by the General Assembly of member states at the 2005 World Summit. The goals and targets are interrelated, forming a coherent whole. The MDGs represented an agreement among countries to achieve the MDGs by 2015 and "create an environment—at the national and global levels alike—which is conducive to development and the elimination of poverty" (UN General Assembly, 2000, section III, para. 2).

The eight MDG goals were subdivided into 21 targets, each with measurable health and economic indicators (these can be accessed at: mdgs.un.org/unsd/mdg/Default .aspx). Detailed descriptions of the MDGs and the specific targets for achieving each goal are available on the UNICEF website (www.unicef.org/statistics/index_24304. html). A conference to review interim progress in meeting the MDG targets was held at the UN in September 2010. A global action plan was adopted to ensure progress toward meeting the eight antipoverty goals by 2015, with special emphasis on promoting women's health and children's health, as well as eradicating hunger and disease. *The Millennium Development Goals Report 2014*, approved in New York on July 7, 2014, summarizes the assessment of global and regional progress toward meeting the MDGs. In comparison with the initial 2000 assessment, improvement across all goals was achieved by 2014, but continued work is required to fully meet the 2015 and post-2015 development agenda (UN Department of Economic and Social Affairs, n.d.).

Since the MDGs were established, UN member countries have achieved significant progress on several MDG indicators. China and India have reported the greatest gains

BOX 12.5

UN MILLENNIUM DEVELOPMENT GOALS FOR IMPROVING THE HEALTH STATUS OF COUNTRIES

1. Eradicate extreme poverty and hunger.

2. Achieve universal primary education.

3. Promote gender equality and empower women.

4. Reduce child mortality.

5. Improve maternal health.

6. Combat HIV/AIDS, malaria, and other diseases.

7. Ensure environmental sustainability.

8. Develop a global partnership for development.

Source: From World Health Organization. (2019b). Millennium Development Goals (MDGS). Retrieved from https://www.who.int/news-room/fact-sheets/detail/millennium-development-goals-(mdgs)

in reducing poverty, and Brazil has achieved most of the eight goals. Nepal remains the world's poorest country. However, increased spending in maternal and child health by Nepal resulted in a 50% reduction in maternal mortality between 1998 and 2006. Developing countries still had 21% of their populations living on less than $1.25 a day in 2010 (UN Economic and Social Council, n.d.). With the USAID investment in global health program collaboration to meet the MDGs, substantial gains were made in macro population health indicators. Sub-Saharan Africa reports that 43 million more children are in primary education since 1999; child mortality has declined by 35% since 1994, malaria deaths have decreased by 30% since 2004, and 2 billion people have access to clean drinking water (UN Economic and Social Council, n.d.). Continued progress on the MDGs and sustaining the progress that has been made requires ongoing collaboration among nations, global organizations, intergovernmental agencies, local government, and community participation.

The eight MDGs—which range from halving extreme poverty rates to halting the spread of HIV/AIDS and providing universal primary education—formed a blueprint agreed to by all the world's countries and all of the world's leading development institutions. They have galvanized unprecedented efforts to meet the needs of the world's poorest. The UN is also working with governments, civil society, and other partners to build on the momentum generated by the MDGs and carry on with an ambitious post-2015 development agenda.

As the MDGs era came to a conclusion with the end of 2015, WHO responded with the official launch of the bold and transformative 2030 Agenda for Sustainable Development (Sustainable Development Goals [SDGs]) adopted by world leaders in September 2015 at the UN). The new Agenda calls on countries to begin efforts to achieve 17 SDGs by 2030. "The seventeen sustainable development goals are our shared vision of humanity and a social contract between the world's leaders and the people," said UN Secretary-General Ban Ki-moon. "They are a to-do list for people and planet, and a blueprint for success" (UN, n.d.b, p. 3; see Box 12.6).

Implications for Advanced Practice Nursing

Nursing has become increasingly more active in global health programs by expanding interprofessional and interdependent collaborations. Global health is an essential component in APRN education and practice. Many schools of nursing have formed GHIs to strengthen culturally sensitive nursing education domestically. APRNs work as educators, policy makers, and clinicians in a variety of communities, with different cultural and ethnic groups, as well as with populations that spend extended time in other countries, such as veterans (National League for Nursing [NLN], n.d.a). Such programs promote a

---

BOX 12.6

THE UNITED NATIONS' SDGs

1. No poverty
2. Zero hunger
3. Good health and well-being
4. Quality education
5. Gender equality
6. Clean water and sanitation
7. Affordable and clean energy
8. Decent work and economic growth
9. Industry, innovation, and infrastructure
10. Raise your voice against discrimination
11. Sustain cities and communities
12. Responsible production and consumption
13. Climate action
14. Life below waters (clean oceans)
15. Life on land (environmental protection)
16. Peace, justice, and strong institutions (use your right to elect your county and community leaders)
17. Partnerships for the goals (SDGs in action)

SDG, sustainable development goals.

Source: From United Nations. (n.d.c). *About the sustainable development goals.* Retrieved from https://www.un.org/sustainabledevelopment/sustainable-development-goals

deeper understanding, in APRN practice, of the complex political, economic, and social factors that affect an individual's health in a community context.

In the future, doctorally prepared nurses will find themselves more and more often in the position of being asked to form strategic partnerships with public and private organizations to strengthen health systems and to deliver culturally competent healthcare. In 2004, the NLN formed the International Nursing Education, Services and Accreditation (INESA) joint taskforce with the NLN Accreditation Commission (NLNAC). In 2013 the NLNAC became the Accreditation Commission for Education in Nursing (ACEN). INESA coordinates exchanges between nurse educators from the United States and around the world, and supports the Nursing Education Network of the ICN (NLN, n.d.b). INESA also promotes educating nurses as an ethnic and culturally diverse workforce to meet the challenge of a worldwide nursing shortage and increased migration across nations. The ACEN serves as a consultant on accreditation issues of nursing education programs in different countries (ACEN, 2019).

International activities have expanded for nursing faculty to include curriculum development, international collaboration in presentations and publications, consulting in hospital administration, and clinical expertise. Applying U.S. models, concepts, and theories of nursing practice in other nations may not be appropriate or feasible, given varying cultural values and beliefs. Many nursing interventions, practices, licensure requirements, and policies are context-specific and cannot be transferred across cultures. APRNs, as primary care providers, should develop awareness of political and cultural issues that influence individual behaviors, lifestyle, risk factors, and clinical care (Aiken et al., 2008). The multilevel global health model for APRN practice emphasizes cultural sensitivity in engaging in comparative effectiveness programs and interdisciplinary, interprofessional educational interchanges (Kulage, Hickey, Honig, Johnson, & Larson, 2014). APRNs play a leadership role in implementing transcultural changes in healthcare, disseminating science within nursing practice, and collaborating with global partners, such as the WHO.

WHO Collaborating Centers

WHO has formed Collaborating Centers with 10 schools of nursing in the United States (WHO, n.d.b). These collaborating centers bring together experts to solve problems in nursing; to address chronic and communicable diseases, nutrition, mental health, and other areas; and to share data, outcomes, and resolutions with UN member countries. The U.S. schools of nursing have agreed to produce a variety of outputs as part of their collaboration agreement with WHO (Box 12.7). The U.S. Schools of Nursing WHO Collaborating Centers each focus on such specific themes as clinical training in health promotion, nursing knowledge implementation and dissemination, international nursing development in primary healthcare, and clinical training in home care nursing.

These collaboration initiatives (Table 12.1) promote the work of U.S. nurses in (a) international NGOs focusing on health, (b) best practices in achieving the MDGs

BOX 12.7

WHO EVALUATION TERMS OF REFERENCE OUTPUTS BETWEEN U.S. SCHOOLS OF NURSING COLLABORATING CENTERS AND WHO

- Health-workforce information and knowledge base strengthened, and country capacities for policy analysis, planning, implementation, information-sharing, and research built up

- Technical support provided to member states, with a focus on those facing severe health-workforce difficulties in order to improve the production, distribution, skill mix, and retention of the health workforce

- Human resource policies and practices in place to attract and retain top talent, promote learning and professional development, manage performance, and foster ethical behavior

- Management and organization of integrated, population-based health-service delivery through public and nonpublic providers and networks improved, reflecting the primary healthcare strategy; scaling up coverage, equity, quality, and safety of personal and population-based health services; and enhancing health outcomes

WHO, World Health Organization.

Source: From World Health Organization. (n.d.b). *World Health Organization Collaborating Centres.* Retrieved from http://apps.who.int/whocc/List.aspx?cc_code=USA&

and SDGs, (c) capacity building of nursing human resources, (d) capacity building in nursing education for primary care, (e) training in disease prevention methods, and (f) supporting nurse educational programs in home care and self-management of chronic diseases (WHO, n.d.b). These issues are important for the APRN to consider when planning effective health delivery programs focusing on the individual and community levels, and ensuring that a safety net includes culturally competent health interventions.

The U.S. Surgeon General's Goals of 2000 identified three broad areas that influence population health status and that require public policy and nursing intervention: (a) health practices or health promotion (decreasing risk factors, personal habits such as smoking, lack of physical exercise, poor diet, alcohol abuse), (b) ecological factors or health protection (decreasing occupational and environmental toxic exposures, decreasing accidents), and (c) medical care factors or preventive health services (increasing access to services such as prenatal care, infant programs, family planning, hypertension control) (Campbell, 2004). These goals are reiterated in the macro population health indicators of *Healthy People 2020* and the MDGs and SDGs of the UN, and progress has already been made in measuring and addressing these concepts of health inequity and inequality. The APRN can further contribute to the monitoring of inequity in health, as a part of population health practice. With nurse leadership, the lessons learned from the application of effective health strategies in different countries can be shared with an interprofessional team in the United States (McNeal, 2013) and international communities.

TABLE 12.1 WHO Collaborating Centers With Schools of Nursing, United States (Active Until 2015–2017)

INSTITUTION	TITLE	TERMS OF REFERENCE
University of Michigan, Ann Arbor, Michigan	WHO Collaborating Centre for Research and Clinical Training in Health Promotion Nursing	• Collaborate with WHO/PAHO to disseminate/share critical information and connect and systematize experiences and good practices of health promotion. • Collaborate with WHO/PAHO to build nursing and local institutional capacity to implement and evaluate individual, family, and community health-promotion interventions. • Collaborate with WHO/PAHO to strengthen nursing/midwifery and local health services education and practice in health promotion. • Collaborate with WHO/PAHO to develop and support nurses' capacity to conduct and implement research on health promotion.
Johns Hopkins School of Nursing, Baltimore, Maryland	WHO Collaborating Centre for Nursing Information, Knowledge Management and Sharing	• Collaborate with PAHO/WHO to facilitate and promote equitable access to information and scientific knowledge via the GANM for the promotion and support of global nursing and midwifery communities of practice and other ICT-supported activities. • Collaborate with PAHO/WHO to contribute to the growth, development, and deployment of learning and informed online environments to address the social determinants of health and improve nursing, health, and healthcare globally.
University of Alabama at Birmingham (UAB) Birmingham, Alabam	WHO Collaborating Centre for International Nursing	• Collaborate with PAHO/WHO to strengthen nursing and midwifery through the development of educational programs and resources to enhance the health of vulnerable families and children. • Collaborate with PAHO and WHO to enhance utilization and dissemination of knowledge resources to strengthen nursing and midwifery capacity, focusing on the health of children and families.
University of Illinois at Chicago, Chicago, Illinois	WHO Collaborating Centre for International Nursing Development in Primary Healthcare	• To collaborate with WHO/PAHO in the dissemination of WHO/PAHO primary healthcare program-based research findings and best practices to address Millennium Development Goals among policy makers, healthcare providers, and consumers. • To collaborate with WHO/PAHO in the facilitation of multidisciplinary research focused on primary healthcare education and practice with special emphasis on capacity building of nursing human resources. • To collaborate with WHO/PAHO in developing education mechanisms to develop nursing and other human resources for health for multidisciplinary global primary healthcare practice, education, and research within the PAHO region.
Case Western Reserve University, Cleveland, Ohio	WHO Collaborating Centre for Research and Clinical Training in Home Care Nursing	• Collaborate with AMRO to strengthen the development of nursing human resources and other healthcare workers in home care focused on self-management of noncommunicable diseases. • Collaborate with AMRO to develop educational programs for nurses and other healthcare workers for the self-management of noncommunicable diseases in the home and community settings. • Collaborate with AMRO to promote and conduct research to support home care and self-management of NCD.

AMRO, Regional Activities in the Americas; GANM, Global Alliance for Nursing and Midwifery; ICT, information, communication and technology; NCD, noncommunicable diseases; PAHO, Pan American Health Organization; WHO, World Health Organization.

Source: From World Health Organization. (n.d.b). *World Health Organization Collaborating Centres.* Retrieved from http://apps.who.int/whocc/List.aspx?cc_code=USA&

SUMMARY

The doctorally prepared APRN is well positioned to contribute to the scientific international discourse on subjects related to national and global health initiatives. This chapter has described the seven domains of the global health core competency model developed by the ASPPH in collaboration with the AACN, and has shown the interrelationship of this model to the AACN DNP Essentials V through VII. It is well recognized that the health of a nation is predicated on its ability to have far-reaching influence on the health status of populations around the world. Although U.S. healthcare expenditures are now nearly 20% of the GDP, healthcare outcomes have not improved with rising healthcare costs. Fragmentation of care, lack of access, third-party payer systems, hospital administrative costs, and expense of health-related technologies all have been cited as reasons for the escalating cost of healthcare in this country. Furthermore, with the increase in the immigrant population within the United States and the resultant heightened cross-national border transmission of disease, nursing doctoral programs must address and include global healthcare concepts within the curriculum of study.

Moving beyond the notion that health outcomes are singularly related to the behaviors of the individual, several documents and reports disseminated by the Commission on Social Determinants of Health have changed the focus of the discussion on health outcomes to include those factors associated with the contextual environment in which the individual resides. The constructs of social determinants of health, MDGs, and SDGs serve to provide a useful framework on which the APRN can design and implement strategies to address the multifactorial, sociopolitical, economic, ecological, and cultural underpinnings that influence and shape population health. Similarly, the theoretical construct for the Multilevel Model of Global Health supports the approach to analyze and evaluate risk factors and treatment effectiveness at both the individual and community levels. Enhanced knowledge and understanding of the impact of GHIs on health outcomes for communities around the world will provide the APRN with the tools needed to contribute to the national and international dialogues related to population health.

EXERCISES AND DISCUSSION QUESTIONS

Exercise 12.1 You are the executive director for a nurse-managed clinic in an underserved community. A large segment of the community population consists of foreign-born immigrants and refugees from African countries, including Liberia. As the APRN in this leadership role, what resources would you use to develop policies and procedures for the management of an Ebola exposure? Ebola outbreak? What strategies would you implement to develop evidence-based guidelines for practice?

Exercise 12.2 As the program director for an APRN doctoral program of study, you are asked to develop the syllabus for a course on population and global health. Develop the course description, objectives, and weekly topical outline for a course titled "Current and Emerging Trends in Population-Based Global Health."

Exercise 12.3 As an APRN you have been requested to present a paper at a national nursing conference on the design, implementation, and evaluation of a community health clinic. The audience consists of advanced practice clinicians and academicians. List the objectives for the presentation. How would you include the eight recommendations of the IOM Report "The Future of Nursing"? Develop the outline for the presentation to include concepts related to social determinants of health, healthcare access, data collection, and analyses and healthcare outcome evaluation.

Exercise 12.4 One of the important components of the role of the APRN is to influence public policy and to interface with law makers and elected officials in the design and implementation of rules and regulations impacting the health of a nation. Toward that end, how might you develop guidelines for a public policy brief on a current health issue?

REFERENCES

Aiken, L. M., Pelter, M. M., Carlson, V., Marshall, A. P., Cross, R., McKinley, S., & Dracup, K. (2008). Effective strategies for implementing a multicenter international clinical trial. *Journal of Nursing Scholarship, 40*(2), 101–108. doi:10.1111/j.1547-5069.2008.00213.x

Accreditation Commission for Education in Nursing. (2019). Home page. Retrieved from https://www.acenursing.org

American Association of Colleges of Nursing. (2006). *The essentials of doctoral education for advanced practice nursing.* Retrieved from http://www.aacn.nche.edu/publications/position/DNPEssentials.pdf

American Association of Colleges of Nursing. (2019). *Nursing infection control education network project.* Retrieved from https://www.aacnnursing.org/Academic-Nursing/Prevention

American Medical Association. (2014). *AMA assembles Ebola resources for physicians and public: Ebola resource center.* Retrieved from https://www.ama-assn.org/delivering-care/public-health/ama-assembles-ebola-resources-physicians-and-public

Association of Faculties of Medicine of Canada. (n.d.). *Intervening in individuals or populations?* AFMC Primer on Population Health. Retrieved from https://ubccpd.ca/sites/ubccpd.ca/files/AFMC%20Primer%20on%20Population%20Health%202014-12-23%20%282%29.pdf

Association of Schools and Programs of Public Health. (2018). *Global health concentration competencies for the MPH degree.* Retrieved from http://www.aspph.org/educate/models/masters-global-health

Campbell, I. M. (1995). Planning of national primary health care and prevention programs. In E. Gallagher & J. Subedi (Eds.), *Global perspectives on health care* (pp. 174–197). Englewood Cliffs, NJ: Prentice-Hall.

Campbell, I. M. (2004). A multilevel evaluation model for health disparity reduction and cultural competency intervention. *Hispanic Health Care International, 1*(3), 1–10.

Campbell, I. M. (2006). An essay on the need to expand and integrate nursing practice educational horizons with information technology and interdisciplinary collaboration [Editorial]. *Journal of Nursing Informatics, 10*(1), Online. Retrieved from http://ojni.org/10%201/irina.htm

Centers for Disease Control and Prevention. (2017). *Global health—Polio eradication.* Retrieved from http://www.cdc.gov/polio

Centers for Disease Control and Prevention. (2019). *Measles cases and outbreaks.* Retrieved from https://www.cdc.gov/measles/cases-outbreaks.html

Healthy People 2020. (2019). *Global health.* Retrieved from http://www.healthypeople.gov/2020/topics-objectives/topic/global-health

Henry J. Kaiser Family Foundation. (2016). *Americans' views on the U.S. role in global health.* Retrieved from https://www.kff.org/global-health-policy/poll-finding/americans-views-on-the-u-s-role-in-global-health

Henry J. Kaiser Family Foundation. (2018). *The U.S. government and international family planning and reproductive health efforts.* Retrieved from https://www.kff.org/global-health-policy/fact-sheet/the-u-s-government-and-international-family-planning-reproductive-health-efforts/#footnote-270769-12

Himmelstein, D. U., Jun, M., Busse, R., Chevreul, K., Geissler, A., Jeurissen, P., . . . Woolhandler, S. (2014). A comparison of hospital administrative costs in eight nations: U.S. costs exceed all others by far. Health Affairs, 33(9), 1586–1594. doi:10.1377/hlthaff.2013.1327

International Council of Nurses. (2019). *International classification for nursing practice*. Retrieved from https://www.icn.ch/what-we-do/projects/ehealth/icnp-download/icnp-download

Kulage, K. M., Hickey, K. T., Honig, J. C., Johnson, M. P., & Larson, E. L. (2014). Establishing a program of global initiatives for nursing education. *Journal of Nursing Education, 53*(7), 371–378. doi:10.3928/01484834-20140617-02

Lorenzoni, L., Belloni, A., & Sassi, F. (2014). Health-care expenditure and health policy in the USA versus other high-spending OECD countries. *The Lancet, 384*(9937), 83–92. doi:10.1016/s0140-6736(14)60571-7

Madden, R., Sykes, C., Ustun, T. B., National Centre for Classification in Health, Australia, Australian Institute of Health and Welfare, and WHO. (n.d.). *The WHO family of international classifications: Definitions, scope and purpose*. Retrieved from http://www.who.int/classifications/en

McKeehan, I. V. (2000). A multilevel city health profile of Moscow. *Social Science and Medicine, 51*(9), 1295–1312. doi:10.1016/s0277-9536(00)00093-9

McNeal, G. J. (2014). Shifting the paradigm: An academic public–private partnership to form a virtual nurse managed clinic. *ABNF Journal, 25*(2), 31–32.

National League for Nursing. (n.d.a). *Faculty preparation for global experiences toolkit*. Retrieved from http://www.nln.org/docs/default-source/default-document-library/toolkit_facprepglobexp5a3fb25c-78366c709642ff00005f0421.pdf

National League for Nursing. (n.d.b). Accrediting Commission. Retrieved from http://www.nlnac.org

OECD. (n.d.a). *History*. Retrieved from http://www.oecd.org/about/history

OECD. (n.d.b). *OECD health statistics 2018*. Retrieved from http://www.oecd.org/els/health-systems/health-data.htm

OECD. (2017a). *Work on health*. Retrieved from http://www.oecd.org/health/Health-Brochure.pdf

OECD. (2017b). *Health at a glance 2017: OECD indicators*. Retrieved from https://www.oecd.org/united-states/Health-at-a-Glance-2017-Key-Findings-UNITED-STATES.pdf

OECD. (2018). *OECD work on health*. Retrieved from http://www.oecd.org/health/Health-Brochure.pdf

Pew Research Center. (2017). *Key facts about refugees to the U.S.* Retrieved from http://www.pewresearch.org/fact-tank/2017/01/30/key-facts-about-refugees-to-the-u-s

Pew Research Center. (2018). *U.S. unauthorized immigrant total dips to lowest level in a decade*. Retrieved from http://www.pewhispanic.org/2018/11/27/u-s-unauthorized-immigrant-total-dips-to-lowest-level-in-a-decade

Prentice, T., Reinders, L. T., & World Health Report Team. (2007). *A safer future: Global health security in the 21st century*. (WHO World Health Report). Retrieved from http://www.who.int/whr/2007/whr07_en.pdf

SabaCare. (2018). *Clinical care classification system*. Retrieved from http://www.SabaCare.com

Title 42 – The Public Health and Welfare. (2013). Retrieved from http://www.gpo.gov/fdsys/search/pagedetails.action?collectionCode=USCODE&searchPath=Title+42&oldPath=Title+42&isCollapsed=true&selectedYearFrom=2013&ycord=1665&browsePath=Title+42%2F-1&granuleId=USCODE-2013-title42-toc&packageId=USCODE-2013-title42&colelapse=true&fromBrowse=true

United Nations. (n.d.a). *The universal declaration of human rights*. Retrieved from http://www.un.org/en/documents/udhr

United Nations. (n.d.b). *We can end poverty*. Retrieved from http://www.un.org/millenniumgoals

United Nations. (n.d.c). *About the sustainable development goals*. Retrieved from https://www.un.org/sustainabledevelopment/sustainable-development-goals

United Nations Department of Economic and Social Affairs. (n.d.). *Millennium development goals report 2014*. Retrieved from http://www.un.org/en/development/desa/publications/mdg-report-2014.html

United Nations Economic and Social Council. (n.d.). *Millennium development goals and post-2015 development agenda*. Retrieved from http://www.un.org/en/ecosoc/about/mdg.shtml

United Nations General Assembly. (2000). United Nations millennium declaration. Retrieved from http://www.un.org/millennium/declaration/ares552e.htm

USAID. (2016). *USAID's global health strategic framework*. Retrieved from https://www.usaid.gov/sites/default/files/documents/1864/gh_framework2012.pdf

USAID. (2017). *Afghanistan and Pakistan*. Retrieved from http://www.usaid.gov/where-we-work/afghanistan-and-pakistan

USAID. (2018). *What we do*. Retrieved from https://www.usaid.gov/what-we-do/global-health/health-systems-strengthening

USAID. (2019). *Fiscal year (FY) 2019 development and humanitarian assistance budget*. Retrieved from https://www.usaid.gov/sites/default/files/documents/1869/USAID_FY2019_Budget_Fact-sheet.pdf

U.S. Citizenship and Immigration Services. (2017). *Refugees*. Retrieved from http://www.uscis.gov/humanitarian/refugees-asylum/refugees

U.S. Department of State – Bureau of Consular Affairs. (2018). *Ebola information for travelers*. Retrieved from https://travel.state.gov/content/travel/en/international-travel/before-you-go/your-health-abroad/ebola.html

United States Senate Committee on Appropriations. (2014). *Chairwoman Mikulski opening statement at full committee hearing on Ebola response*. Retrieved from https://www.appropriations.senate.gov/news/minority/chairwoman-mikulski-opening-statement-at-full-committee-hearing-on-ebola-response

The White House. (2014). *Fact sheet: U.S. response to the Ebola epidemic in West Africa*. Retrieved from http://www.whitehouse.gov/the-press-office/2014/09/16/fact-sheet-us-response-ebola-epidemic-west-africa

World Health Organization. (n.d.a). *WHO global competency model*. Retrieved from https://www.who.int/employment/competencies/WHO_competencies_EN.pdf

World Health Organization. (n.d.b). *World Health Organization Collaborating Centres*. Retrieved from http://apps.who.int/whocc/List.aspx?cc_code=USA&

World Health Organization. (2007). *Overview*. Retrieved from http://www.who.int/whr/2010/media_centre/en

World Health Organization. (2018a). *Global health observatory data*. Retrieved from https://www.who.int/gho/mortality_burden_disease/en

World Health Organization. (2018b). *Classifications*. Retrieved from https://www.who.int/classifications/network/en

World Health Organization. (2019a). Collaborations and Partnerships. Retrieved from https://www.who.int/about/collaborations/en

World Health Organization. (2019b). Millennium Development Goals (MDGS). Retrieved from https://www.who.int/news-room/fact-sheets/detail/millennium-development-goals-(mdgs)

INTERNET RESOURCES

Association of Schools and Programs of Public Health: https://s3.amazonaws.com/ASPPH_Media_Files/Docs/APPENDIX+A-Final_2018-07-16.pdf

Centers for Disease Control and Prevention: www.cdc.gov/vaccines/pubs/pinkbook/meas.html

CDC, Epidemiology and Prevention of Vaccine-Preventable Diseases, CDC, Epidemiology and Prevention of Vaccine-Preventable Diseases, Measles: www.cdc.gov/vaccines/pubs/pinkbook/meas.html

WHO Global Competency Model: https://www.who.int/employment/competencies/WHO_competencies_EN.pdf

INDEX